Drug Metabolism, Pharmacokinetics and Bioanalysis

Drug Metabolism, Pharmacokinetics and Bioanalysis

Special Issue Editors

Hye Suk Lee
Kwang-Hyeon Liu

MDPI • Basel • Beijing • Wuhan • Barcelona • Belgrade

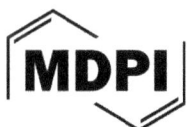

MDPI

Special Issue Editors

Hye Suk Lee
The Catholic University of Korea
Korea

Kwang-Hyeon Liu
Kyungpook National University
Korea

Editorial Office
MDPI
St. Alban-Anlage 66
4052 Basel, Switzerland

This is a reprint of articles from the Special Issue published online in the open access journal *Pharmaceutics* (ISSN 1999-4923) in 2018 (available at: https://www.mdpi.com/journal/pharmaceutics/special_issues/dmpk_and_bioanalysis)

For citation purposes, cite each article independently as indicated on the article page online and as indicated below:

LastName, A.A.; LastName, B.B.; LastName, C.C. Article Title. *Journal Name* **Year**, *Article Number*, Page Range.

ISBN 978-3-03897-916-6 (Pbk)
ISBN 978-3-03897-917-3 (PDF)

Contents

About the Special Issue Editors

Hye Suk Lee acquired her B.S., MS, and Ph.D. degrees at the College of Pharmacy, Sungkyunkwan University, Korea. She has worked as a senior researcher in Toxicology Research Center, Korea Research Institute of Chemical Technology. She also served as professor in College of Pharmacy, Wonkwang University, Korea from 1995 to 2010, and she was a dean of College of Pharmacy, Wonkwang University from 2003 to 2005. In 2011, she moved to College of Pharmacy, The Catholic University of Korea and was a dean of College of Pharmacy from 2014 to 2016. She is currently a director of BK21 Plus Team for Creative Leader Program for Pharmacomics-Based Future Pharmacy since 2013. Dr. Lee has published 210 peer-reviewed articles, and her research has focused on pharmacokinetics and metabolism, drug interaction, and forensic analytical toxicology. She serves on the Editorial members of *Pharmaceutics* (SCIE), *Bioanalysis* (SCIE), *Mass Spectrometry Letters* (SCOPUS), and *Integrative Medicine Research* (SCOPUS).

Kwang-Hyeon Liu acquired his B.S. degree in agricultural chemistry in 1990 from Seoul National University in Suwon, Korea and a Ph.D. in agricultural biotechnology in 1999 from the same university. He then joined BK21 Agricultural Biotechnology, Seoul National University where he was a postdoctoral fellow. He joined Inje University College of Medicine in 2003 and served as a member of the faculty in the Department of Pharmacology. After eight years, he moved to Kyungpook National University in 2011, where he currently serves as a Professor in the College of Pharmacy. While at Inje University and Kyungpook National University, much of his research has focused on drug metabolism/bioanalysis, pharmacokinetics, pharmacometabolomics, and lipidomics, and he has published close to 160 peer-reviewed articles. Currently, Dr. Liu's research is supported by the National Research Foundation of Korea, Korea Healthcare Technology R&D Project, and Kyungpook National University. He is currently a Director of BK21 Plus KNU Multi-Omics based Creative Drug Research Team, having started in this position in 2016, and is the dean of college of pharmacy, KNU. Dr. Liu is a Founding Member of the Korean Society of Metabolomics and serves on the Editorial Board of *Xenobiotica* (SCI) and *Mass Spectrometry Letters* (SCOPUS).

Preface to "Drug Metabolism, Pharmacokinetics and Bioanalysis"

Drug metabolism, pharmacokinetics, and drug interaction studies have been extensively carried out in order to secure the druggability and safety of new chemical entities throughout the development of new drugs. Recently, drug metabolism by phase I and II drug metabolizing enzymes and transport by drug transporters have been studied. A combination of biochemical advances in the function and regulation of drug metabolizing enzymes and automated analytical technologies are revolutionizing drug metabolism research. There are also potential drug–drug interactions with co-administered drugs due to inhibition and/or induction of drug metabolizing enzymes and drug transporters. In addition, drug interaction studies have been actively performed to develop substrate cocktails that do not interfere with each other and simultaneous analytical method of substrate drugs and their metabolites using high-performance liquid chromatography–tandem mass spectrometry.

This Special Issue serves to highlight current progress in drug metabolism, pharmacokinetics, drug interactions, and bioanalysis. Fifteen outstanding research articles and one review article cover the topics of, first, the bioanalytical method development of adalimumab, anthraquinones, chlorogenic acid, ethyl glucuronide, globotriaosylceramide, and procainamide, second, the pharmacokinetics of antigastric ulcer agents, anti-Parkinson's drug candidate, and pharmaceutical excipient, third, the drug–drug interaction studies of memantine and cimetidine, and metformin and red ginseng extracts, fourth, the reaction phenotyping studies of loxoprofen and osthenol, fifth, the bioavailability study of eurycomanone, and sixth, drying technologies for the stability and bioavailability of biopharmaceuticals.

We expect that this Special Issue will provide insights into drug metabolism and pharmacokinetic studies and contribute to the advancement of the relevant research areas.

Hye Suk Lee, Kwang-Hyeon Liu
Special Issue Editors

pharmaceutics

MDPI

Review

Drying Technologies for the Stability and Bioavailability of Biopharmaceuticals

Fakhrossadat Emami [1], Alireza Vatanara [1,*], Eun Ji Park [2] and Dong Hee Na [2,*]

[1] College of Pharmacy, Tehran University of Medical Sciences, Tehran 1417614411, Iran;
    f-emami@razi.tums.ac.ir
[2] College of Pharmacy, Chung-Ang University, Seoul 06974, Korea; 1978ej@naver.com
*   Correspondence: vatanara@tums.ac.ir (A.V.); dhna@cau.ac.kr (D.H.N.);
    Tel.: +98-21-6698-0445 (A.V.); +82-2-820-5677 (D.H.N.)

Received: 30 June 2018; Accepted: 13 August 2018; Published: 17 August 2018

Abstract: Solid dosage forms of biopharmaceuticals such as therapeutic proteins could provide enhanced bioavailability, improved storage stability, as well as expanded alternatives to parenteral administration. Although numerous drying methods have been used for preparing dried protein powders, choosing a suitable drying technique remains a challenge. In this review, the most frequent drying methods, such as freeze drying, spray drying, spray freeze drying, and supercritical fluid drying, for improving the stability and bioavailability of therapeutic proteins, are discussed. These technologies can prepare protein formulations for different applications as they produce particles with different sizes and morphologies. Proper drying methods are chosen, and the critical process parameters are optimized based on the proposed route of drug administration and the required pharmacokinetics. In an optimized drying procedure, the screening of formulations according to their protein properties is performed to prepare a stable protein formulation for various delivery systems, including pulmonary, nasal, and sustained-release applications.

Keywords: biopharmaceuticals; drying technology; protein stability; bioavailability; pharmacokinetics

1. Introduction

The intrinsic instability of protein molecules is currently the predominant challenge for biopharmaceutical scientists [1–3]. Because of their higher molecular weights and diversity of composition, therapeutic proteins have much more complicated structures than conventional chemical drugs [3–5]. Exposure to some environmental stresses, such as pH extremes, high temperatures, freezing, light, agitation, sheer stress, and organic solvents, can cause protein instability [4,5]. Since proteins can be degraded easily during manufacturing and storage, some strategies are suggested to improve protein stability, including the addition of stabilizers, protein modification with biocompatible molecules, nanomedicine, and nano- or micro-particle technology [6–13].

Drying strategies that process and dehydrate proteins to produce more stable protein formulations in the solid state are frequently used for biopharmaceuticals that are insufficiently stable in aqueous solutions [14–16]. Solid dosage forms of proteins are less prone to shear-related denaturation and precipitation during manufacturing and storage [1,15,17,18]. Because water molecules can induce mobilization of therapeutic proteins and other additives, liquid formulations of proteins are more susceptible to unfavorable physicochemical degradation. Consequently, water removal and embedding of proteins in a glassy matrix are good approaches for improved storage against physicochemical protein degradation [1,5,18].

Dried therapeutic protein powders have shown good storage stability at room temperature ($\leq 25\,^\circ C$), and dehydration is an easy and economical approach [19,20]. Dehydration is not only a drying procedure for improving protein shelf-life, but may also be used for engineering protein particles for various routes of administration. Dried biopharmaceutical powders have gained popularity as inhalation preparations for pulmonary, nasal, and sustained drug-delivery systems [21,22]. Numerous reviews of drying strategies have been published [23,24]. However, most of these reviews focus on small molecules, and reviews of using drying methods to improve stability or pharmacokinetic properties of therapeutic proteins are relatively few [25,26]. Because proteins are sensitive to environmental stresses, the techniques available for producing dried biopharmaceuticals are limited by factors such as production time, temperature, and various process-related stresses [26]. The features and drawbacks of each drying procedure should be considered for rational selection of a drying method to improve the stability of therapeutic proteins for different drug administration applications [27]. In this review, the drying techniques of biopharmaceuticals are discussed, with focus on the selection of appropriate drying methods for improving stability and desired pharmacokinetic properties of biopharmaceuticals. Stabilizers for protein formulations and applications of dried-powder formulations to local or systemic drug delivery are also highlighted.

2. Drying Techniques

Generally, drying involves three steps, which may be operated simultaneously. First, energy is transferred from an external source to water or dispersion medium in the product. The second step is phase transformation of the liquid phase to a vapor or solid phase. Finally, the transfer of vapor generated away from the pharmaceutical product occurs. The characteristics of dried particles can be effectively influenced by process parameters, such as temperature, pressure, relative humidity, and gas feed rate, besides characteristics of protein formulations, such as composition and type of excipients, concentration of solutes, viscosity, and type of solvent [28] (Table 1). Drying based on the mechanism of removing water can be classified into subgroups. Drying can be performed using an evaporation mechanism, such as vacuum dying or foam drying; evaporation and atomization pathways such as spray drying (SD); sublimation mechanisms such as freeze drying (FD) and spray freeze drying; and supercritical fluid drying methods using a precipitation mechanism [27]. The most common drying techniques, namely freeze drying, spray drying, spray freeze drying, and supercritical fluid drying will be discussed in this review.

2.1. Freeze Drying (FD)

The most common drying method for therapeutic proteins is FD [14,26,29], which has been used for many therapeutic proteins, including insulin dry powder for inhalation (Afrezza®, MannKind Corporation, Valencia, CA, USA) [14]. Since water molecules can induce mobilization of protein solution, protein stability can be improved by water removal and embedding of proteins in a glassy matrix through lyophilization [5]. FD is based on sublimation, where solid materials are directly transformed to the gaseous phase. The FD process involves the following three steps: freezing, primary drying, and secondary drying [1,5,18,30,31].

Freeze-dried proteins have greater storage stability than proteins in liquid dosage forms; however, this process applies freezing and dehydration stresses to the proteins, which may result in the alteration of protein structure [31–33]. Upon drying, the hydration shell surrounding the protein, which provides a protective effect, is removed. In addition, the protein solution becomes saturated because of ice crystal formation during the freezing process. The solute concentration, pH change, and ionic strength changes are formulation variables that should be considered for a stable protein formulation (Table 1) [1,33]. Recent infrared spectroscopic analyses have shown that acute freezing and dehydration stresses of lyophilization can induce protein unfolding [29,34]. To develop a successful protein formulation using an FD procedure, physical properties, such as glass transition temperature (T_g) and residual moisture content, and operational parameters, such as pH and cooling rate, should be considered [29].

Furthermore, a hydrophilic molecule can be incorporated into the protein formulation as a lyoprotectant to overcome protein denaturation and preserve stability during lyophilization [1,17]. Stabilizers can protect proteins during freezing (cryoprotectants) and lyophilization (lyoprotectants) through water replacement and hydrogen bond formation (Table 2) [1,18,30,35]. Moreover, excipients have the potential to provide a glassy matrix to decrease protein-protein interactions and reduce protein mobility in a solid dosage form [36]. In summary, optimization of process variables and proper combinations of additives as stabilizers are requirements for stable freeze-dried products [35–37].

Liao et al. investigated the effect of excipients, such as glycerol, sucrose, trehalose, and dextran, on the stability of freeze-dried lysozymes using second derivative Fourier transform infrared (FTIR) spectroscopy [17]. They showed that the combination of trehalose and sucrose could raise the T_g of freeze-dried lysozymes, leading to the stabilization of lysozyme in freeze-dried formulations. This study indicated that the T_g of freeze-dried formulations and the protein stability during lyophilization were dependent on the excipient type and excipient to enzyme mass ratio. A recent study by Tonnis et al. [38] showed the influence of size and molecular flexibility of sugars on the stability of freeze-dried proteins, including insulin, hepatitis B surface antigen, lactate dehydrogenase, and β-galactosidase. Among freeze-dried proteins prepared in the presence or absence of disaccharide (trehalose) or oligosaccharide (inulin, 4 kDa; dextran, 6 kDa; dextran 70 kDa), those prepared in the presence of the smallest sugar (trehalose) showed high stability although trehalose-containing formulations had the lowest T_g. In addition, the flexible oligosaccharide inulin was more stable than the rigid oligosaccharide dextran 6 kDa or 70 kDa. The combination of polysaccharide dextran 70 kDa and trehalose greatly increased the T_g of the formulation and improved the stability of proteins, as compared to formulations containing dextran alone. The flexible oligosaccharide inulin (4 kDa) provided better stabilization than the similarly sized but molecularly rigid oligosaccharide dextran 6 kDa. This study indicated that the combination of trehalose and dextran has an additive effect owing to the interaction potential of trehalose (water replacement) and enhanced T_g of dextran (glassy state).

Table 1. Comparison of characteristics of different drying technologies. Table adopted from [15,21,23,24,39,40].

Drying Procedure	Process Parameters	Stress	Advantages	Limitations	Typical Powder Characteristics
Freeze drying	• Solute concentration • Cooling temperature • Freezing rate • Drying temperature • Drying pressure	• Crystallization • pH changes • Dehydration stress • Ionic strength change • Interfacial stress (ice-liquid) • Ice crystal formation	• Elevated temperature not required for drying • Accurately dosed • Controlled moisture content • Short reconstitution time • Appealing physical form • Homogenous dispersion • Good for materials sensitive to air or O_2	• No particle engineering • Expensive set up • Long processing time • Complex process • Maintenance cost • Exposure to ice-water interface • Few months for large objects	• Intact cake • High surface area • Uniform color • Consistency • Elegant cake appearance • High strength to prevent cracking, powdering, or collapse
Spray drying	• Solute concentration • Feed flow rate • Hot air flow rate (Inlet and outlet) • Additive solubility • Inlet temperature	• Thermal stress • Atomization stress • Mechanical stress • Interfacial stress (air-liquid) • Dehydration stress	• Simple • Convenient system • Cost effectiveness • One step (Short process time) • Scalability • Repeatability • Particle engineering • Good aerosolization	• Yield (50–70%) • Unsuitable for materials sensitive to air • Non-aseptic	• Fine powder • Hollow particle • Shrinkage • Toughening • Spherical, ellipsoid, toroid, or dimpled shape
Spray freeze drying	• Solute concentration • Feed flow rate • Solid content	• Atomization stress • Interfacial stress (air-liquid) • Freezing stress • Interfacial stress (ice-liquid) • Dehydration stress	• Fast freezing • Particle engineering • High yield • Excellent aerosolization • Aseptic drying	• Three steps (Time consuming) • High cost • Fragile particles • Complex • Inconvenient (require liquid N_2)	• Spherical, porous particle • Light weight • Smooth surface • Very low density • High surface area
Supercritical fluid drying	• Solute concentration • Feed flow rate • Co-solvent flow rate • SCF flow rate • Temperature • Pressure • Nozzle size	• Atomization stress • Dehydration stress	• Fast process • Particle engineering • Mild process condition (mild temperature) • Aseptic drying • Scalability	• Exposure to organic solvent • Special set-up • High cost	• Spherical • Smooth surface

2.2. Spray Drying (SD)

SD is the most common particle engineering method that generates solid (particulate) proteins for pharmaceutical applications [41]. SD as a single-step process may provide dried protein particles with the required size and morphology [30,42]. SD technology comprises atomization, drying, and separation of particles. Protein solution is sprayed through nozzles into a drying chamber. Droplet formation and subsequent dehydration is performed very rapidly in a hot drying medium. The resulting protein powders are transferred into a cyclone (Figure 1). Owing to the short procedure time, SD is a mild technique for producing stable protein powders for inhalation and other applications [1,42–45].

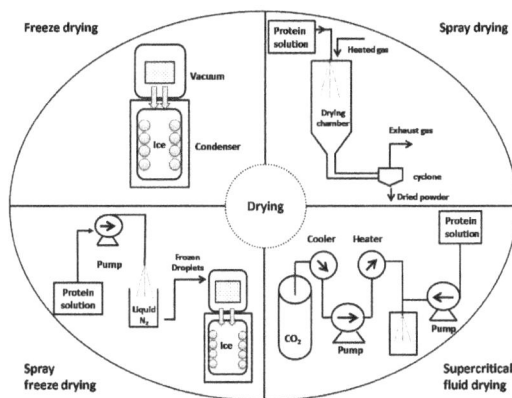

Figure 1. Schematic illustration of drying methods using freeze drying (FD), spray drying (SD), spray freeze drying (SFD), and supercritical fluid drying (SCFD) technologies.

Peclet number (Pe), which is the proportion of droplet evaporation rate and the diffusional motion of solutes in the SD method, can determine the morphology and density of the final particles that are either dense or hollow. The solute concentration, feeding flow rate, flow rate of hot air, solubility of additives through effects on evaporation rate, as well as inlet temperature are adjustable process parameters in the SD method. Large molecules with low diffusional coefficients having low solubility and high density, such as albumin and growth hormone, can prompt surface saturation at high temperatures. In addition, high surface-active agents such as leucine and trileucine would be located on particle surface and saturate the surface rapidly. Thus, for proteins and high surface-active agents, the solutes cannot diffuse to the center of droplets (Pe > 1) and generate hollow particles with low density that are suitable for pulmonary drug delivery [46]. Because of thermo-sensitivity of proteins, the loss of hydration layer in contact with hot air, as well as exposure to air/liquid interface at the droplet surface during atomization may cause degradation. Moreover, this engineering technique may induce shear stress in protein structure during the atomization step (Table 1) [1,2,5,44]. Excipients used as stabilizers may provide a functional shield surrounding the protein and prevent exposure of the protein to the interfacial surface or hot atmosphere [36]. The rational choice of stabilizers and optimization of the process variables are essential approaches to guarantee protein stability and achieve the desired particle properties.

Schule et al. studied the biophysical and conformational stability of spray-dried antibody-mannitol formulations [47] and concluded that antibody formulations during storage stability tests showed some levels of aggregates when measured by size-exclusion chromatography (SEC). FTIR analysis demonstrated that despite antibody aggregation during the SD process, the secondary structure of the antibody was conserved. Furthermore, their data suggested that the unfolding of protein structure was reversible and through reconstitution, the unfolded form of antibody formulation was refolded to a native form.

Ajmera et al. studied the SD of catalase formulations in the presence of some amino acids [1]. The ability of hydrophilic and hydrophobic amino acids to serve as protective agents during the SD of catalase was evaluated. The mean particle size of the spray-dried powder was estimated to be in the range of 3.3–4.8 μm, and amino acids have shown different stabilizing efficacies against the stresses induced by the SD technique. Spray-dried catalase, in comparison with the liquid form, showed greater stability. Arginine and histidine preserved the stability of enzyme formulations during SD. Due to its small size and surface activity, arginine exhibited fast diffusion to the droplet surface during droplet formation. Thus, arginine was localized at the droplet surface and protected the enzyme from air-liquid interface adsorption. Furthermore, hydrogen bond formation between amino acids and proteins in solid dosage forms plays a key role in the suppression of dehydration stress (water replacement). Charged hydrophilic amino acids, such as arginine and histidine, could form hydrogen bonds with catalase because of the presence of protonated nitrogen. X-ray diffraction (XRD) measurements have clearly shown that spray-dried pure catalase assumes a crystalline structure, while the enzyme remains in an amorphous state in the presence of histidine, and combination with arginine shifts its structure to a semi-amorphous state. A catalase-methionine formulation resulted in a crystalline product, which provided no protective effects. Despite its crystalline structure, glycine interacted with proteins as a water substitute and serves as a good stabilizer. Furthermore, a combination of arginine and glycine provides synergistic stabilizing effects and offers a potentially stable catalase powder preparation.

Li et al. prepared an inhalable protein formulation comprising 67% (w/w) sodium carboxymethylcellulose (Na-CMC) and 33% (w/w) alkaline phosphatase using SD [48]. They concluded that spray-dried alkaline phosphatase particles exhibited smooth surfaces. Particles with smooth surfaces are cohesive, which enhances the inter-particulate interactions and protein aggregation, causing low aerosol performance. Na-CMC as a polysaccharide in alkaline phosphatase formulations dried by SD may produce wrinkled protein particles. The roughness of protein surfaces may suppress unnecessary interactions and protein degradation. Spray-dried alkaline phosphatase-Na-CMC formulations maintained their stability immediately after preparation or following storage for three months, and subsequent protein powders produced in this manner have shown excellent aerodynamic performance.

2.3. Spray Freeze Drying (SFD)

Another effective and versatile technique for transforming protein solution into dried particles is SFD, which is the combination of traditional FD and SD processes. Atomization, fast freezing, and drying by ice sublimation are the three phases of SFD process (Figure 1). SFD is a method for preparing lyophilized protein powders with spherical microparticles [49].

Atmospheric freezing, spray freezing with compressed carbon dioxide, spray freezing into a vapor over a cryogenic liquid, and spray freezing into a liquid are different types of SFD methods [50–52]. SFD involves the atomization of protein solution via a nozzle at extremely low temperatures, and has potential applications for thermo-labile active pharmaceutical ingredients. Because of the critically low temperature, the atomized droplets are rapidly frozen. SFD methods may immobilize the protein and avoid exposure to air-water interface. The frozen micronized droplets are sublimated using a lyophilizer under vacuum to prepare a dried powder.

In SFD, the liquid solution is sprayed into a vapor via a nozzle using a cryogenic fluid, such as liquid nitrogen [43,44,53–55]. The chemical composition, protein solution concentrations, atomization rate, freezing rate, as well as the temperature of cryogenic liquid have key roles in determining the density and particle size distribution of spray freeze-dried powders [50]. Supercooling phenomena using a cryogenic liquid in SFD may reduce the undesirable effects of ice crystallization, pH shift values, as well as phase separation of the drug and excipient that have existence in FD. Moreover, since freezing is very rapid, there is not sufficient time for molecular rearrangements. Biopharmaceuticals are embedded amorphously in the excipients, minimizing the probability of protein crystallization and subsequent phase separation between the active pharmaceutical ingredient and stabilizers [56]. Furthermore,

SFD can create such powders with the required density and particle size distributions for different pharmaceutical applications. Therefore, SFD is more advantageous than traditional FD [4,44,50].

Rogers et al. prepared spray freeze-dried insulin in the presence of tyloxapol and lactose as lyoprotectants [57]. Spray freeze-dried insulin in the presence of surfactant and sugar as lyoprotectants showed improved stability. The concentration of the covalent dimer of insulin in spray freeze-dried pure insulin preparations is only slightly higher than that of the unprocessed bulk insulin. Spray freeze-dried insulin with or without lyoprotectants showed little degradation, indicating that such preparations are as stable as the unprocessed native insulin. Maa et al. showed that SFD powders of influenza vaccines have superior stability compared with liquid formulations [58]. Processing other proteins such as rhDNase, anti-IgE monoclonal antibodies [21], calcitonin [53], and parathyroid hormone [44] using SFD provided stable dried powders with appropriate particle sizes and good flow properties.

Spray freeze-dried powders may be produced for different drug delivery system applications. Specific physical characteristics such as particle size distribution, density, surface area, and volume are required, depending on their application [50]. SFD typically produces highly porous particles with a high percentage of fine particle fraction (FPF) and proper aerodynamic behavior for pulmonary delivery [44]. In addition, spray freeze-dried particles have applications for needle-free intradermal injection system, nasal, colonic, and ophthalmic drug delivery, as well as in processing for microencapsulation platforms [50]. Spray freeze-dried particles with a geometric diameter of 7–42 μm and very low density, representing an aerodynamic diameter of 1–5 μm, could be effective in pulmonary drug delivery systems. However, for nasal delivery and intradermal injection systems, particles with geometric diameters of 25–70 μm and 34–50 μm are required, respectively [50].

2.4. Supercritical Fluid Drying (SCFD)

Supercritical fluid drying (SCFD) is an attractive alternative drying method, because dehydration can be rapidly accomplished in the absence of extreme temperatures. SCFD may produce large amounts of dried biopharmaceuticals with adjustable particle sizes and morphology [59]. SCF uses a material such as ethylene, methanol, or carbon dioxide above its critical temperature and pressure. The critical temperature of a liquid is the temperature at which its vapor cannot be liquefied, no matter how much pressure is applied. The pressure that is needed to condense a gas at its critical temperature defines its critical pressure. SCF exhibits the appropriate characteristics of gas and liquid, including penetration of gas and solubility of liquids. Density, viscosity, and diffusivity of SCF above its critical point are in the range of the gas and liquid states of the solvent. SCFD is a versatile process that can adjust the density of SCF and the solubility of a solute through modulation of pressures and temperatures used in the procedure.

Carbon dioxide is a non-toxic, non-inflammable, and relatively cheap fluid, with mild critical temperature (31 °C) and pressure (73 bar) for SCFD processes. Supercritical carbon dioxide ($scCO_2$) may be used as a solvent or non-solvent in several SCFD applications, such as particle formation, chemical extraction, and purification. Rapid expansion of a supercritical solvent (RESS) and particles from a gas-saturated solution (PGSS) are two types of drying using $scCO_2$ as a solvent. Gas anti-solvent (GAS), supercritical anti-solvent process (SAS), and solution-enhanced dispersion system (SEDS) processes are examples of anti-solvent $scCO_2$ drying [15]. In previous studies, two theories explain the use of SCF for drying of protein products. In the first theory, SCFD is based on the anti-solvent and water extraction of SCF for protein formulations. Because of water extraction, the protein would be concentrated and precipitated. The concentrated protein solution is dried through the extraction of remaining water molecules using SFD. In the second theory, SCF is used as a propellant to enhance the atomization rate. In this process, SCF is dissolved at high pressure and the protein solution and SCF pass through a two-fluid nozzle, where the feed solution is atomized by the SCF, allowing a short drying procedure [60]. By monitoring the spraying gas flow rate, solution flow rate, solution concentration, nozzle size, temperature, pressure, and solvent, uniform spherical particles with distinct particle sizes and acceptable flow properties may be achieved [15,22].

Table 2. Studies of solid protein formulations prepared by different drying methods in the presence of stabilizers.

Process	Proteins/Peptides	Stabilizers	Mechanism of Stabilization	Applications		References
				Stability Improvement	Drug Delivery	
Freeze drying	IgG	Trehalose, Sucrose, PEG	Glassy state, Water replacement	✓	—	[61,62]
	Lysozyme	PEG, Glycerol, Sucrose, Trehalose, Dextran	Water replacement	✓	—	[17]
	BSA	Glucose, Sucrose, Maltose,	Glassy state, Water replacement	✓	—	[63]
	Anti-IgE antibody	Trehalose, Maltotriose / Histidine, Arginine, Glycine, Aspartic acid	Glassy state	✓	—	[18]
Spray drying	IgG	Trehalose, Sucrose, Leucine, Glycine, Lysine, Phenylalanine	Glassy state, Water replacement	✓	Pulmonary	[42,45,47]
	Trastuzumab		Glassy state, Water replacement	✓		[2]
	Anti-IgE	Trehalose, HPβCD, βCD	Glassy state, Water replacement	✓	Pulmonary	[21]
	Mab, rhDNase	Mannitol, Trehalose, Sucrose	Water replacement, Inhibit interfacial adsorption	—		[64]
	Catalase	Arginine, Glycine, Histidine		✓		[1]
	Influenza vaccine	HEPES buffer, Phosphate buffer	Buffer	—	Pulmonary	[64]
	Alkaline phosphatase	Sodium carboxy methylcellulose	Glassy state, Water replacement	✓	Pulmonary	[48]
	Erythropoietin	Dextran	Glassy state, Water replacement	—	Sustained release	[65]
Spray freeze drying	IgG	Leucine, Phenylalanine, Glycine, Trehalose	Water replacement	—	Sustained release	[52]
	BSA	Ammonium sulfate, Mannitol, Trehalose	Reduction specific surface area	✓	Pulmonary	[36]
	Anti-IgE	Mannitol, Trehalose, Sucrose	Glassy state, Water replacement	✓	Pulmonary	[21]
	Mab, rhDNase	Trehalose, HPβCD, Leucine, Citric acid	Water replacement, Inhibit interfacial adsorption	—	Pulmonary	[44]
	PTH	Trehalose, HPβCD, Maltose, Tween80	Glassy state, Water replacement, Inhibit interfacial adsorption	✓	Pulmonary	[53]
	Calcitonin	HEPES buffer, Phosphate buffer	Inhibit interfacial adsorption	✓	Pulmonary	[64]
	Influenza vaccine	Dextran, Mannitol, Trehalose, Arginine	Buffer	—	Epidermal	[58]
	Influenza vaccine	Trehalose, Lactose	Glassy state, Water replacement	✓	Enhance solubility	[57]
	Insulin	Trehalose		✓	Nasal	[19]
	Anthrax vaccine			✓		
Supercritical fluid drying	IgG	Trehalose, HPβCD	Glassy state, Water replacement	✓	—	[66]
	Lysozyme	Trehalose, Sucrose	Glassy state, Water replacement	✓	—	[22,59]
	Lysozyme, Myoglobin	Trehalose, Sucrose		✓	—	[67]
	Insulin	TMC, Dextran	Carrier	✓	Pulmonary	[68]

Immunoglobulin G (IgG), polyethylene glycol (PEG), hydroxypropyl β cyclodextrin (HPβCD), β cyclodextrin (βCD), bovine serum albumin (BSA), N-trimethyl chitosan (TMC), recombinant human DNase (rhDNase).

2.5. Comparison of the Physical Characteristics of Dried Powders

As shown in Figure 2, immunoglobulin G (IgG) formulations prepared using different drying methods with trehalose as a stabilizer represent different particle morphologies. The diversity in the size and morphology of particles in SEM micrographs could be explained by the particle formation procedure used in different drying techniques [64,69].

The most common drying method for proteins and peptides is FD, which produces a dry cake. Intact cakes have very low residual moisture content with great long-term stability. FD powders of protein formulations after reconstitution can be used for parenteral drug delivery [33]. However, the use of FD for particle-based formulations, such as those for pulmonary drug delivery, is limited because it is not a direct particle formation method [37]. For particle formation, additional procedures to break the cake are necessary. Such additional processes may reduce the production yield and lead to poor control of critical particle properties, such as particle size, size distribution, density, and morphology [41].

SD is a well-established particle engineering process producing fine powders with smooth or shrunken surfaces. Generally, SD powders exhibit hollow particles with a dimpled shape. SD methods typically provide small particles between 2–10 μm and an FPF between 20–70%, respectively. Particles with low density have potential for use in pulmonary or nasal drug delivery applications [42,45]. SD processes can be used for microencapsulation of biopharmaceuticals as a controlled-release system [65]. Solid proteins prepared using the SFD method have specific morphological characteristics, namely presence of numerous pores on the surface and within the microparticles. Cross-sections of SFD particles have shown an internal porous structure similar to a honeycomb [59]. Compared with spray-dried particles, SFD particles showed higher sphericity and porosity, resulting in relatively low densities appropriate for inhalation [69]. When atomized with the same combination of feed solution, SFD produced a smaller aerodynamic diameter in comparison with SD particles because of their high porosity and relatively lower density. Small aerodynamic diameter means high FPF and good aerosol performance [50].

Saluja et al. used SD and SFD powders of influenza subunit vaccine with inulin as a stabilizer for inhalation [64]. SD techniques produced particles with a small median volume diameter (<5 μm), but SFD generated particles with a larger volume median diameter (>10 μm). Although these particles have different physical sizes, they have an acceptable aerodynamic size in the range of 1–5 μm for pulmonary drug delivery based on their bulk densities. SFD, rather than SD, is recommended for proteins sensitive to elevated temperatures [50].

Maa et al. reported that the same formulation of rhDNase and anti-IgE antibody prepared by SFD and SD resulted in different particle morphologies [21]. Differing morphologies observed in SEM images of the same protein formulation is indicative of particles with different sizes and densities. Although the diameter of SFD particles is approximately doubled (3.3 μm for SD vs. 7.7 μm for SFD), the FPF increased from 27% to 50%, which reflects an improved aerodynamic performance of SFD powder. These observations suggest that superior aerodynamic behavior by SFD particles is probably correlated with small aerodynamic size. Consequently, SFD powders, in comparison with SD powders, are reported to possess higher FPF and lower aerodynamic diameter, which result in higher aerosolization efficiency [52]. Because of rapid evaporation of water in the drying chamber, SD particles had smaller sizes resulting from particle shrinkage. With the SFD technique, immediately after atomization, droplets were frozen and solid ice crystals were produced throughout the frozen droplet. During lyophilization, the ice crystals sublimate, and particles with an interconnected porous structure are formed. SFD particles can maintain approximately 80% of their droplet size and therefore result in large-sized particles with high sphericity [50,64,69]. Low particle density can compensate for the large geometric diameter. However, particles with low density have lower mechanical strength and are more fragile, and are therefore more susceptible to degradation [70].

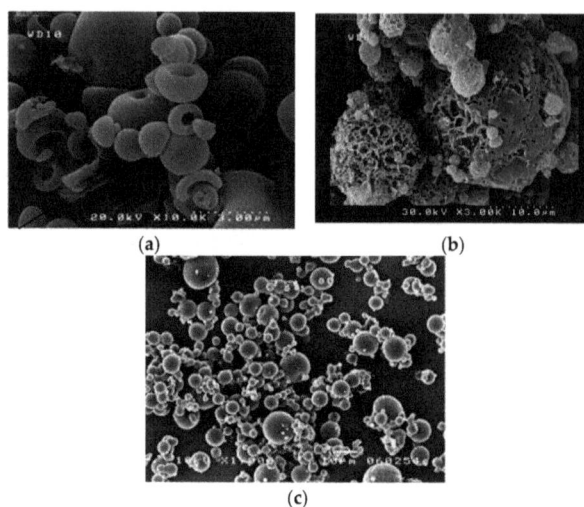

Figure 2. Scanning electron micrographs of dried IgG formulations produced using different drying methods: (a) SD [42], (b) SFD [52], and (c) SCFD methods [66].

Unlike FD, the SFD method can adjust particle size, thereby producing better dispersibility. By managing morphological parameters, dense protein particles may be obtained for intradermal injection applications [58], and low-density particles can be used for nasal [19] and pulmonary drug delivery [44,53]. In addition, supercooling in SFD is advantageous for reducing the unfavorable effects of freezing-induced concentration of proteins that are present in FD. Furthermore, fast freezing during SFD may provide amorphous matrices that can trap proteins in a solid matrix and preserve protein stability [50].

Jovanovic et al. prepared dried IgG powder using an SCFD procedure, in which the product showed decreased aggregation at lower temperature [66]. They evaluated the stability of the antibody using trehalose and hydroxypropyl-β-cyclodextrin (HPβCD) as stabilizers. The occurrence of IgG aggregation in IgG formulations with lower pH values was also reported. Conversely, IgG-sugar formulations in the presence of ethanol as a co-solvent are less stable.

Consequently, all these techniques were useful for improving protein storage stability. These drying methods may be beneficial when the combinining of drying and particle engineering in one process is desired for preparation of dried protein powders.

3. Stabilizers for Dried-Powder Protein Formulations

Although proteins are formulated in a solid dosage form to maintain shelf-life stability, proteins are susceptible to various physicochemical degradations upon drying and in solid form [20]. According to the stress conditions encountered in each drying method, different degradation pathways may occur simultaneously. Various physical instabilities, such as unfolding, adsorption, denaturation, aggregation, and precipitation, may occur during the drying process. Deamination, oxidation, β-elimination, hydrolysis, racemization, isomerization, and disulfide exchange are irreversible reactions that are considered chemical degradations for biopharmaceuticals [71,72]. Physicochemical parameters such as moisture content, temperature, crystallinity of the formulation, and additives have a significant impact on these unfavorable reactions [20]. In addition, the protein sequence, hydrophobicity, isoelectric point (pI), and carbohydrate content play key roles in the susceptibility of proteins to inactivation. Degradation of protein products may result in reduced bioactivity with increased immunogenicity [20,73].

The stresses faced during drying procedures and in solid dosage forms remain a considerable challenge in biopharmaceutical development [18]. Rational selection of stabilizers may help preserve protein stability against stress-induced degradation [20]. The commonly used excipients are listed in five groups, namely proteins (BSA), amino acids (glycine, alanine), polyols (polyethylene glycol), carbohydrates (glucose, lactose, sucrose, trehalose), and others (surfactants, polymers, salts) [35], in Table 3. Cryoprotectants can preserve protein stability in solution and during freezing by preferential exclusion. Higher glass transition temperatures of protein formulations are required to provide stability to protein products. Moreover, lyoprotectants can provide thermodynamic stability of proteins during freeze-drying and dehydration process [17]. In instances where one stabilizer does not act as both a cryoprotectant and lyoprotectant, a combination of stabilizers may be beneficial to protect the proteins against FD-induced stresses [18]. As reported, protective agents can physically preserve protein stability via several mechanisms (Table 3). Among all stabilization pathways, water replacement and the glassy state hypothesis are more prevalent. Addition of excipients for stabilization may be required to stabilize proteins by either a thermodynamic stabilization pathway or by a kinetic mechanism [74].

3.1. The Water Replacement Hypothesis

Water plays a critical role in maintaining the native structure of proteins. During dehydration, water is removed and thermodynamic equilibrium between the native and unfolded state of the protein shifts to an unstable form. During drying, some stabilizers in the protein formulation can maintain the native protein conformation. These additives may enhance the free energy of protein unfolding reactions. Stabilizers with functional hydroxyl groups, such as carbohydrate and polyol, have the potential to form hydrogen bonds with bioactive proteins and substitute for the removed water molecules (anhydrobiosis). The hydrogen bonds formed between the carbohydrate and active protein are responsible for ameliorating dehydration stress in the solid state. As mentioned, this pathway can guarantee thermodynamic protein stability during the dying process [20,74].

3.2. The Glassy Matrix Hypothesis

The glassy matrix hypothesis is another mechanism that has a considerable effect on the kinetics of protein denaturation reactions. Because of molecular mobility, protein formulations are prone to chemical degradation, including protein aggregation and unfolding reactions. Some excipients, such as high molecular weight carbohydrates, may provide a rigid, glassy matrix that suppresses undesirable degradation reactions (glass dynamic hypothesis). Protein molecules can embed in a solid glassy matrix, which limits global mobility. Since protein mobility in a solid dosage form is restricted, possible protein-protein interactions are slowed, and the stability of proteins are preserved [20,74].

3.3. Reducing Surface Adsorption

Surfactants such as polysorbate 20 can localize at the interfacial surface owing to high surface activity. Thus fewer proteins are localized at particle surfaces and inhibit protein degradation [1].

Table 3. Additives used as stabilizers during drying procedures.

Stabilizers		Stabilization		References
		Mechanism	Process	
Proteins	Human or Bovine serum albumin	Water replacement (Hydrogen bonding)	Freezing Dehydration Thermal stress	[1,18,52,74]
Amino acids	Glycine, Alanine, Histidine, Leucine Phenylalanine, Arginine, Aspartic acid	Water replacement Bulking agent Buffering agent Prevent protein-protein interactions		
Polyols	Polyethylene glycol, Mannitol, Sorbitol	Water replacement Glassy state Increase matrix density	Freezing Dehydration	[74]
Carbohydrate (reducing and non-reducing sugar)	Fructose, Glucose, Lactose, Maltose, Maltodextrin Trehalose, Sucrose, Inulin, Dextran	Water replacement Glassy state (reduce global protein mobility) Reduce local protein mobility Protein-sugar interactions	Freezing Dehydration Thermal stress	[20,52,74]
Buffer and Salt	HEPES buffer, Citrate buffer, Phosphate buffer saline, Ammonium sulfate	Buffering agent	Freezing	[64]
Surfactant	Polysorbate 20, 80, Oleic acid, Sodium glycolate	Prevent surface adsorption (Reduce interfacial stress) Prevent protein-protein interactions (Prevent intermolecular interactions) Slow dissolution rate	Shear stress Interfacial stress Freezing Reconstitution	[20,74]
Polymers and Polysaccharides	Cyclodextrin, Dextran, PLGA, Hydroxy propyl β-cyclodextrin, Na-Carboxy methylcellulose	Glassy state	Freezing	[20]
Metals	Zinc	Reduce surface area	Freezing Interfacial stress	[36]

4. Delivery and Pharmacokinetics of Dried-Powder Proteins

4.1. Pulmonary Delivery

The most predominant application of dried-powder protein formulations is for pulmonary delivery. In the pulmonary delivery of proteins, mucocilliary clearance, phagocytosis by macrophages, and alveolar proteolytic enzymes are critical biological barriers to local and systemic delivery. In systemic delivery, passage of the alveolar capillary membrane, proteases in blood circulation, renal clearance, and hepatic clearance are restricting factors that decrease the bioavailability of protein drugs [14].

4.1.1. Local Delivery

Dried protein inhalation has been used as a topical drug delivery method for treating respiratory diseases. Direct drug delivery to the site of action provides high drug concentrations in the lung while reducing systemic blood circulation exposure to the drug, allowing safe therapies with high efficacies. The IL-4/IL-13 antagonist, IgG1, and an anti-IgE monoclonal antibody (Omalizumab®) have been administered as dried powder inhaler preparations for asthma, chronic obstructive pulmonary disease (COPD), or other related lung diseases [75]. For local administration, some important biological barriers should be considered to provide optimal therapeutic efficacy. Alveolar macrophage clearance of inhaled proteins is dependent on particle size, which can be decreased using both nanoparticles (diameter < 0.3 μm) and large particles (geometric diameter > 6 μm) [14]. Using SD method, insulin-loaded phospholipid/chitosan nanoparticles have been incorporated into microspheres in the presence of mannitol. Insulin-loaded microspheres have shown spherical morphology with suitable aerodynamic behavior as an inhalation preparation (aerodynamic diameter: 2–3 μm, density: 0.4–0.5 g/cm^3) [76]. Edwards et al. showed that the in vivo sustained release of insulin in rats was achieved after inhalation of large porous particles (diameter > 5 μm, density < 0.4 g/cm^2) prepared from poly(lactide-co-glycolide) (PLGA) [77]. Large porous insulin particles were inspired deep into the lungs and escaped pulmonary macrophage clearance mechanisms with a decreased immune response. Inhalation of larger porous insulin particles compared with smaller non-porous particles results in higher systemic bioavailability and suppression of systemic glucose levels for a longer period. This study showed that pulmonary protein delivery might provide highly efficient delivery of inhaled drugs into the systemic blood circulation. Additionally, large porous particles present better aerosolization efficiency. Higher aerosolization efficiency results in a decreased possibility of deposition losses before particle entry into the intrapulmonary airways, thereby enhancing the systemic concentration of an inhaled drug. Because of the relatively smaller surface areas of dried powders of large porous particles, less inter-particulate interaction occurs, resulting in decreased aggregation. Large porous particles based on a dipalmitoyl phosphatidylcholine (DPPC) combination as a dried powder inhaler preparation has revealed good characteristics for pulmonary delivery of peptides and proteins, such as parathyroid hormone, insulin, heparin, and human growth hormone. Moreover, in the presence of DPPC, the protein particles might have the potential for sustained release as an inhalant [14]. Among microparticles, hybrid large porous particles that have been prepared by the accumulation of nanoparticles using SD method are advantageous. The drug delivery and release patterns of nanoparticles combined with proper flow properties and aerosolization potential of large porous particles result in greater therapeutic effects of inhaled drugs [78].

Another clearance mechanism is the proteolytic enzymes present in the lung, which can degrade biomacromolecules by proteolysis. The addition of a protease inhibitor such as nafamostat, bacitracin, a trypsin inhibitor, chymostatin, leupeptin, bestatin, or aprotonin to the inhaled protein formulation may be useful for protecting proteins and leads to concentration enhancement [79,80]. When inhalable insulin was co-administered with nafamostat and bacitracin, its relative bioavailability increased, indicating that the proteins escaped from lung protease clearance [81,82].

4.1.2. Systemic Delivery

Besides local inhalation therapies, pulmonary delivery of calcitonin, parathyroid hormone, and insulin (Exubera® and Afrezza®) was developed for the treatment of osteoporosis, growth deficiency, and diabetes, respectively [71]. Systemic protein delivery through inhalation has been suggested to be a very promising alternative to parenteral delivery of proteins, and features the unique combination of a highly dispersed dosage form and an extended surface area to access the blood circulatory system [71]. Specific obstacles must be considered when a therapeutic protein is intended for systemic administration, because a sufficient proportion of drug molecule is required to be absorbed via the alveolar epithelium. For systemic administration of proteins, it is necessary to prevent degradation by blood clearance pathways, such as blood proteolytic enzymes, hepatic metabolism, and renal clearance to achieve an appropriate circulatory drug level leading to sufficient systemic bioavailability [14]. A major challenge to crossing the alveolar capillary membrane is the relative impermeability of the membrane to biomacromolecules. Macromolecule absorption through the double-layered phospholipid membrane by simple diffusion is limited by high molecular weight and hydrophilic nature of proteins. The absorption rates of macromolecules into the blood circulation are usually inversely related to molecular weight, with higher molecular weights leading to a higher T_{max} and lower C_{max} and partition coefficients [83]. There are some strategies to improve protein adsorption through the capillary membrane from the lungs into the blood. Absorption enhancers, such as surfactants, bile salts, cyclodextrins, citric acid, chitosan, and lipid-based carriers (liposomes), are suggested pathways to address the absorption issue [14].

4.2. Nasal Delivery

There is growing interest in the solid dosage forms of vaccines, which eliminate preservatives and the cold chain circulation for shipping and storage, while preserving protein stability at ambient temperature. Nasal delivery of vaccine formulations may be a good alternative to conventional vaccines [19]. Garmise et al. [84] demonstrated that an SFD powder of influenza virus increased local residence time and subsequently enhanced mucosal and systemic antibody production for nasal vaccination. Muco-adhesive compounds were characterized for their effects on the nasal residence time of vaccine powders in rats compared with in vitro data and stimulated immune responses. In vitro studies and in vivo imaging experiments revealed that sodium alginate and carboxy-methyl-cellulose powder combinations could enhance residence time in Brown Norway rats. It was concluded that nasal administration of dry powder influenza vaccine, especially in the presence of sodium alginate, could enhance serum and mucosal antibody responses. Furthermore, nasal delivery is an attractive vaccine platform for inoculating against other mucosal-transmitted diseases. Recently, Cho et al. [85] prepared a nasal powder formulation of salmon calcitonin (sCT) in the presence of a stabilizer (inulin or trehalose) and an absorption enhancer (chitosan, sodium taurocholate, or βCD) to improve its bioavailability. Dried powder inhalers of sCT were prepared by SD and novel SCF-assisted spray drying (SCF-SD). The in vivo absorption test in rats showed that spray-dried and SCF-spray-dried sCT powders increased the bioavailability of the peptide drug when compared with the nasal administration of unprocessed sCT, which was attributed to the absorption enhancer. Among the three absorption enhancers, chitosan-containing formulation showed the highest bioavailability, which was thought to be due to its properties of mucoadhesion or effects on tight junction to decrease mucociliary clearance. In addition, SCF-spray-dried sCT exhibited higher nasal absorption than spray-dried sCT in all formulations owing to the smaller size of particles. This study showed that SCF-SD method would be a promising approach for nasal delivery of dried powder inhaler of sCT.

4.3. Sustained-Release Delivery

Despite the high bioavailability of parenteral protein delivery, frequent injections result in poor patient compliance. Microsphere depot delivery system is designed to release the drug in a sustained manner over an extended period for systemic or local delivery. Spray freeze-dried BSA nanoparticles are encapsulated into PLGA microspheres to allow sustained release and to reduce the burst release pattern. The porous, solid protein particles break up into sub-micrometer particles followed by encapsulation into PLGA microspheres using anhydrous double emulsion techniques. In SFD, because of fast freezing and the absence of interfacial interactions, denaturation and aggregation of BSA were minimized, and the integrity and conformational stability of encapsulated BSA were preserved. The reduced burst release of BSA is attributed to the uniform distribution of protein nanoparticles in PLGA microspheres, which could be used as a sustainable delivery vehicle for biopharmaceuticals. Protein-PEG complexes are prepared by solubilizing BSA and recombinant human growth hormone (rhGH) in the methylene chloride phase. The organic phase containing PLGA and PEG/protein complexes was atomized through SD to prepare PLGA microparticles encapsulating proteins with good stability [86]. They exhibited sustained release profiles of BSA and rhGH and the released protein from the microsphere preserved their stability without aggregation. The protein microencapsulation method may prove to be a good platform for sustained delivery of therapeutic proteins that are not soluble in organic solvents. Cleland et al. [87] prepared PLGA microspheres containing recombinant human vascular endothelial growth factor (rhVEGF). The protein formulation was first sprayed into liquid nitrogen using an ultrasonic atomizer to produce rhVEGF PLGA microspheres. The SFD protein powder was added to a PLGA solution to prepare microspheres with a 9% *w/w* loading efficiency. SEC and mitogenic receptor-IgG binding affinity analyses showed that the stability and efficacy of rhVEGF were preserved through the SFD procedure. A study conducted by Al-Qadi et al. [88] presented a dried powder inhaler comprising microencapsulated insulin-loaded chitosan nanoparticles. The developed system was evaluated in rats to evaluate its potential for systemic delivery of insulin. The insulin-loaded chitosan nanoparticles were prepared by ionotropic gelation, followed by co-spray drying of nanoparticles with mannitol. Dried powder inhaler of insulin showed proper aerodynamic behavior for pulmonary delivery. The assessment of plasma glucose levels following intratracheal administration to rats showed that the microencapsulated insulin-loaded chitosan nanoparticles provided a sustained release of insulin with a more pronounced hypoglycemic effect than the insulin solution. This presents a good example of sustained release dried formulations for local or systemic delivery.

4.4. Enhancing Solubility and Bioavailability of Cyclosporine A

Cyclosporine A (CsA) is a cyclic undecapeptide drug used for the prevention of allograft rejection after lung transplantation [37]. As CsA has poor water-solubility, approaches to improve its solubility, bioavailability, and therapeutic efficacy have been designed. The solid dispersion of amorphous CsA in a methylcellulose-based matrix showed higher solubility than the physical mixture of the drug and methylcellulose. Additionally, an inhalable dry-emulsion preparation of CsA in the presence of glycerol monooleate as a surfactant showed better dissolution behavior and improved bioavailability compared with the native drug and its amorphous solid dispersion. The polymer-based amorphous solid dispersion of CsA as a dry powder inhaler revealed improved pharmacodynamic behavior as well as fewer side-effects [37]. Chiou et al. used a liquid impinging jet procedure to precipitate CsA nanoparticles with lecithin and lactose as stabilizing agents, followed by SD to produce nanoparticles for inhalation [89]. The aerosol performance of powders was evaluated using an Aeroliser® dry powder inhaler with multi-stage liquid impinging jets. Nanomatrix powders exhibited appropriate flow properties (with a fine particle fraction of approximately 55%) and corresponding aerosol behavior. They demonstrated that the combination of precipitation with SD procedure has the potential to allow the design of protein particles with improved pharmacokinetics. Yamasaki et al. demonstrated that inhalable CsA nanoparticles in a mannitol-based matrix improved the dissolution of the drug [90]. CsA nanosuspensions were prepared using anti-solvent precipitation and subsequently, the micro aggregates were achieved using an SD procedure. The combination of amorphous CsA and crystalline mannitol showed similar drug content to the theoretical doses. The inclusion of mannitol as a wetting agent improved the dissolution rate of the drug, without significant impact on aerosol performance.

This study indicated that the proper combination of drug and excipients could provide enhanced dissolution rate, with improved bioavailability of hydrophobic drugs, such as CsA.

4.5. Pharmacokinetics of Inhaled Insulins

In 2006, Exubera® (Pfizer Inc., New York, NY, USA; Nektar Therapeutics, San Carlos, CA, USA) became the first inhaled insulin preparation approved by the US Food and Drug Administration (FDA) and European Medicines Evaluation Agency (EMEA). The Exubera® device involves dispersion of insulin dry powder into aerosolized insulin within a large chamber, followed by patient inhalation. Exubera® was delivered in a dry powder formulation containing amorphous insulin, glycine, mannitol, and sodium citrate as stabilizers. The dry powder of matrix particles was prepared using an SD method. The resulting powder, with low moisture content, showed good storage stability at room temperature for two years [91]. The onset of action was more rapid (32 min vs. 48 min, respectively) for Exubera® than for subcutaneously injected (s.c.) insulin, and was comparable to lispro insulin. Furthermore, the duration of action of Exubera® was longer than the duration of lispro (387 min vs. 313 min) and comparable to s.c. insulin [92]. However, after one year of commercialization, Exubera® was withdrawn in 2007 because of its low bioavailability and enhanced treatment-related cost [92,93]. Some previous studies demonstrated the equivalence of Exubera® to regular s.c. insulin in both type I and type II diabetes patients [94,95].

Another inhaled insulin product Afrezza® (MannKind Corporation, Valencia, CA, USA) reached the market in 2014 and is currently the only inhaled insulin available in the market [91]. The formulation is based on Technosphere™ drug carrier technology, in which insulin is trapped and microencapsulated in small precipitated particles during self-assembly [96,97]. The precipitates are freeze-dried, but leaves small residual amounts of water [98]. Afrezza® is a drug–device product containing a Technosphere insulin (TI) inhalation powder in single-use dose cartridges, which are administered with an inhaler. The particle size is 2–3 μm, with an internal porosity of approximately 70%, and once inhaled, it dissolves in the pH-neutral environment of the deep lung and rapidly releases insulin into the systemic blood circulation. TI inhalers mimic rapid-acting s.c. insulin analogs with a C_{max} of 15 min [91,98]. Pfützner and Forst compared the pharmacokinetics of 100 IU of Afrezza®, 10 IU with regular s.c. insulin, and 5 IU of i.v. insulin in healthy subjects [96]. Afrezza® demonstrated very rapid absorption, with a mean T_{max} of 13 min vs. 121 min for regular s.c. insulin. In addition, Afrezza® provided significantly higher bioavailability and faster absorption than Exubera® (bioavailability relative to s.c. regular insulin of 26% and 10% respectively, and T_{max} of 13 min vs. 45 min). Afrezza® still presents a much greater bioavailability than any other inhaled insulin formulations introduced to date. The observed pharmacokinetic profile could be explained by the highly efficient delivery of Afrezza® particles to the deep lung (owing to the smaller particle size of Afrezza®). Because they are very small and porous, particles can be dissolved rapidly and provide high local concentrations of insulin that can be rapidly absorbed in the alveolae [98].

5. Future Perspectives and Conclusions

The development of therapeutic proteins has increased rapidly owing to their high therapeutic efficacy. Since the advent of human insulin in 1982, over hundreds of recombinant proteins have been developed and monoclonal antibody therapeutics market increased exponentially. Structurally modified proteins, such as PEGylated proteins and fusion proteins, and antibody-drug conjugate for cancer therapy have been recently available as therapeutics [99–101]. Biopharmaceuticals are available as liquid or solid dosage forms. In general, proteins have greater stability in the solid state than in the liquid state [33,41]. To achieve the desirable stability of proteins in formulations, solid-state dosage form is preferred to liquid-state dosage form, because it can provide a better shelf-life in storage. Numerous drying technologies, including FD, SD, SFD, and SCFD, have been used for dried protein formulations, and they have become an important method for the manufacture, storage, and delivery of protein-based biopharmaceuticals [14,25,26,37]. However, dried protein formulations still have challenges of stability and further optimization for desirable pharmacokinetic properties [3,83].

Currently, many dried protein powders have been produced through SD methods and other drying methods are still used only at the laboratory scale. In the future, drying methods at the laboratory scale must be scaled up for biopharmaceutical product development. Thus, modification of the existing drying technologies may be required. Achieving higher level of control of drying process parameters and performing under milder conditions may contribute to the improvement of stability and quality of biopharmaceuticals.

Dried powder inhaler preparations have mainly focused on local drug delivery systems for treating pulmonary diseases. However, these dosage forms also have a potential for systemic administration of therapeutic proteins, as demonstrated by the approved inhaled insulin products (Exubera® and Afrezza®) [91]. Inhalation delivery of proteins can be a good choice for systemic delivery of protein drugs because pulmonary administration generally leads to higher bioavailability of protein drugs than other nonparenteral administrations, such as nasal or transdermal delivery [14]. Pulmonary route leads to rapid drug absorption owing to large surface area, low thickness of the epithelium, and rich blood supply, and avoids hepatic first-pass metabolism [83].

Since the development of pulmonary protein administration has shown significant progress, it can be predicted that soon the inhalation of proteins may become the first practical alternative to parenteral delivery. Clinical trials, as well as experimental studies have demonstrated that insulin as an inhaler possesses similar pharmacokinetic properties to that of s.c. injection of regular insulin, and even better properties than those observed with s.c. administration of rapid-acting insulin analogs. Substitution of injection with inhalation would be preferred by patients. However, there is no improvement with respective developments. If inhaled insulin becomes successful for diabetic therapy in terms of bioavailability and treatment cost, it will most probably create opportunities for the use of other biopharmaceuticals as inhalation preparations. Recently, other proteins and peptides have been studied for treating diabetes through the pulmonary route [100,102]. The major concerns regarding the long-term application of protein inhalers, such as insulin, are the development of insulin-antibodies and lung safety issues, which should be considered in future studies. Additionally, there are not sufficient studies considering the economic aspects of healthcare systems.

In conclusion, the successful solid dosage form of protein formulations in the presence of stabilizing agents could be achieved using several drying technologies. Cryoprotectants and lyoprotectants can maintain the stability and bioactivity of biopharmaceuticals. In each drying method, critical process parameters should first be optimized. Finally, screening of formulations based on protein properties is performed to determine the optimal stable protein/stabilizer combinations for a sustained-release, pulmonary, or nasal formulation.

Author Contributions: F.E. wrote the paper as the primary author. E.J.P. contributed to part of the text. D.H.N. and A.V. conceived the design of the article, supervised its writing, and had editorial responsibility. All the authors approved the final manuscript.

Funding: This research received no external funding.

Acknowledgments: This work was supported by the National Research Foundation of Korea (NRF) grants funded by the Ministry of Science and ICT (NRF-2018R1A2B3004266) and by the Technology Innovation Program (20000265, Stabilization platform of high concentration and stable liquid injection based on physical properties of biomaterials) funded by the Ministry of Trade, Industry & Energy (MOTIE, Korea).

Conflicts of Interest: The authors declare no conflict of interest.

References

1. Ajmera, A.; Scherliess, R. Stabilisation of proteins via mixtures of amino acids during spray drying. *Int. J. Pharm.* **2014**, *463*, 98–107. [CrossRef] [PubMed]
2. Ramezani, V.; Vatanara, A.; Najafabadi, A.R.; Shokrgozar, M.A.; Khabiri, A.; Seyedabadi, M. A comparative study on the physicochemical and biological stability of IgG 1 and monoclonal antibodies during spray drying process. *DARU J. Pharm. Sci.* **2014**, *22*, 31. [CrossRef] [PubMed]
3. Cicerone, M.T.; Pikal, M.J.; Qian, K.K. Stabilization of proteins in solid form. *Adv. Drug Deliv. Rev.* **2015**, *93*, 14–24. [CrossRef] [PubMed]
4. Daugherty, A.L.; Mrsny, R.J. Formulation and delivery issues for monoclonal antibody therapeutics. *Adv. Drug Deliv. Rev.* **2006**, *58*, 686–706. [CrossRef] [PubMed]
5. Kumar, V.; Sharma, V.K.; Kalonia, D.S. In situ precipitation and vacuum drying of interferon alpha-2a: Development of a single-step process for obtaining dry, stable protein formulation. *Int. J. Pharm.* **2009**, *366*, 88–98. [CrossRef] [PubMed]
6. Na, D.H.; Youn, Y.S.; Lee, I.B.; Park, E.J.; Park, C.J.; Lee, K.C. Effect of molecular size of pegylated recombinant human epidermal growth factor on the biological activity and stability in rat wound tissue. *Pharm. Dev. Technol.* **2006**, *11*, 513–519. [CrossRef] [PubMed]
7. Lee, W.; Park, E.J.; Kwak, S.; Lee, K.C.; Na, D.H.; Bae, J.-S. Trimeric peg-conjugated exendin-4 for the treatment of sepsis. *Biomacromolecules* **2016**, *17*, 1160–1169. [CrossRef] [PubMed]
8. Park, E.J.; Tak, T.H.; Na, D.H.; Lee, K.C. Effect of PEGylation on stability of peptide in poly(lactide-*co*-glycolide) microspheres. *Arch. Pharm. Res.* **2010**, *33*, 1111–1116. [CrossRef] [PubMed]
9. Na, D.H.; DeLuca, P.P. PEGylation of octreotide: I. Separation of positional isomers and stability against acylation by poly(D,L-lactide-*co*-gycolide). *Pharm. Res.* **2005**, *22*, 736–742. [CrossRef] [PubMed]
10. Kim, Y.; Park, E.J.; Na, D.H. Recent progress in dendrimer-based nanomedicine. *Arch. Pharm. Res.* **2018**, *41*, 571–582. [CrossRef] [PubMed]
11. Szlachcic, A.; Zakrzewska, M.; Otlewski, J. Longer action means better drug: Tuning up protein therapeutics. *Biotechnol. Adv.* **2011**, *29*, 436–441. [CrossRef] [PubMed]
12. Mohtashamian, S.; Boddohi, S. Nanostructured polysaccharide-based carriers for antimicrobial peptide delivery. *J. Pharm. Investig.* **2017**, *47*, 85–94. [CrossRef]
13. Kim, C.H.; Lee, S.G.; Kang, M.J.; Lee, S.; Choi, Y.W. Surface modification of lipid-based nanocarriers for cancer cell-specific drug targeting. *J. Pharm. Investig.* **2017**, *47*, 203–227. [CrossRef]
14. Depreter, F.; Pilcer, G.; Amighi, K. Inhaled proteins: Challenges and perspectives. *Int. J. Pharm.* **2013**, *447*, 251–280. [CrossRef] [PubMed]
15. Maltesen, M.J.; Van De Weert, M. Drying methods for protein pharmaceuticals. *Drug Discov. Today Technol.* **2008**, *5*, e81–e88. [CrossRef] [PubMed]
16. Smales, C.M.; James, D.C. *Therapeutic Proteins: Methods and Protocols*; Springer: Berlin, Germany, 2005; Volume 308.
17. Liao, Y.H.; Brown, M.B.; Martin, G.P. Investigation of the stabilisation of freeze-dried lysozyme and the physical properties of the formulations. *Eur. J. Pharm. Biopharm.* **2004**, *58*, 15–24. [CrossRef] [PubMed]
18. Tian, F.; Sane, S.; Rytting, J.H. Calorimetric investigation of protein/amino acid interactions in the solid state. *Int. J. Pharm.* **2006**, *310*, 175–186. [CrossRef] [PubMed]
19. Wang, S.H.; Kirwan, S.M.; Abraham, S.N.; Staats, H.F.; Hickey, A.J. Stable dry powder formulation for nasal delivery of anthrax vaccine. *J. Pharm. Sci.* **2012**, *101*, 31–47. [CrossRef] [PubMed]
20. Mensink, M.A.; Frijlink, H.W.; van der Voort Maarschalk, K.; Hinrichs, W.L. How sugars protect proteins in the solid state and during drying (review): Mechanisms of stabilization in relation to stress conditions. *Eur. J. Pharm. Biopharm.* **2017**, *114*, 288–295. [CrossRef] [PubMed]
21. Maa, Y.-F.; Nguyen, P.-A.; Sweeney, T.; Shire, S.J.; Hsu, C.C. Protein inhalation powders: Spray drying vs. spray freeze drying. *Pharm. Res.* **1999**, *16*, 249–254. [CrossRef] [PubMed]
22. Nuchuchua, O.; Every, H.A.; Hofland, G.W.; Jiskoot, W. Scalable organic solvent free supercritical fluid spray drying process for producing dry protein formulations. *Eur. J. Pharm. Biopharm.* **2014**, *88*, 919–930. [CrossRef] [PubMed]
23. Walters, R.H.; Bhatnagar, B.; Tchessalov, S.; Izutsu, K.; Tsumoto, K.; Ohtake, S. Next generation drying technologies for pharmaceutical applications. *J. Pharm. Sci.* **2014**, *103*, 2673–2695. [CrossRef] [PubMed]

24. Weers, J.G.; Miller, D.P. Formulation design of dry powders for inhalation. *J. Pharm. Sci.* **2015**, *104*, 3259–3288. [CrossRef] [PubMed]

25. Langford, A.; Bhatnagar, B.; Walters, R.; Tchessalov, S.; Ohtake, S. Drying of biopharmaceuticals: Recent developments, new technologies and future direction. *Jpn. J. Food Eng.* **2018**, *19*, 15–24.

26. Langford, A.; Bhatnagar, B.; Walters, R.; Tchessalov, S.; Ohtake, S. Drying technologies for biopharmaceutical applications: Recent developments and future direction. *Dry. Technol.* **2018**, *36*, 677–684. [CrossRef]

27. Abdul-Fattah, A.M.; Kalonia, D.S.; Pikal, M.J. The challenge of drying method selection for protein pharmaceuticals: Product quality implications. *J. Pharm. Sci.* **2007**, *96*, 1886–1916. [CrossRef] [PubMed]

28. Guerrero, M.; Albet, C.; Palomer, A.; Guglietta, A. Drying in pharmaceutical and biotechnological industries. *Food Sci. Technol. Int.* **2003**, *9*, 237–243. [CrossRef]

29. Shukla, S. Freeze drying process: A review. *Int. J. Pharm. Sci. Res.* **2011**, *2*, 3061.

30. Faghihi, H.; Khalili, F.; Amini, M.; Vatanara, A. The effect of freeze-dried antibody concentrations on its stability in the presence of trehalose and hydroxypropyl-β-cyclodextrin: A box–behnken statistical design. *Pharm. Dev. Technol.* **2017**, *22*, 724–732. [CrossRef] [PubMed]

31. Roy, I.; Gupta, M.N. Freeze-drying of proteins: Some emerging concerns. *Biotechnol. Appl. Biochem.* **2004**, *39*, 165–177. [CrossRef] [PubMed]

32. Tang, X.; Pikal, M.J. Design of freeze-drying processes for pharmaceuticals: Practical advice. *Pharm. Res.* **2004**, *21*, 191–200. [CrossRef] [PubMed]

33. Lim, J.Y.; Kim, N.A.; Lim, D.G.; Kim, K.H.; Choi, D.H.; Jeong, S.H. Process cycle development of freeze drying for therapeutic proteins with stability evaluation. *J. Pharm. Investig.* **2016**, *46*, 519–536. [CrossRef]

34. Pieters, S.; De Beer, T.; Kasper, J.C.; Boulpaep, D.; Waszkiewicz, O.; Goodarzi, M.; Tistaert, C.; Friess, W.; Remon, J.P.; Vervaet, C.; et al. Near-infrared spectroscopy for in-line monitoring of protein unfolding and its interactions with lyoprotectants during freeze-drying. *Anal. Chem.* **2012**, *84*, 947–955. [CrossRef] [PubMed]

35. Oetjen, G.W. *Freeze-Drying*; Wiley: Hoboken, NJ, USA, 2004.

36. Costantino, H.R.; Firouzabadian, L.; Wu, C.; Carrasquillo, K.G.; Griebenow, K.; Zale, S.E.; Tracy, M.A. Protein spray freeze drying. 2. Effect of formulation variables on particle size and stability. *J. Pharm. Sci.* **2002**, *91*, 388–395. [CrossRef] [PubMed]

37. Chen, L.; Okuda, T.; Lu, X.-Y.; Chan, H.-K. Amorphous powders for inhalation drug delivery. *Adv. Drug Deliv. Rev.* **2016**, *100*, 102–115. [CrossRef] [PubMed]

38. Tonnis, W.; Mensink, M.; De Jager, A.; Van Der Voort Maarschalk, K.; Frijlink, H.; Hinrichs, W. Size and molecular flexibility of sugars determine the storage stability of freeze-dried proteins. *Mol. Pharm.* **2015**, *12*, 684–694. [CrossRef] [PubMed]

39. Pilcer, G.; Amighi, K. Formulation strategy and use of excipients in pulmonary drug delivery. *Int. J. Pharm.* **2010**, *392*, 1–19. [CrossRef] [PubMed]

40. Sosnik, A.; Seremeta, K.P. Advantages and challenges of the spray-drying technology for the production of pure drug particles and drug-loaded polymeric carriers. *Adv. Colloid Interface Sci.* **2015**, *223*, 40–54. [CrossRef] [PubMed]

41. Ameri, M.; Maa, Y.-F. Spray drying of biopharmaceuticals: Stability and process considerations. *Dry. Technol.* **2006**, *24*, 763–768. [CrossRef]

42. Faghihi, H.; Vatanara, A.; Najafabadi, A.R.; Ramezani, V.; Gilani, K. The use of amino acids to prepare physically and conformationally stable spray-dried IgG with enhanced aerosol performance. *Int. J. Pharm.* **2014**, *466*, 163–171. [CrossRef] [PubMed]

43. Maa, Y.-F.; Sellers, S.P. Solid-state protein formulation. In *Therapeutic Proteins Methods Protocols*; Humana Press: New York, NY, USA, 2005; pp. 265–285.

44. Poursina, N.; Vatanara, A.; Rouini, M.R.; Gilani, K.; Rouholamini Najafabadi, A. Systemic delivery of parathyroid hormone (1–34) using spray freeze-dried inhalable particles. *Pharm. Dev. Technol.* **2017**, *22*, 733–739. [CrossRef] [PubMed]

45. Ramezani, V.; Vatanara, A.; Najafabadi, A.R.; Gilani, K.; Nabi-Meybodi, M. Screening and evaluation of variables in the formation of antibody particles by spray drying. *Powder Technol.* **2013**, *233*, 341–346. [CrossRef]

46. Vehring, R. Pharmaceutical particle engineering via spray drying. *Pharm. Res.* **2008**, *25*, 999–1022. [CrossRef] [PubMed]

47. Schüle, S.; Frieß, W.; Bechtold-Peters, K.; Garidel, P. Conformational analysis of protein secondary structure during spray-drying of antibody/mannitol formulations. *Eur. J. Pharm. Biopharm.* **2007**, *65*, 1–9. [CrossRef] [PubMed]
48. Li, H.Y.; Song, X.; Seville, P.C. The use of sodium carboxymethylcellulose in the preparation of spray-dried proteins for pulmonary drug delivery. *Eur. J. Pharm. Sci.* **2010**, *40*, 56–61. [CrossRef] [PubMed]
49. Wanning, S.; Suverkrup, R.; Lamprecht, A. Jet-vortex spray freeze drying for the production of inhalable lyophilisate powders. *Eur. J. Pharm. Sci.* **2017**, *96*, 1–7. [CrossRef] [PubMed]
50. Wanning, S.; Süverkrüp, R.; Lamprecht, A. Pharmaceutical spray freeze drying. *Int. J. Pharm.* **2015**, *488*, 136–153. [CrossRef] [PubMed]
51. Rogers, T.L.; Johnston, K.P.; Williams, R.O., 3rd. Solution-based particle formation of pharmaceutical powders by supercritical or compressed fluid CO_2 and cryogenic spray-freezing technologies. *Drug Dev. Ind. Pharm.* **2001**, *27*, 1003–1015. [CrossRef] [PubMed]
52. Emami, F.; Vatanara, A.; Najafabadi, A.R.; Kim, Y.; Park, E.J.; Sardari, S.; Na, D.H. Effect of amino acids on the stability of spray freeze-dried immunoglobulin G in sugar-based matrices. *Eur. J. Pharm. Sci.* **2018**, *119*, 39–48. [CrossRef] [PubMed]
53. Poursina, N.; Vatanara, A.; Rouini, M.R.; Gilani, K.; Najafabadi, A.R. The effect of excipients on the stability and aerosol performance of salmon calcitonin dry powder inhalers prepared via spray freeze drying process. *Acta Pharm.* **2016**, *66*, 207–218. [CrossRef] [PubMed]
54. Rahmati, M.R.; Vatanara, A.; Parsian, A.R.; Gilani, K.; Khosravi, K.M.; Darabi, M.; Najafabadi, A.R. Effect of formulation ingredients on the physical characteristics of salmeterol xinafoate microparticles tailored by spray freeze drying. *Adv. Powder Technol.* **2013**, *24*, 36–42. [CrossRef]
55. Parsian, A.R.; Vatanara, A.; Rahmati, M.R.; Gilani, K.; Khosravi, K.M.; Najafabadi, A.R. Inhalable budesonide porous microparticles tailored by spray freeze drying technique. *Powder Technol.* **2014**, *260*, 36–41. [CrossRef]
56. Rogers, T.L.; Nelsen, A.C.; Hu, J.; Brown, J.N.; Sarkari, M.; Young, T.J.; Johnston, K.P.; Williams, R.O. A novel particle engineering technology to enhance dissolution of poorly water soluble drugs: Spray-freezing into liquid. *Eur. J. Pharm. Biopharm.* **2002**, *54*, 271–280. [CrossRef]
57. Rogers, T.L.; Hu, J.; Yu, Z.; Johnston, K.P.; Williams, R.O. A novel particle engineering technology: Spray-freezing into liquid. *Int. J. Pharm.* **2002**, *242*, 93–100. [CrossRef]
58. Maa, Y.F.; Ameri, M.; Shu, C.; Payne, L.G.; Chen, D. Influenza vaccine powder formulation development: Spray-freeze-drying and stability evaluation. *J. Pharm. Sci.* **2004**, *93*, 1912–1923. [CrossRef] [PubMed]
59. Jovanovic, N.; Bouchard, A.; Sutter, M.; Van Speybroeck, M.; Hofland, G.W.; Witkamp, G.J.; Crommelin, D.J.; Jiskoot, W. Stable sugar-based protein formulations by supercritical fluid drying. *Int. J. Pharm.* **2008**, *346*, 102–108. [CrossRef] [PubMed]
60. Jovanović, N.; Bouchard, A.; Hofland, G.W.; Witkamp, G.-J.; Crommelin, D.J.; Jiskoot, W. Stabilization of proteins in dry powder formulations using supercritical fluid technology. *Pharm. Res.* **2004**, *21*, 1955–1969. [CrossRef] [PubMed]
61. Garidel, P.; Pevestorf, B.; Bahrenburg, S. Stability of buffer-free freeze-dried formulations: A feasibility study of a monoclonal antibody at high protein concentrations. *Eur. J. Pharm. Biopharm.* **2015**, *97*, 125–139. [CrossRef] [PubMed]
62. Mohammad Zadeh, A.H.; Rouholamini Najafabadi, A.; Vatanara, A.; Faghihi, H.; Gilani, K. Effect of molecular weight and ratio of poly ethylene glycols' derivatives in combination with trehalose on stability of freeze-dried IgG. *Drug Dev. Ind. Pharm.* **2017**, *43*, 1945–1951. [CrossRef] [PubMed]
63. Imamura, K.; Ogawa, T.; Sakiyama, T.; Nakanishi, K. Effects of types of sugar on the stabilization of protein in the dried state. *J. Pharm. Sci.* **2003**, *92*, 266–274. [CrossRef] [PubMed]
64. Saluja, V.; Amorij, J.P.; Kapteyn, J.C.; de Boer, A.H.; Frijlink, H.W.; Hinrichs, W.L. A comparison between spray drying and spray freeze drying to produce an influenza subunit vaccine powder for inhalation. *J. Control. Release* **2010**, *144*, 127–133. [CrossRef] [PubMed]
65. Bittner, B.; Morlock, M.; Koll, H.; Winter, G.; Kissel, T. Recombinant human erythropoietin (rhEPO) loaded poly (lactide-*co*-glycolide) microspheres: Influence of the encapsulation technique and polymer purity on microsphere characteristics. *Eur. J. Pharm. Biopharm.* **1998**, *45*, 295–305. [CrossRef]
66. Jovanovic, N.; Bouchard, A.; Hofland, G.W.; Witkamp, G.J.; Crommelin, D.J.; Jiskoot, W. Stabilization of IgG by supercritical fluid drying: Optimization of formulation and process parameters. *Eur. J. Pharm. Biopharm.* **2008**, *68*, 183–190. [CrossRef] [PubMed]

67. Jovanovic, N.; Bouchard, A.; Hofland, G.W.; Witkamp, G.J.; Crommelin, D.J.; Jiskoot, W. Distinct effects of sucrose and trehalose on protein stability during supercritical fluid drying and freeze-drying. *Eur. J. Pharm. Sci.* **2006**, *27*, 336–345. [CrossRef] [PubMed]

68. Amidi, M.; Pellikaan, H.C.; de Boer, A.H.; Crommelin, D.J.; Hennink, W.E.; Jiskoot, W. Preparation and physicochemical characterization of supercritically dried insulin-loaded microparticles for pulmonary delivery. *Eur. J. Pharm. Biopharm.* **2008**, *68*, 191–200. [CrossRef] [PubMed]

69. Ali, M.E.; Lamprecht, A. Spray freeze drying for dry powder inhalation of nanoparticles. *Eur. J. Pharm. Biopharm.* **2014**, *87*, 510–517. [CrossRef] [PubMed]

70. Mueannoom, W.; Srisongphan, A.; Taylor, K.M.; Hauschild, S.; Gaisford, S. Thermal ink-jet spray freeze-drying for preparation of excipient-free salbutamol sulphate for inhalation. *Eur. J. Pharm. Biopharm.* **2012**, *80*, 149–155. [CrossRef] [PubMed]

71. Filipe, V.; Hawe, A.; Carpenter, J.F.; Jiskoot, W. Analytical approaches to assess the degradation of therapeutic proteins. *TrAC Trends Anal. Chem.* **2013**, *49*, 118–125. [CrossRef]

72. Song, J.G.; Lee, S.H.; Han, H.-K. The stabilization of biopharmaceuticals: Current understanding and future perspectives. *J. Pharm. Investig.* **2017**, *47*, 475–496. [CrossRef]

73. Wang, W.; Singh, S.; Zeng, D.L.; King, K.; Nema, S. Antibody structure, instability, and formulation. *J. Pharm. Sci.* **2007**, *96*, 1–26. [CrossRef] [PubMed]

74. Chang, L.L.; Pikal, M.J. Mechanisms of protein stabilization in the solid state. *J. Pharm. Sci.* **2009**, *98*, 2886–2908. [CrossRef] [PubMed]

75. Hertel, S.P.; Winter, G.; Friess, W. Protein stability in pulmonary drug delivery via nebulization. *Adv. Drug Deliv. Rev.* **2015**, *93*, 79–94. [CrossRef] [PubMed]

76. Grenha, A.; Remuñán-López, C.; Carvalho, E.L.; Seijo, B. Microspheres containing lipid/chitosan nanoparticles complexes for pulmonary delivery of therapeutic proteins. *Eur. J. Pharm. Biopharm.* **2008**, *69*, 83–93. [CrossRef] [PubMed]

77. Edwards, D.A.; Hanes, J.; Caponetti, G.; Hrkach, J.; Ben-Jebria, A.; Eskew, M.L.; Mintzes, J.; Deaver, D.; Lotan, N.; Langer, R. Large porous particles for pulmonary drug delivery. *Science* **1997**, *276*, 1868–1872. [CrossRef] [PubMed]

78. Tsapis, N.; Bennett, D.; Jackson, B.; Weitz, D.A.; Edwards, D. Trojan particles: Large porous carriers of nanoparticles for drug delivery. *Proc. Natl. Acad. Sci. USA* **2002**, *99*, 12001–12005. [CrossRef] [PubMed]

79. Hussain, A.; Arnold, J.J.; Khan, M.A.; Ahsan, F. Absorption enhancers in pulmonary protein delivery. *J. Control. Release* **2004**, *94*, 15–24. [CrossRef] [PubMed]

80. Siekmeier, R.; Scheuch, G. Treatment of systemic diseases by inhalation of biomolecule aerosols. *J. Physiol. Pharmacol.* **2009**, *60*, 15–26. [PubMed]

81. Okumura, K.; Iwakawa, S.; Yoshida, T.; Seki, T.; Komada, F. Intratracheal delivery of insulin absorption from solution and aerosol by rat lung. *Int. J. Pharm.* **1992**, *88*, 63–73. [CrossRef]

82. Todo, H.; Okamoto, H.; Iida, K.; Danjo, K. Improvement of stability and absorbability of dry insulin powder for inhalation by powder-combination technique. *Int. J. Pharm.* **2004**, *271*, 41–52. [CrossRef] [PubMed]

83. Hu, X.; Yang, F.F.; Liao, Y.H. Pharmacokinetic Considerations of inhaled pharmaceuticals for systemic delivery. *Curr. Pharm. Des.* **2016**, *22*, 2532–2548. [CrossRef] [PubMed]

84. Garmise, R.J.; Staats, H.F.; Hickey, A.J. Novel dry powder preparations of whole inactivated influenza virus for nasal vaccination. *AAPS PharmSciTech* **2007**, *8*, 2–10. [CrossRef] [PubMed]

85. Cho, W.; Kim, M.-S.; Jung, M.-S.; Park, J.; Cha, K.-H.; Kim, J.-S.; Park, H.J.; Alhalaweh, A.; Velaga, S.P.; Hwang, S.-J. Design of salmon calcitonin particles for nasal delivery using spray-drying and novel supercritical fluid-assisted spray-drying processes. *Int. J. Pharm.* **2015**, *478*, 288–296. [CrossRef] [PubMed]

86. Mok, H.; Park, T.G. Water-free microencapsulation of proteins within PLGA microparticles by spray drying using PEG-assisted protein solubilization technique in organic solvent. *Eur. J. Pharm. Biopharm.* **2008**, *70*, 137–144. [CrossRef] [PubMed]

87. Cleland, J.L.; Duenas, E.T.; Park, A.; Daugherty, A.; Kahn, J.; Kowalski, J.; Cuthbertson, A. Development of poly-(D,L-lactide-coglycolide) microsphere formulations containing recombinant human vascular endothelial growth factor to promote local angiogenesis. *J. Control. Release* **2001**, *72*, 13–24. [CrossRef]

88. Al-Qadi, S.; Grenha, A.; Carrión-Recio, D.; Seijo, B.; Remuñán-López, C. Microencapsulated chitosan nanoparticles for pulmonary protein delivery: In vivo evaluation of insulin-loaded formulations. *J. Control. Release* **2012**, *157*, 383–390. [CrossRef] [PubMed]

89. Chiou, H.; Chan, H.-K.; Heng, D.; Prud'homme, R.K.; Raper, J.A. A novel production method for inhalable cyclosporine a powders by confined liquid impinging jet precipitation. *J. Aerosol Sci.* **2008**, *39*, 500–509. [CrossRef]

90. Yamasaki, K.; Kwok, P.C.L.; Fukushige, K.; Prud'homme, R.K.; Chan, H.-K. Enhanced dissolution of inhalable cyclosporine nano-matrix particles with mannitol as matrix former. *Int. J. Pharm.* **2011**, *420*, 34–42. [CrossRef] [PubMed]

91. Cavaiola, T.S.; Edelman, S. Inhaled insulin: A breath of fresh air? A review of inhaled insulin. *Clin. Ther.* **2014**, *36*, 1275–1289. [CrossRef] [PubMed]

92. Rave, K.; Bott, S.; Heinemann, L.; Sha, S.; Becker, R.H.; Willavize, S.A.; Heise, T. Time-action profile of inhaled insulin in comparison with subcutaneously injected insulin lispro and regular human insulin. *Diabetes Care* **2005**, *28*, 1077–1082. [CrossRef] [PubMed]

93. Bailey, C.J.; Barnett, A.H. Inhaled insulin: New formulation, new trial. *Lancet* **2010**, *375*, 2199–2201. [CrossRef]

94. Quattrin, T.; Bélanger, A.; Bohannon, N.J.; Schwartz, S.L. Efficacy and safety of inhaled insulin (Exubera) compared with subcutaneous insulin therapy in patients with type 1 diabetes: Results of a 6-month, randomized, comparative trial. *Diabetes Care* **2004**, *27*, 2622–2627. [CrossRef] [PubMed]

95. Skyler, J.S.; Weinstock, R.S.; Raskin, P.; Yale, J.-F.; Barrett, E.; Gerich, J.E.; Gerstein, H.C. Use of inhaled insulin in a basal/bolus insulin regimen in type 1 diabetic subjects: A 6-month, randomized, comparative trial. *Diabetes Care* **2005**, *28*, 1630–1635. [CrossRef] [PubMed]

96. Pfützner, A.; Forst, T. Pulmonary insulin delivery by means of the technosphere™ drug carrier mechanism. *Expert Opin. Drug Deliv.* **2005**, *2*, 1097–1106. [CrossRef] [PubMed]

97. Cassidy, J.P.; Amin, N.; Marino, M.; Gotfried, M.; Meyer, T.; Sommerer, K.; Baughman, R.A. Insulin lung deposition and clearance following technosphere® insulin inhalation powder administration. *Pharm. Res.* **2011**, *28*, 2157–2164. [CrossRef] [PubMed]

98. Angelo, R.; Rousseau, K.; Grant, M.; Leone-Bay, A.; Richardson, P. Technosphere® insulin: Defining the role of technosphere particles at the cellular level. *J. Diabetes Sci. Technol.* **2009**, *3*, 545–554. [CrossRef] [PubMed]

99. Swierczewska, M.; Lee, K.C.; Lee, S. What is the future of PEGylated therapies? *Expert Opin. Emerg. Drugs* **2015**, *20*, 531–536. [CrossRef] [PubMed]

100. Park, E.J.; Lim, S.M.; Lee, K.C.; Na, D.H. Exendins and exendin analogs for diabetic therapy: A patent review (2012–2015). *Expert Opin. Ther. Pat.* **2016**, *26*, 833–842. [CrossRef] [PubMed]

101. Kim, Y.; Park, E.J.; Na, D.H. Antibody-drug conjugates for targeted anticancer drug delivery. *J. Pharm. Investig.* **2016**, *46*, 341–349. [CrossRef]

102. Li, X.; Huang, Y.; Huang, Z.; Ma, X.; Dong, N.; Chen, W.; Pan, X.; Wu, C. Enhancing stability of exenatide-containing pressurized metered-dose inhaler via reverse microemulsion system. *AAPS PharmSciTech* **2018**, *19*, 2499–2508. [CrossRef] [PubMed]

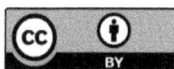

pharmaceutics

MDPI

Article

Pharmacokinetic Properties of Acetyl Tributyl Citrate, a Pharmaceutical Excipient

Hyeon Kim [1,†], Min Sun Choi [1,†], Young Seok Ji [1], In Sook Kim [1], Gi Beom Kim [1], In Yong Bae [1], Myung Chan Gye [2,*] and Hye Hyun Yoo [1,*]

[1]   Institute of Pharmaceutical Science and Technology and College of Pharmacy, Hanyang University, Ansan, Gyeonggi-do 15588, Korea; kimhyeon2000@nate.com (H.K.); chm2456@hanyang.ac.kr (M.S.C.); wldudtjr23@hanyang.ac.kr (Y.S.J.); kis@hanyang.ac.kr (I.S.K.); shbn13@naver.com (G.B.K.); iybae722@naver.com (I.Y.B.)
[2]   Department of Life Science, Institute of Natural Sciences, Hanyang University, Seoul 04763, Korea
*   Correspondence: mcgye@hanyang.ac.kr (M.C.G.); yoohh@hanyang.ac.kr (H.H.Y.); Tel.: +82-10-400-5804 (H.H.Y.)
†   These authors contributed equally to this work.

Received: 14 August 2018; Accepted: 6 October 2018; Published: 8 October 2018

Abstract: Acetyl tributyl citrate (ATBC) is an (the Food and Drug Administration) FDA-approved substance for use as a pharmaceutical excipient. It is used in pharmaceutical coating of solid oral dosage forms such as coated tablets or capsules. However, the information of ATBC on its pharmacokinetics is limited. The aim of this study is to investigate the pharmacokinetic properties of ATBC using liquid chromatography–tandem mass spectrometric (LC–MS/MS) analysis. ATBC was rapidly absorbed and eliminated and the bioavailability was 27.4% in rats. The results of metabolic stability tests revealed that metabolic clearance may have accounted for a considerable portion of the total clearance of ATBC. These pharmacokinetic data would be useful in studies investigating the safety and toxicity of ATBC.

Keywords: acetyl tributyl citrate; pharmaceutical excipient; pharmacokinetics; metabolic stability; plasma

1. Introduction

Plasticizers are chemicals which are added into polymeric materials to increase their flexibility and workability. They are also used in polymers for pharmaceutical applications such as drug carriers and coatings. In the chemical industry, many kinds of plasticizers are utilized. However, for pharmaceutical application, the use of only several kinds of plasticizers has been approved as it requires low toxicity and migration. Pharmaceutically used plasticizers can be categorized into hydrophobic and hydrophilic groups [1]. The hydrophobic plasticizers include acetyl tributyl citrate (ATBC), acetyl triethyl citrate, castor oil, diacetylated monoglycerides, dibutyl sebacate, diethyl phthalate, triacetin, tributyl citrate, and triethyl citrate. The hydrophilic plasticizers include clycerin, polyethylene glycols, polyethylene glycols monomethyl ether, propylene glycol, and sorbitol sorbitan solution.

Among the plasticizers mentioned above, ATBC is a biodegradable plasticizer formed by the esterification of citric acid. ATBC is used in pharmaceutical coating of solid oral dosage forms such as coated tablets or capsules. According to the online (the Food and Drug Administration) FDA database, some oral drugs contain 0.56~57.55 mg of ATBC [2]. For example, Cardizem CD (a coated capsule for extended release containing diltiazem hydrochloride) contains ATBC; if the maximum dose of Cardizem CD (480 mg) is given to patients, they may be exposed to approximately 20 mg of ATBC per day [2].

Generally, citric acid trimesters are known to be very safe. The toxicity of ATBC has been investigated thoroughly in animals. Research showed that the acute oral LD50 for ATBC in mice or rats was greater than 25 g/kg and that ATBC was not associated with any significant reproductive toxicity in mice or rats [3]. The European Commission stated that the no-observed adverse effect level of ATBC was 100 mg/kg bw/day (C7/GF/csteeop/ATBC/080104 D(04)). The European Food Safety Authority has given ATBC a tolerable daily intake value of 1.0 mg/kg bodyweight [4]. Based on these reports, ATBC is considered toxic only at very high concentrations. However, one study reported that ATBC induced intestinal Cytochrome P450 3A4 (CYP3A4) at a relatively low concentration (about 4.02 µg/mL) [2]. In addition, studies published recently suggested that ATBC may affect female reproduction at a low dose [5]. Therefore, human exposure to ATBC levels needs to be monitored, and a better understanding of the pharmacokinetics of ATBC is needed.

There is a report on the safety of ATBC which evaluated the absorption, metabolism, and excretion profiles of ATBC using 14C-labeled compounds [2]. This report provides the overall pharmacokinetic properties of ATBC but the detailed pharmacokinetic information on ATBC, an unchanged form, is unavailable.

Many studies have described analytical methods for the determination of ATBC in plastic materials. These analytical methods include gas chromatography–mass spectrometry (GC–MS), GC with a flame ionization detector, high-performance liquid chromatography (HPLC) with an ultraviolet/visible spectroscopic detector, HPLC with an evaporative light scattering detector, and nuclear magnetic resonance spectroscopy [6–9]. Recently, a liquid chromatography–tandem mass spectrometric (LC–MS/MS) method has been reported [10]. However, there are no analytical methods for the determination of ATBC in biological samples.

In the present study, we developed an analytical method for the pharmacokinetic analysis of ATBC using liquid chromatography–tandem mass spectrometry (LC–MS/MS). Based on the developed method, we investigated the pharmacokinetic properties of ATBC in vitro and in vivo.

2. Materials and Methods

2.1. Chemicals and Materials

ATBC (>98%), acetyl triethyl citrate (ATEC, internal standard) and PMSF (esterase inhibitor) were purchased from Sigma-Aldrich (St. Louis, MO, USA). HPLC grade water was generated using a Milli-Q purification system (Millipore, Bedford, MA, USA). HPLC grade methanol (MeOH) and acetonitrile (ACN) was purchased from J.T. Baker (Phillipsburg, NJ, USA). Blank plasma was collected in a heparin tube from male Sprague-Dawley rats. All chemicals and solvents were of analytical grade.

2.2. Preparation of Calibration and Quality Control Standards

A stock solution (5 mg/mL) of ATBC was prepared in 70% acetonitrile. The stock solution was stored at −20 °C and brought to room temperature before use. Working standard solutions were prepared to final concentrations ranging from 0.1 µg/mL to 10 µg/mL with acetonitrile. An internal standard (IS, ATEC) solutions (5 mg/mL) was prepared at 5 mg/mL and further diluted to a concentration of 100 ng/mL in methanol. Calibration samples (10, 50, 100, 200, 500 and 1000 ng/mL) were prepared by spiking 90 µL of rat plasma with the appropriate working standard solution of the 10 µL. Four levels of quality control (QC) samples were prepared at 10, 30, 400 and 800 ng/mL in the same way as the calibration standards. All the prepared plasma samples were stored at −20 °C until use. Calibration standards and QC samples were added with 3 volumes of the IS solution for protein precipitation, vortex-mixed for 30 s, and centrifuged at 12000 rpm for 5 min at 4 °C. The supernatant was collected and transferred to an LC vial for LC-MS/MS analysis.

2.3. Analytical Method Validation

The method was validated according to the US Food and Drug Administration Bioanalytical Method Validation Guidance [11,12]. The selectivity was evaluated by comparing the chromatograms of six individual blank plasmas with corresponding standard-spiked plasma samples. Calibration curves were constructed by plotting the peak area ratios of the analyte to the IS versus the analyte concentrations. The equation model was obtained by weighted least squares linear regression analysis. The lower limit of quantification (LLOQ) was determined as the lowest concentration with a relative standard deviation (RSD) of <20% and with 80–120% accuracy. The intra- and inter-day accuracy and precision were evaluated by analyzing replicates (n = 5 for intra-day; n = 3 for inter-day) of spiked plasma samples at concentrations of 10, 30, 400 and 800 ng/mL. The extraction recovery was defined by comparing the peak area of the pre-spiked extracted sample with that of the post-spiked extracted sample. The effect of plasma matrix was evaluated by comparing the peak area of the post-spiked extracted sample with that of the neat solution. Six different lots of blank plasma were evaluated. The stability of the analyte was determined: Freeze and thaw, bench-top, long-term, and post-preparative stability.

2.4. Pharmacokinetics Study in Rats

The developed and validated method was applied to a pharmacokinetic study of ATBC in rats after oral administration. Male Sprague-Dawley rats (8 weeks, 257 ± 20 g) were purchased from Orient Bio (Seongnam, Korea) and maintained at a temperature of 23 ± 3 °C with a 12 h light-dark cycle and moisture (55 ± 15% relative humidity) controlled room. Before dosing, the rats had fasted for 12 h and had free access to water. The rats were administered ATBC in 30% PEG intravenously (10 mg/kg) and orally (500 mg/kg). Blood samples (200 µL) were collected from the carotid artery into tubes containing heparin: Esterase inhibitor (1 M PMSF) was used to prevent degradation in rat plasma. Blood samples were collected at 1, 2, 5, 10, 15, and 30 min and 1, 2, 4, 6, 10, and 24 h for IV injection and 5, 15, 30, and 45 min and 1, 2, 4, 6, 8, 10, and 24 h for oral administration. Plasma samples, obtained by centrifuging blood at 12,000 rpm for 5 min at 4 °C. The supernatant plasma (50 µL) was collected in a separate microtube and treated with 150 µL methanol with IS (100 ng/mL of ATEC). The samples were vortexed and centrifuged at 12,000 rpm for 5 min. The supernatant was analyzed using LC-MS/MS. All animal procedures were approved by the Institutional Animal Care and Use Committee of Hanyang University (2016-0235A).

2.5. Pharmacokinetics Analysis

The pharmacokinetic parameters of ATBC were calculated by using the noncompartmental analysis of the Phoenix WinNonlin Enterprise Program v5.3 (Pharsight Inc., St. Louis, MO, USA). Data were shown as mean ± standard deviation. The following pharmacokinetic parameter were calculated. Maximum plasma concentration (Cmax) and the time to reach maximum (Tmax) were determined directly from the measured data. The elimination half-life ($t_{1/2}$) was calculated as $0.693/\lambda z$. The terminal elimination rate constant (λz) was determined by linear least-squares regression of the terminal portion of the logged plasma concentration-time curve. The area under the plasma concentration-time curve (AUC) from time 0 to the time of the last measurable concentration (AUC0 → t) was calculated using the log-linear trapezoidal rule. In the IV dosing data, the distribution volumes (Vd) based on the terminal phase and the total-body clearance (Cl) were obtained directly from the experimental data.

2.6. Metabolic Stability Assay

ATBC was incubated at 37 °C for 0, 30, 60, and 120 min in rat and human plasma and liver microsomes. The detailed procedures are described in previously published reports [13]. In addition, to characterize the enzymes which may be involved in microsomal metabolism of ATBC, ATBC was incubated at 37 °C for 60 min with cDNA expressed human CYP isoforms. The final concentration of each CYP isozyme was 0.05 nmol/mL. After incubation, the sample was treated as described in 2.4. All experiments were performed in triplicate. The concentration of ATBC was measured using LC-MS/MS analysis.

2.7. LC-MS/MS Conditions

The LC/MS/MS system consisted of a 6460 triple quadrupole mass spectrometer (Agilent Technologies, Santa Clara, CA, USA) coupled with the Agilent 1260 infinity HPLC system. The column temperature was maintained at 30 °C using a thermostatically controlled column oven. The mobile phases consisted of 0.1% formic acid in DW (solvent A) and 0.1% formic acid in 90% ACN (solvent B). A gradient elution was performed at a flow rate of 0.3 mL/min and initiated with 10% of mobile phase B, increased to 100% for 1 min and held for 3 min and restored to the initial percentage for 2 min to re-equilibrate. Chromatographic separation was achieved with a Kinetex C18 (2.1 mm × 50 mm, 2.6 μm; Phenomenex). The electrospray ionization (ESI) source was operated in positive mode. Multiple reaction monitoring (MRM) was employed. The precursor-product ion pairs used were 403.2 $m/z \rightarrow$ 129.0 m/z for ATBC and 319.1 $m/z \rightarrow$ 157.0 m/z for ATEC. The fragmentor voltages were 80 V and 70 V, and the collision energy were 20 V and 10 V for ATBC and ATEC, respectively. The product ion spectrum of ATBC and ATEC is presented with its chemical structure in Figure 1a,b.

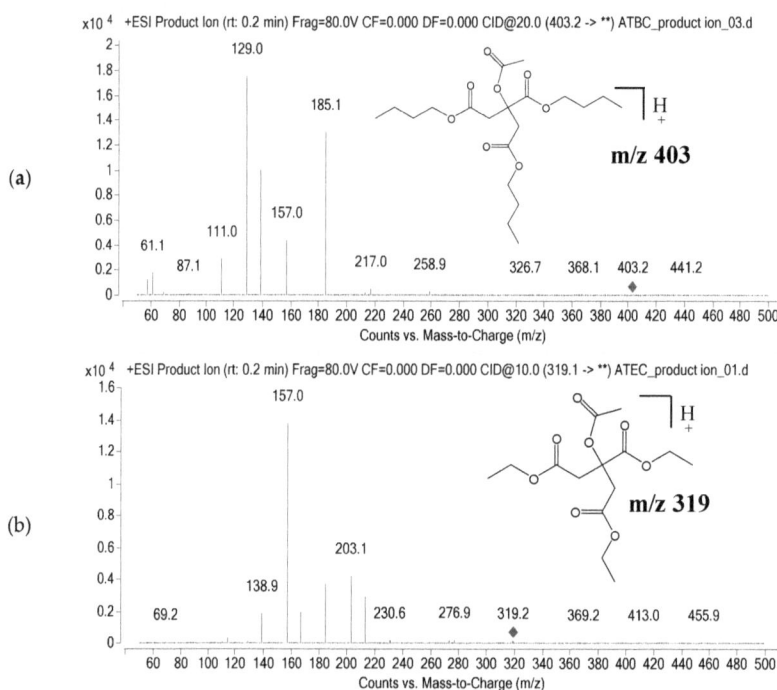

Figure 1. Product ion mass spectrum of (**a**) Acetyl tributyl citrate (ATBC) and (**b**) Internal standard (IS) (ATEC, acetyl triethyl citrate).

3. Results

3.1. Analytical Method Validation

ATBC has three ester bonds in its structure. Generally, compounds with esters are susceptible to hydrolysis in plasma, making it difficult to analyze ATBC in plasma samples [14,15]. Accordingly, pretreatment is required to ensure the stability of ATBC in plasma samples. We utilized phenylmethylsulfonyl fluoride (PMSF) as an esterase inhibitor in the pretreatment step, which enabled an accurate and reproducible analysis of ATBC in plasma.

3.1.1. Selectivity

Typical chromatograms of blank plasma, blank plasma spiked with ATBC (10 ng/mL) and ATEC (IS; 100 ng/mL), and rat plasma samples 15 min after PO administration of ATBC are shown in Figure 2. The retention times of ATBC and ATEC (IS) were 3.5 min and 2.7 min, respectively. As shown in Figure 2, endogenous plasma components did not interfere with the retention times of the analyte and IS.

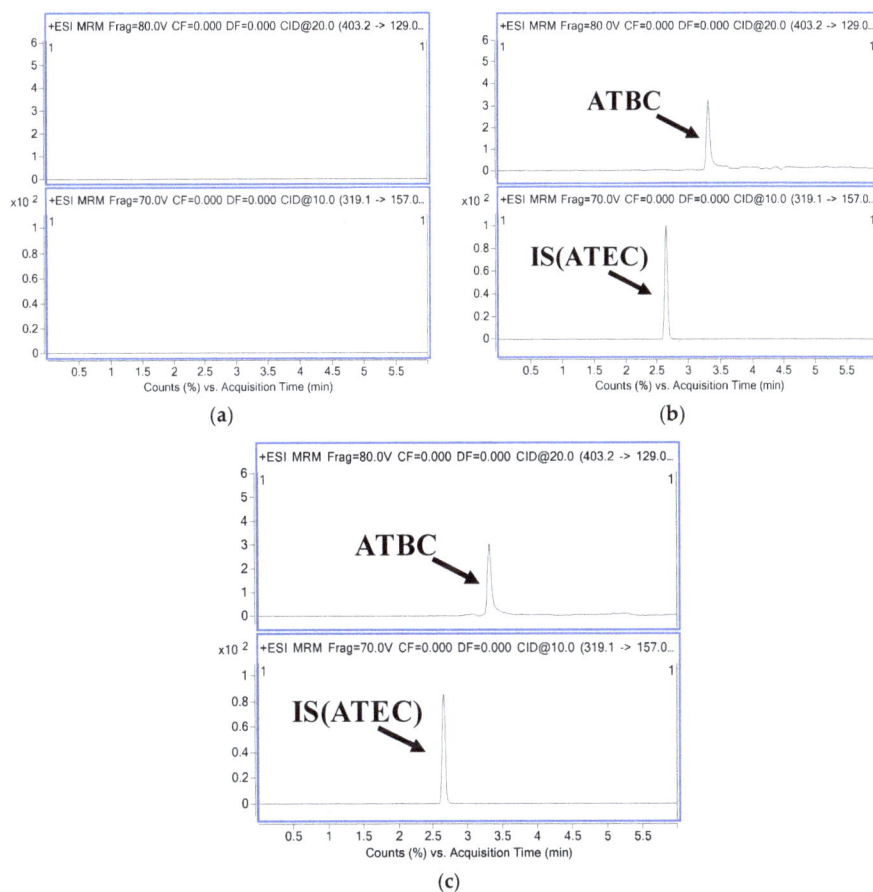

Figure 2. Representative multiple reaction monitoring (MRM) chromatograms of ATBC and IS (ATEC) in rat plasma. (**a**) blank plasma; (**b**) The lower limit of quantification (LLOQ) of ATBC at 10 ng/mL and IS at 100 ng/mL; (**c**) plasma sample at 10 h after oral (PO) administration of 500 mg/kg of ATBC.

3.1.2. Linearity

Calibration curves using six concentration levels (10, 50, 100, 200, 500 and 1000 ng/mL) with eight replicates each were constructed to evaluate the calibration model. The regression coefficient ($r2$) was ≥ 0.990. The accuracy and precision of the calibration standard curves were reliable (less than $\pm 15\%$ RSD) for all the concentration points tested.

3.1.3. Accuracy and Precision

The results for intra-day and inter-day precision and accuracy in plasma QC samples at concentrations of 10, 30, 400, and 800 ng/mL are summarized in Table 1. The intra- and inter-day precision was within 11.4%. The intra-day accuracy was 90.7–117.6%, whereas the inter-day accuracy was 100.2–103.4%.

Table 1. Intra- and inter-day accuracy and precision for the determination of acetyl tributyl citrate (ATBC) in rat plasma.

Nominal Conc. (ng/mL)	Intra-Day (*n* = 5)			Inter-Day (*n* = 5)		
	Measured Conc. (ng/mL)	Accuracy (%)	Precision (%)	Measured Conc. (ng/mL)	Accuracy (%)	Precision (%)
10	11.8	117.6	6.8	10.3	103.4	11.4
30	31.2	103.8	5.4	31.2	104.1	5.0
400	405.1	101.3	4.9	411.7	102.9	4.8
800	725.9	90.7	11.4	801.3	100.2	6.2

3.1.4. Extraction Recovery and Matrix Effect

The mean extraction recovery of ATBC from rat plasma was $85.5 \pm 9.0\%$ and $93.8 \pm 12.0\%$ at concentrations of 30 and 800 ng/mL, respectively (Table 2). The mean matrix effects of ATBC were $42.1 \pm 4.9\%$ and $54.3 \pm 1.2\%$ at concentrations of 30 and 800 ng/mL, respectively.

3.1.5. Stability

The stability of ATBC in plasma was investigated under various sample preparation and storage conditions. The resulting data are summarized in Table 3. In rat plasma samples, ATBC was stable for 8 h at room temperature (>94.1%, *n* = 5), and it was stable for 14 days at $-20\,^{\circ}\text{C}$ (>99.9%, *n* = 5). It was also stable for at least three freeze-thaw cycles at $-20\,^{\circ}\text{C}$ (>103.8%, *n* = 5). Furthermore, the prepared samples were stable when stored for 12 h at $4\,^{\circ}\text{C}$ in an autosampler (>103.2%, *n* = 5).

Table 2. Stability of ATBC in rat plasma.

	Recovery (% Remained)	
Stability	Concentration (ng/mL)	
	30	800
Short-term (Room temperature for 8 h)	94.1 ± 7.6	94.9 ± 8.9
Long-term ($-20\,^{\circ}\text{C}$ for 14 days)	100.6 ± 11.5	99.9 ± 14.5
Freeze-thaw ($-20\,^{\circ}\text{C}$, 3 cycles)	103.8 ± 10.7	104.2 ± 8.2
Auto-sampler ($4\,^{\circ}\text{C}$ for 24 h)	106.8 ± 12.1	103.2 ± 10.8

3.2. Pharmacokinetic Study

The developed method was successfully applied in a study of the pharmacokinetic parameters of ATBC in rat plasma after IV and oral administration. Plasma concentration-time curves are shown in Figure 3. The main pharmacokinetic parameters of ATBC are summarized in Table 3. After IV administration, ATBC was rapidly eliminated, with a clearance of 75.7 L/h/kg. As ATBC seems to follow two compartment model, initial (α) and final (β) excretion half-lives were calculated. To calculate initial and final phase half-lives, the first four points and the last three points were used respectively. When orally administered, ATBC was rapidly absorbed, with a Tmax of 0.4 h. The AUC of ATBC was 201.3 ng·h/mL when administered IV (10 mg/kg), and it was 2757.1 ng·h/mL when administered orally (500 mg/kg). Based on the dose normalized AUC, bioavailability was 27.4%.

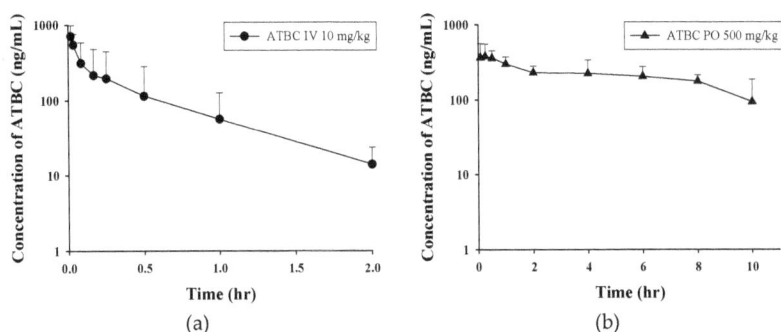

Figure 3. Plasma concentration-time profile of ATBC after (**a**) IV administration of 10 mg/kg of ATBC and (**b**) PO administration of 500 mg/kg to rats. Data were expressed as mean ± SD.

Table 3. Pharmacokinetic parameters after intravenous (IV) and oral (PO) administration of ATBC to rats.

Parameter	ATBC	
	IV (10 mg/kg, *n* = 5)	PO (500 mg/kg, *n* = 6)
$t_{1/2\alpha}$ (h)	0.02 ± 0.01	-
$t_{1/2\beta}$ (h)	0.58 ± 0.31	-
AUC (ng·h/mL)	201.3 ± 215.3	2757.1 ± 726.3
Tmax (h)	-	0.4 ± 0.3
Cmax (ng/mL)	-	478.7 ± 170.9
Vz (L/kg)	80.4 ± 47.4	-
Cl (L/h/kg)	75.7 ± 64.4	-
F (%)	-	27.4

To better understand the pharmacokinetic behavior of ATBC, we tested the metabolic stability of ATBC in plasma and liver microsomes (Figure 4). In rat plasma, ATBC disappeared rapidly and remained less than 10% of the dose 1 h after incubation. The mean half-life was calculated to be 0.23 h and 0.21 h at 1 μM and 10 μM, respectively. This result was expectable and therefore we applied the esterase inhibitor in the sample preparation procedure. However, in human plasma, ATBC was fairly stable and the mean percentage of remaining was more than 80%. According to Bahar et al., there is species difference of plasma esterase expression and activity [16]. For example, paraoxonase and butyrylcholinesterase were highly expressed in humans and dogs, whereas carboxylesterase was only abundant in rabbits, mice, and rats. Thus, carboxylesterase is considered involved in hydrolysis of ATBC and accordingly, our results are well agreed with this. Therefore, such species difference should be considered for extrapolation of human pharmacokinetic parameters from the present data with rats.

Meanwhile, the liver microsomal stability of ATBC was comparable between rats and humans; ATBC was easily metabolized in both microsomes. The mean half-life in rat liver microsomes was 0.27 h and 0.64 h at 1 μM and 10 μM, respectively. The mean half-life in human liver microsomes was 0.26 h and 0.37 h at 1 μM and 10 μM, respectively. Based on these findings, hepatic metabolism may play an important role in determining the systemic exposure of ATBC in humans.

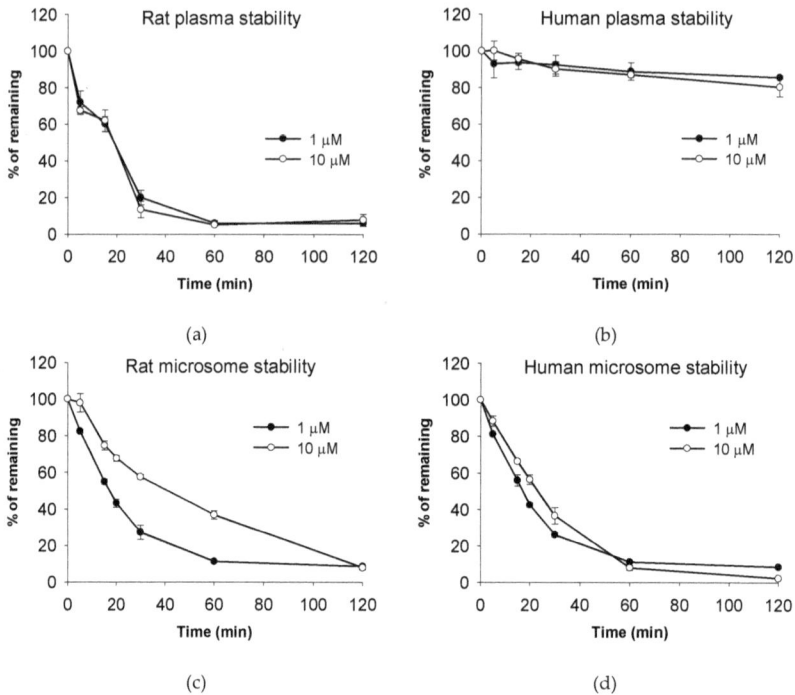

Figure 4. Metabolic stability of ATBC in plasma and liver microsomal fractions. (**a**) Rat plasma; (**b**) human plasma; (**c**) rat liver microsomes; (**d**) human liver microsomes. Data were expressed as mean $\pm$ SD ($n = 3$).

As described above, ATBC is fairly stable in human plasma, but easily metabolized in human liver microsomes. This indicates that liver microsomal enzymes may contribute substantially to ATBC metabolism in humans. To characterize the enzymes which may be involved in microsomal metabolism of ATBC, ATBC was incubated with human recombinant CYP supersomes and the stability was investigated. Figure 5 shows that all the CYP isozymes tested may be involved in the metabolism of ATBC. In particular, CYP 2C19 and CYP3A4 showed a high metabolic activity for ATBC.

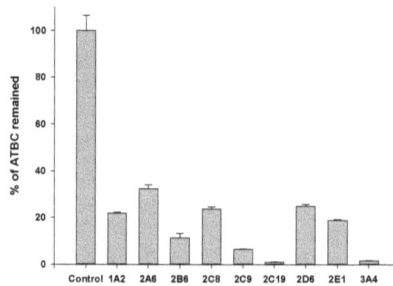

Figure 5. Metabolic stability of ATBC in human recombinant CYP supersomes. Data were expressed as mean $\pm$ SD ($n = 3$). ATBC was tested at 10 μM. Control: blank incubation matrix (all except for CYPs).

4. Discussion

According to a report on the safety of ATBC, approximately 99% of 14C-ATBC orally administered to rats was excreted in urine (59–70%), feces (25–36%), and expired air (2%) within 48 h [3]. As reported in previous research, the metabolism of ATBC occurred rapidly in the present study. The metabolites mentioned in the previous report included acetyl citrate, monobutyl citrate, acetyl monobutyl citrate, dibutyl citrate, and acetyl dibutyl citrate [3]. Thus, the metabolites are mainly generated via hydrolysis and any significant toxic issues are not expected based on their chemical structures. However, inter-species differences in the pharmacokinetics and metabolism of ATBC need to be considered as the human profile may be different from the rat profile.

The IV plasma concentration patterns indicate that ATBC may follow the two compartment pharmacokinetic model. Thus, it suggests that ATBC is distributed to certain tissues at a slower rate. The pharmacokinetics of ATBC in oral administration was investigated at a somewhat higher dose (500 mg/kg) considering its detectability. In the plasma concentration profile of oral administration, the elimination appears to be nonlinear at some stages with individual variation in curve patterns. Thus, the elimination half-life for oral administration could not be calculated. This could be because the saturation in the processes of absorption, metabolism or elimination of ATBC takes place at a high dose. Therefore, the possibility of erroneous measurement of oral bioavailability should be considered.

Rasmussen et al. investigated the effects of in vitro exposure to ATBC on ovarian antral follicle growth and viability [17]. At a dose of 0.01 µg/mL, ATBC increased the number of nongrowing follicles and terminal deoxynucleotidyl transferase dUTP nick end labeling (TUNEL)-positive area in treated follicles, pointing to the possibility that ATBC may disrupt antral follicle function at low concentrations. They also tested the effects of oral exposure to ATBC on female reproduction in mice [5]. Oral administration of ATBC at a dose of 10 mg/kg/day for 15 days decreased the number of primordial, primary and secondary follicles present in the ovary. These findings give rise to concern that low levels of ATBC may be harmful to ovarian function and affect female reproduction.

The findings in the aforementioned literature highlight the need to investigate possible toxic effects of ATBC at low dosages. A previous toxicological study found no adverse effects of ATBC (systemic toxicity or reproductive toxicity) at a relatively high dose (~1000 mg/kg/day) in animal models and concluded that ATBC was a safe alternative to phthalates. However, attention should still be paid to the safety of ATBC as it is extensively used in coating materials for tablets, capsules, and granules for masking the taste of medication or controlling drug release [18]. According to the FDA report, some patients may intake up to 60 mg of ATBC per day as a pharmaceutical excipient [2]. In this context, the pharmacokinetics of ATBC should be necessarily studied for its safe use. In addition, the exposure level of ATBC in plasma or other biofluids needs to be investigated.

5. Conclusions

We investigated the pharmacokinetic properties of ATBC in vitro and in vivo. ATBC was rapidly absorbed and eliminated and the bioavailability was 27.4%. Metabolic clearance may play an important role in determining the systemic exposure of ATBC. This is the first report to demonstrate the pharmacokinetic study of ATBC using LC-MS/MS. Our findings would be useful in studies investigating the safety and toxicity of ATBC.

Author Contributions: Contributed to the research design: H.H.Y., M.C.G.; Conducted experiments: H.K., M.S.C., I.S.K., Y.S.J., G.B.K., I.Y.B.; Contributed to data analysis and interpretation: H.K.; Contributed to the preparation of the manuscript: H.K., I.S.K., H.H.Y.

Funding: This work was supported by the National Research Foundation of Korea (NRF) grant by the Korea government (NRF-2015M3C8A6A06012996 and NRF-2017R1A2B4001814).

Conflicts of Interest: The authors declare no conflict of interest.

References

1.	Snejdrova, E.; Dittrich, M. Pharmaceutically used plasticizers. In *Recent Advances in Plasticizers*; Mohammad, L., Ed.; IntechOpen: Rijeka, Croatia, 2012; pp. 45–68.

2. Takeshita, A.; Igarashi-Migitaka, J.; Nishiyama, K.; Takahashi, H.; Takeuchi, Y.; Koibuchi, N. Acetyl tributyl citrate, the most widely used phthalate substitute plasticizer, induces cytochrome P450 3A through steroid and xenobiotic receptor. *Toxicol. Sci.* **2011**, *123*, 460–470. [CrossRef] [PubMed]
3. Johnson, W., Jr. Final report on the safety assessment of acetyl triethyl citrate, acetyl tributyl citrate, acetyl trihexyl citrate, and acetyl trioctyl citrate. *Int. J. Toxicol.* **2002**, *21*, 1–17. [PubMed]
4. Gordon, L.R. *Food Packaging: Principles and Practice*, 3rd ed.; CRC Press: Boca Raton, FL, USA, 2013; pp. 624–626.
5. Rasmussen, L.M.; Sen, N.; Liu, X.; Craig, Z.R. Effects of oral exposure to the phthalate substitute acetyl tributyl citrate on female reproduction in mice. *J. Appl. Toxicol.* **2017**, *37*, 668–675. [CrossRef] [PubMed]
6. Gimeno, P.; Thomas, S.; Bousquet, C.; Maggio, A.F.; Civade, C.; Brenier, C.; Bonnet, P.A. Identification and quantification of 14 phthalates and 5 non-phthalate plasticizers in PVC medical devices by GC-MS. *J. Chromatogr. B Anal. Technol. Biomed. Life Sci.* **2014**, *949–950*, 99–108. [CrossRef] [PubMed]
7. Radaniel, T.; Genay, S.; Simon, N.; Feutry, F.; Quagliozzi, F.; Barthelemy, C.; Lecoeur, M.; Sautou, V.; Decaudin, B.; Odou, P. Quantification of five plasticizers used in PVC tubing through high performance liquid chromatographic-UV detection. *J. Chromatogr. B Anal. Technol. Biomed. Life Sci.* **2014**, *965*, 158–163. [CrossRef] [PubMed]
8. Bourdeaux, D.; Yessaad, M.; Chennell, P.; Larbre, V.; Eljezi, T.; Bernard, L.; Sautou, V. Analysis of PVC plasticizers in medical devices and infused solutions by GC-MS. *J. Pharm. Biomed. Anal.* **2016**, *118*, 206–213. [CrossRef] [PubMed]
9. Bernard, L.; Bourdeaux, D.; Pereira, B.; Azaroual, N.; Barthelemy, C.; Breysse, C.; Chennell, P.; Cueff, R.; Dine, T.; Eljezi, T.; et al. Analysis of plasticizers in PVC medical devices: Performance comparison of eight analytical methods. *Talanta* **2017**, *162*, 604–611. [CrossRef] [PubMed]
10. Kim, H.; Kim, G.B.; Choi, M.S.; Kim, I.S.; Gye, M.C.; Yoo, H.H. Liquid chromatography-tandem mass spectrometric analysis of acetyl tributyl citrate for migration testing of food contact materials. *Microchem. J.* **2018**, *139*, 475–479. [CrossRef]
11. Food and Drug Administration. Guidance for Industry: Bioanalytical Method Validation. 2018. Available online: https://www.fda.gov/downloads/drugs/guidances/ucm070107.pdf (accessed on 10 June 2018).
12. Kachingwe, B.H.; Uang, Y.S.; Huang, T.J.; Wang, L.H.; Lin, S.J. Development and validation of an LC-MS/MS method for quantification of NC-8 in rat plasma and its application to pharmacokinetic studies. *J. Food. Drug Anal.* **2018**, *26*, 401–408. [CrossRef] [PubMed]
13. Rehman, S.U.; Kim, I.S.; Choi, M.S.; Luo, Z.; Yao, G.; Xue, Y.; Zhang, Y.; Yoo, H.H. Evaluation of Metabolic stability of kinsenoside, an antidiabetic candidate, in rat and human liver microsomes. *Mass Spectrom. Lett.* **2015**, *6*, 48–51. [CrossRef]
14. Di, L.; Kerns, E.H.; Hong, Y.; Chen, H. Development and application of high throughput plasma stability assay for drug discovery. *Int. J. Pharm.* **2005**, *297*, 110–119. [CrossRef] [PubMed]
15. Rehman, S.U.; Kim, I.S.; Choi, M.S.; Luo, Z.; Yao, G.; Xue, Y.; Zhang, Y.; Yoo, H.H. Development of a hydrophilic interaction liquid chromatography-tandem mass spectrometric method for the determination of kinsenoside, an antihyperlipidemic candidate, in rat plasma and its application to pharmacokinetic studies. *J. Pharm. Biomed. Anal.* **2016**, *120*, 19–24. [CrossRef] [PubMed]
16. Bahar, F.G.; Ohura, K.; Ogihara, T.; Imai, T. Species difference of esterase expression and hydrolase activity in plasma. *J. Pharm. Sci.* **2012**, *101*, 3979–3988. [CrossRef] [PubMed]
17. Rasmussen, L.M.; Sen, N.; Vera, J.C.; Liu, X.; Craig, Z.R. Effects of in vitro exposure to dibutyl phthalate, mono-butyl phthalate, and acetyl tributyl citrate on ovarian antral follicle growth and viability. *Biol. Reprod.* **2017**, *96*, 1105–1117. [CrossRef] [PubMed]
18. Kennedy, S.W.; Rowe, R.C.; Sheskey, P.J.; Owen, S.C. Acetyltributyl citrate. In *Handbook of Pharmaceutical Excipients*; London Pharmaceutical Press: London, UK, 2006; pp. 10–11.

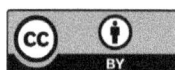

pharmaceutics

MDPI

Article

Pharmacokinetics and Anti-Gastric Ulceration Activity of Oral Administration of Aceclofenac and Esomeprazole in Rats

Tae Hwan Kim [1], Subindra Kazi Thapa [2], Da Young Lee [3], Seung Eun Chung [3], Jun Young Lim [3], Hyeon Myeong Jeong [3], Chang Ho Song [3], Youn-Woong Choi [4], Sang-Min Cho [4], Kyu-Yeol Nam [4], Won-Ho Kang [4], Soyoung Shin [2] and Beom Soo Shin [3],*

[1]   College of Pharmacy, Catholic University of Daegu, Gyeongsan, Gyeongbuk 38430, Korea; thkim@cu.ac.kr
[2]   College of Pharmacy, Wonkwang University, Iksan, Jeonbuk 54538, Korea;
      thapasubindra@gmail.com (S.K.T.); shins@wku.ac.kr (S.S.)
[3]   School of Pharmacy, Sungkyunkwan University, Suwon, Gyeonggi 16419, Korea;
      dayoung717@skku.edu (D.Y.L.); jsehome08@skku.edu (S.E.C.); panacea89@skku.edu (J.Y.L.);
      wise219143@skku.edu (H.M.J.); sky84312@skku.edu (C.H.S.)
[4]   Korea United Pharm. Inc., Seoul 06116, Korea; choi0528@kup.co.kr (Y.-W.C.);
      sweety1723@kup.co.kr (S.-M.C.); kynam@kup.co.kr (K.-Y.N.); kangwonho@kup.co.kr (W.-H.K.)
*   Correspondence: bsshin@skku.edu; Tel.: +82-31-290-7705

Received: 13 August 2018; Accepted: 4 September 2018; Published: 6 September 2018

Abstract: This study examined the effects of esomeprazole on aceclofenac pharmacokinetics and gastrointestinal complications in rats. Aceclofenac alone, or in combination with esomeprazole, was orally administered to male Sprague-Dawley rats. Plasma concentrations of aceclofenac, its major metabolite diclofenac, and esomeprazole were simultaneously determined by a novel liquid chromatography-tandem mass spectrometry method. Gastrointestinal damage was determined by measuring ulcer area and ulcer lesion index of the stomach. Oral administration of aceclofenac induced significant gastric ulceration, which was inhibited by esomeprazole administration. Following concurrent administration of aceclofenac and esomeprazole, overall pharmacokinetic profiles of aceclofenac and metabolic conversion to diclofenac were unaffected by esomeprazole. Aceclofenac metabolism and pharmacokinetics were not subject to significant food effects, whereas bioavailability of esomeprazole decreased in fed compared to fasting conditions. In contrast, the pharmacokinetics of aceclofenac and esomeprazole were significantly altered by different dosing vehicles. These results suggest that co-administration of esomeprazole with aceclofenac may reduce aceclofenac-induced gastrointestinal complications without significant pharmacokinetic interactions. The optimal combination and clinical significance of the benefits of the combination of aceclofenac and esomeprazole need to be further evaluated.

Keywords: aceclofenac; diclofenac; esomeprazole; pharmacokinetics; gastric ulcer

1. Introduction

Aceclofenac is one of the most popular oral nonsteroidal anti-inflammatory drugs (NSAIDs), and has proven effective in the treatment of osteoarthritis [1], rheumatoid arthritis [2], ankylosing spondylitis [3], and pain [4,5]. The absolute oral bioavailability of aceclofenac is 15% in rats [6] due to extensive metabolism. However, metabolism of aceclofenac is species-specific [7]. While aceclofenac is mainly metabolized to 4′-hydroxyaceclofenac in humans, the major metabolite in rats is diclofenac [7]. Aceclofenac and its metabolites exert anti-inflammatory effects by inhibition of prostaglandin E2 (PGE2) production via cyclooxygenases COX-1 and COX-2. Aceclofenac and 4′-hydroxyaceclofenac are selective COX-2 inhibitors with IC50 of 0.77 and 36 μM, respectively. Aceclofenac and 4′-hydroxyaceclofenac have IC50 > 100 μM for COX-1 in human whole blood [8]. In contrast, diclofenac inhibits both COX-1 (IC50 = 0.6 μM) and COX-2 (IC50 = 0.04 μM) [8]. Therefore, although diclofenac is present at lower levels in the plasma following aceclofenac administration in humans, diclofenac may contribute to the pharmacological action of aceclofenac in both humans and rats based on low IC50 values.

In general, selective COX-2 inhibitors exert less adverse effects on the gastrointestinal (GI) tract because COX-1 plays a protective role by stimulating the secretion of mucus and bicarbonate, increasing mucosal blood flow, and promoting epithelial proliferation [9]. Nevertheless, the superior clinical safety of aceclofenac related to GI adverse events is controversial. Aceclofenac was well tolerated, and the incidence of adverse GI events was generally lower than that of other NSAIDs [10]. Several clinical studies have shown that the overall withdrawal rate in aceclofenac recipients was lower than that in patients treated with tenoxicam [11], ketoprofen [2], and diclofenac [12]. Conversely, adverse events associated with aceclofenac use are still observed and include nausea, diarrhea, flatulence, gastritis, constipation, vomiting, and ulcerative stomatitis. No significant differences in GI event rates were reported between aceclofenac and other NSAIDs in individual clinical trials [1–3,11–19]. The number of patients with fecal blood loss did not differ significantly between aceclofenac and similar drugs such as tenoxicam [11,19], diclofenac [12,13], piroxicam [16], or indomethacin [3].

Gastroprotective therapy, such as with proton pump inhibitors (PPIs) in combination with NSAIDs, has been recommended for patients who are at risk for GI complications [20]. Among PPIs, esomeprazole, the S-isomer of omeprazole, has been shown to be useful in the prevention and healing of NSAID-induced gastric injury in clinical studies [21–25]. Nevertheless, co-therapy with NSAIDs and gastroprotective agents often results in poor clinical outcomes due to inadequate dosing and low patient compliance [26,27]. To improve patient compliance and clinical outcomes, a fixed-dose combination of an NSAID (naproxen) and esomeprazole magnesium (VIMOVO®) was approved by the United States FDA in 2010.

Despite relatively low frequency and severity of GI complications with aceclofenac treatment alone, aceclofenac therapy may benefit when combined with esomeprazole. However, potential pharmacokinetic and pharmacodynamic interactions between aceclofenac and esomeprazole are not well characterized. To our knowledge, no reports are available on the effects of esomeprazole on the prevention or healing of aceclofenac-induced GI ulceration in preclinical and clinical studies.

Therefore, the present study evaluated pharmacokinetic interactions between aceclofenac and esomeprazole, as well as effects of esomeprazole on aceclofenac-induced gastric ulceration in rats. Food effects on the pharmacokinetics of aceclofenac and esomeprazole were also studied.

2. Materials and Methods

2.1. Chemicals

Aceclofenac and esomeprazole magnesium dihydrate were supplied by Korea United Pharm. Inc. (Seoul, Korea). Diclofenac, lansoprazole, ammonium formate, sodium bicarbonate, and methylcellulose were purchased from Sigma-Aldrich Co. (St. Louis, MO, USA). HPLC grade acetonitrile, methanol, and distilled water were purchased from J.T. Baker, Inc. (Philipsburg, NJ, USA). Polyethylene glycol (PEG) 200 and citric acid were obtained from Junsei Chemical Co. (Tokyo, Japan), dimethyl sulfoxide (DMSO) was purchased from Kanto Chemical Co. (Tokyo, Japan), and urea was purchased from USB Co. (Cleveland, OH, USA).

2.2. Animals

Male Sprague-Dawley rats (8–10 weeks; body weight 220–282 g) were purchased from Samtako (Osan, Korea) and kept in plastic cages with free access to water and standard rat diet. The rats were maintained at a temperature of $23 \pm 2\,^\circ C$ with a 12 h light-dark cycle and relative humidity of $50 \pm 10\%$. They were acclimatized for at least one week prior to experimentation. All animal care and the protocols were conducted according to the Guidelines for the Care and Use of Animals which was approved by the Catholic University of Daegu (IACUC-2016-006; 29 April 2016) and Wonkwang University (WKU17-02; 10 January 2017).

2.3. Pharmacokinetic Studies

Aceclofenac and esomeprazole were prepared in four different vehicles, i.e., DMSO:PEG200:distilled water = 10:70:20 (vehicle A), 0.5% methylcellulose suspension in distilled water (vehicle B), citric urea buffer which consisted of urea (20 g/mL) and trisodium citrate (10 g/mL) for aceclofenac and 0.5% methylcellulose suspension containing 0.25 mM $NaHCO_3$ for esomeprazole (vehicle C), and DMSO:citric urea buffer = 1:14 solution for aceclofenac and DMSO:citric urea buffer = 1:9 solution for esomeprazole (vehicle D).

The rats were fasted for 12 h prior to the drug administration except for the rats for the fed condition in which the rats were allowed free access to standard rat diet to examine food effect. Aceclofenac and esomeprazole solutions or suspensions were administered to rats by oral gavage. For vehicles A and B, aceclofenac and esomeprazole were dissolved or suspended together in the vehicle and simultaneously administered to rats. For vehicle C, aceclofenac in the citric urea buffer, esomeprazole in 0.5% methylcellulose suspension, and 0.25 mM $NaHCO_3$ were sequentially administered with a 5 min interval. For vehicle D, esomeprazole solution was administered first, and aceclofenac solution was administered 10 min after the esomeprazole dose. Approximately 200 µL of venous blood was collected predose and 0.25, 0.5, 1, 2, 3, 4, 6, 8, 12, 18, and 24 h postdose from the jugular vein. Plasma samples were obtained by centrifugation of the blood samples at $4000 \times g$ for 10 min and stored at $-70\,°C$ until analysis. The stomach was collected for measurement of gastric lesions.

2.4. Measurement of Gastric Lesions

To evaluate the effects of esomeprazole on gastric damage associated with aceclofenac administration, rats were separated into six groups, i.e., control group (blank vehicle D, *n* = 7), positive control group (200 mg/kg of aceclofenac, *n* = 7), and four test groups (200 mg/kg of aceclofenac + 5, 10, 20, or 40 mg/kg of esomeprazole, *n* = 3 or 4). The rats were fasted 24 h before aceclofenac and esomeprazole doses. Esomeprazole solution was administered 10 min prior to aceclofenac (200 mg/kg) administration. At 6 h after the aceclofenac dose, rats were sacrificed, the stomach was excised, and gastric damage was examined. Since this study was conducted by two separate experiments and each experiment has the control and positive control, the number of animals included for the control (*n* = 7) and positive control (*n* = 7) was higher than test groups (*n* = 3–4). Except for the esomeprazole doses, all experimental protocols were identical between the two studies.

The gastric damage by aceclofenac was measured by calculation of ulcerative lesion area and ulcer index. After sacrificing the animal, the stomach was dissected along its greater curvature and fixed on a board. The stomach was then macroscopically examined, and the area of the lesion was quantified using an image analysis program, Image J (National Institutes of Health, Bethesda, MD, USA). The extent of ulceration was also assessed by calculation of an ulcer index according to the method of Andrade et al. [28,29]. Ulcers were first classified as ulcer area < 1 mm^2 (Level I), ulcer area = 1–3 mm^2 (Level II), and ulcer area > 3 mm^2 (Level III), and the ulcer indexes were calculated:

Ulcer index
$$= 1 \times (number\ of\ Level\ I\ ulcer) + 2 \times (number\ of\ Level\ II\ ulcer) + 3 \times (number\ of\ Level\ III\ ulcer)$$

2.5. Liquid Chromatography-Tandem Mass Spectrometry (LC-MS/MS)

Concentrations of aceclofenac, its metabolite, diclofenac, and esomeprazole in the rat plasma were determined by a newly developed LC-MS/MS assay. Calibration samples were prepared by spiking 50 µL of blank rat plasma with 50 µL of the standard aceclofenac, diclofenac, and esomeprazole working standard solutions in methanol followed by addition of 50 µL of the internal standard (IS) solution (lansoprazole, 100 ng/mL in methanol) and 350 µL of methanol as precipitation solvent. The final calibration samples yielded concentrations of 5, 10, 50, 100, 500, 1000, 5000, and 10,000 ng/mL for aceclofenac, 10, 50, 100, 500, 1000, 5000, and 10,000 ng/mL for diclofenac, and 0.25, 0.5, 2.5, 5, 25, 50, 250, and 500 ng/mL for esomeprazole. For plasma sample preparation, 50 μL of the IS and 400 μL of methanol were added to 50 μL of the rat plasma samples. The mixture was then mixed on a vortex mixer for 1 min and centrifuged at 34,220× *g* for 10 min. After centrifugation, 100 μL of the supernatant was diluted with the same volume of 25 mM ammonium formate, and a volume of 2 μL was injected into the LC-MS/MS.

The LC-MS/MS comprised an Agilent 6430 coupled with an Agilent 1200 HPLC system (Agilent, Santa Clara, CA, USA). Chromatographic separations were achieved on a Kinetex C18 column 50 × 2.10 mm i.d., 2.0 μm (Phenomenex, Torrence, CA, USA) with a Security Guard Cartridge (Phenomenex, Torrence, CA, USA). The mobile phase (MP) consisted of a mixture of 25 mM ammonium formate with 0.2% formic acid (MP-A) and acetonitrile (MP-B). The initial condition of 77% MP-A and 23% MP-B was held for 4 min followed by a linear increase of MP-B to 90% in the next 0.3 min. The flow rate of the mobile phase was set at 0.35 mL/min at the initial condition. The composition of 10:90 of MP-A:MP-B was maintained for 1 min, and the flow rate was 0.6 mL/min. The system was brought back to the initial condition of 77% MP-A by a linear gradient in 0.3 min and a flow rate of 0.35 mL/min and maintained for 3 min before the next injection. The column oven temperature was 40 °C. The mass spectrometer was operated using electron spray ionization (ESI) in positive ion mode with a dwell time of 100 ms. The fragmentor voltage was 85 V for aceclofenac, esomeprazole, and the IS, and 80 V for diclofenac. The collision energy was 40 V for aceclofenac, 34 V for diclofenac, 5 V for esomeprazole, and 5 V for the IS. Gas temperature, gas flow rate, and nebulizer gas pressure were set at 350 °C, 10 L/min, and 20 psi, respectively. The transition of the precursors to the product ion was monitored at *m/z* 354.0→214.0 for aceclofenac, 296.0→214.0 for diclofenac, 346.3→198.0 for esomeprazole, and 370.1→252.0 for the IS.

The lower limit of quantification (LLOQ) of the assay was 5 ng/mL, 10 ng/mL, and 0.25 ng/mL for aceclofenac, diclofenac, and esomeprazole, respectively, in the rat plasma. The intra- and inter-day accuracy was 103.0–110.8% for aceclofenac, 95.2–108.8% for diclofenac, and 90.4–111.0% for esomeprazole (*n* = 4, each). The intra- and inter-day precision was below 11.0% for aceclofenac, 12.1% for diclofenac, and 13.2% for esomeprazole (*n* = 4, each). The recovery calculated by comparing the peak area obtained from the standard solution spiked in the blank plasma followed by a protein precipitation process to that obtained from the matrix-free solvent was 97.2 ± 6.8% for aceclofenac, 89.9 ± 5.0% for diclofenac, 109.3 ± 2.0% for esomeprazole, and 107.5 ± 3.1% for the IS (*n* = 3).

2.6. Non-Compartmental Analysis

The non-compartmental pharmacokinetic parameters were estimated by Phoenix® WinNonlin® 6.4 (Certara, Princeton, NJ, USA). These parameters included terminal half-life ($t_{1/2}$), peak plasma concentration (C_{max}) and time to reach C_{max} (T_{max}), areas under the plasma concentration vs. time curve from time zero to the last observation time (AUC_{all}) and from time zero to infinity (AUC_{∞}), and systemic clearance (CL/F).

2.7. Statistical Analysis

The obtained data were analyzed with unpaired *t*-tests for comparisons between two means of unpaired data or one-way analyses of variance followed by Tukey's post hoc test for comparisons among more than two means of unpaired data. Data were expressed as the mean ± standard deviation (SD). The statistical significance level was set at $p < 0.05$ (SPSS Statistics 17.0, SPSS Inc., Chicago, IL, USA).

3. Results

3.1. Effects of Esomeprazole on Aceclofenac Induced Gastric Damage

Figure 1 shows ulcer index and ulcer areas following oral administration of aceclofenac (200 mg/kg) with or without esomeprazole pre-treatments (0, 5, 10, 20, 40 mg/kg). Two separate experiments were conducted, and data from the two studies were pooled together. While minimal gastric ulcers were observed after administration of control vehicle, significantly higher ulcer index and ulcer area were observed following aceclofenac administration at 200 mg/kg. Ulcer index was significantly reduced by administration of esomeprazole (Figure 1A). However, no statistically significant dose-dependent differences across esomeprazole doses of 5–40 mg/kg were observed, and increasing the dose of esomeprazole to 40 mg/kg did not result in an increased reduction of aceclofenac-induced gastric lesions. Both absolute gastric ulcer area (mm^2) and relative ulceration area compared to total stomach area (%) showed a trend similar to the ulcer index. Significantly higher ulcer areas were observed with aceclofenac treatment, with reduction by esomeprazole co-administration at 10 and 20 mg/kg (Figure 1B,C).

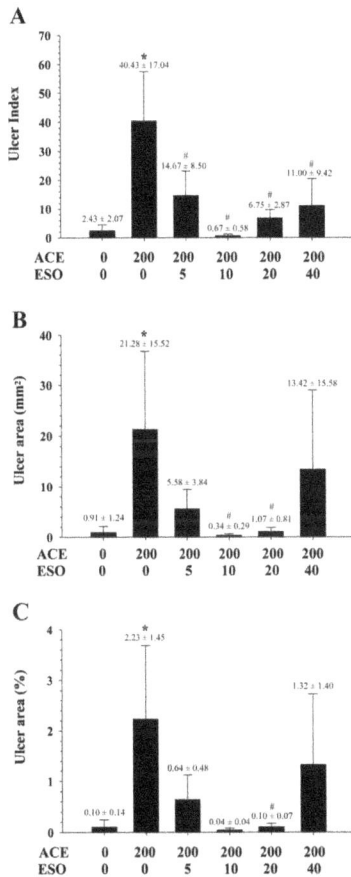

Figure 1. Aceclofenac (ACE) 200 mg/kg-induced gastric ulcers represented by (**A**) ulcer index, (**B**) ulcer area (mm^2), and (**C**) relative ulcer area (%) in the absence or in the presence of pre-treatments with esomeprazole (ESO) 0, 5, 10, 20, 40 mg/kg in rats. Each column represents the mean ± SD. *, $p < 0.05$ vs. control (ACE = 0/ESO = 0 mg/kg); #, $p < 0.05$ vs. ACE = 200/ESO = 0 mg/kg.

3.2. Effects of Esomeprazole on Aceclofenac Pharmacokinetics

Effects of esomeprazole on aceclofenac pharmacokinetics were evaluated after oral administration of aceclofenac (20 mg/kg) in combination with esomeprazole (0, 4, 8 mg/kg) delivered with vehicle C in rats. Average plasma concentration vs. time profiles of aceclofenac, diclofenac, and esomeprazole are shown in Figure 2, and non-compartmental pharmacokinetic parameters are summarized in Table 1. Plasma aceclofenac concentration rapidly increased and reached C_{max} within 0.23 h. Plasma concentration then declined with a mean terminal half-life ($t_{1/2}$) of 0.94–1.39 h. No significant differences in aceclofenac pharmacokinetic parameters were found with esomeprazole co-administration (Table 1).

Diclofenac, a metabolite of aceclofenac, plasma concentrations also rapidly increased following aceclofenac administration to maximum concentrations (C_{max}) of 4.91–10.76 µg/mL with mean T_{max} of 0.23–0.50 h. C_{max} as well as AUC of diclofenac were higher than those of aceclofenac. The $t_{1/2}$ of diclofenac was 3.24–3.84 h. Pharmacokinetic parameters of diclofenac were unaltered by esomeprazole co-administration. The fraction of metabolite formation (AUC_{DIC}/AUC_{ACE}) was also unaltered by esomeprazole administration.

Following oral co-administration of aceclofenac and esomeprazole, esomeprazole plasma concentration rapidly increased and reached C_{max} within 0.15 h, then declined with a $t_{1/2}$ of 3.87–5.67 h (Figure 2C and Table 1). While the $t_{1/2}$ and T_{max} were similar following 4 and 8 mg/kg esomeprazole administration, average C_{max}, AUC_{all}, and AUC_∞ proportionally increased with the dose increase.

Table 1. Non-compartmental pharmacokinetic parameters of aceclofenac, diclofenac, and esomeprazole obtained after oral administration of aceclofenac (20 mg/kg) and esomeprazole (0, 4 and 8 mg/kg) to rats. Parameters include terminal half-life ($t_{1/2}$), peak plasma concentration (C_{max}), time to reach C_{max} (T_{max}), areas under the plasma concentration vs. time curve from time zero to the last observation time (AUC_{all}) and from time zero to infinity (AUC_∞), and systemic clearance (CL/F).

Compound	Parameters	ACE 20/ESO 0 mg/kg (*n* = 4)	ACE 20/ESO 4 mg/kg (*n* = 6)	ACE 20/ESO 8 mg/kg (*n* = 4)
Aceclofenac	$t_{1/2}$ (h)	1.38 ± 0.21	0.94 ± 0.70	1.39 ± 0.72
	T_{max} (h)	0.23 ± 0.20	0.17 ± 0.07	0.19 ± 0.10
	C_{max} (µg/mL)	3.07 ± 1.20	5.12 ± 1.66	5.72 ± 2.55
	AUC_{all} (µg·h/mL)	2.30 ± 0.54	2.54 ± 0.51	2.79 ± 0.61
	AUC_∞ (µg·h/mL)	2.36 ± 0.52	2.57 ± 0.51	2.83 ± 0.60
	CL/F (mL/min/kg)	146.80 ± 32.40	134.77 ± 32.32	121.94 ± 26.32
Diclofenac	$t_{1/2}$ (h)	3.84 ± 0.32	3.82 ± 1.65	3.24 ± 0.98
	T_{max} (h)	0.50 ± 0.30	0.28 ± 0.11	0.23 ± 0.08
	C_{max} (µg/mL)	4.91 ± 3.19	10.76 ± 2.74	8.89 ± 4.98
	AUC_{all} (µg·h/mL)	7.16 ± 1.98	9.44 ± 1.1	8.56 ± 3.32
	AUC_∞ (µg·h/mL)	7.76 ± 2.13	10.1 ± 1.35	8.97 ± 3.24
	AUC_{DIC}/AUC_{ACE}	3.94 ± 1.73	4.64 ± 1.32	3.63 ± 0.97
Esomeprazole	$t_{1/2}$ (h)	-	3.87 ± 2.21	5.67 ± 3.68
	T_{max} (h)	-	0.15 ± 0.14	0.13 ± 0.05
	C_{max} (µg/mL)	-	57.14 ± 25.94	142.75 ± 132.71
	AUC_{all} (µg·h/mL)	-	27.68 ± 13.39	64.02 ± 49.78
	AUC_∞ (µg·h/mL)	-	30.91 ± 12.76	68.71 ± 48.72
	CL/F (mL/min/kg)	-	2442.37 ± 884.54	3087.76 ± 2334.25

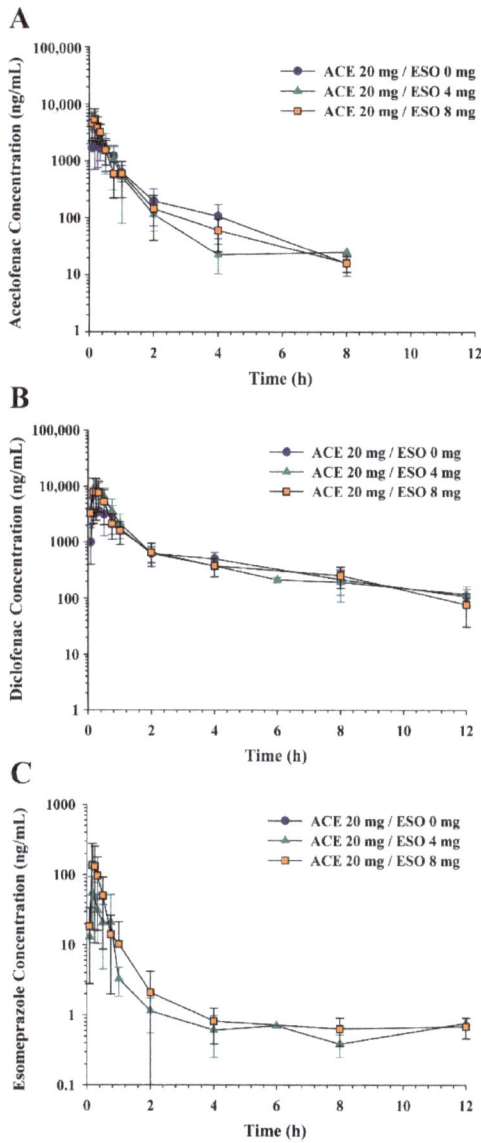

Figure 2. Average plasma concentration-time profiles of (**A**) aceclofenac, (**B**) diclofenac, and (**C**) esomeprazole following oral administration of aceclofenac (20 mg/kg) in combination with esomeprazole (0, 4, 8 mg/kg) in rats. Data represent mean ± SD (*n* = 4–6).

3.3. Effects of Different Dosing Vehicles on the Pharmacokinetics of Aceclofenac and Esomeprazole

Figure 3 summarizes plasma concentration vs. time profiles of aceclofenac, diclofenac, and esomeprazole following administration of aceclofenac and esomeprazole using different dosing vehicles. The non-compartmental pharmacokinetic parameters are summarized in Table 2. Since different doses were used with vehicles A, B, C (aceclofenac 20 mg/kg and esomeprazole 4 mg/kg), and vehicle D (aceclofenac 200 mg/kg and esomeprazole 20 mg/kg), the systemic exposure parameters C_{max} and AUC were normalized by dose and compared. Statistical comparisons were made only for dose-independent parameters, such as $t_{1/2}$, T_{max}, C_{max}/D, AUC/D, and CL/F.

For aceclofenac, significant differences were found for $t_{1/2}$, C_{max}/D, and AUC_{all}/D depending on the vehicle. Drug $t_{1/2}$ was longer when vehicle B (0.5% methylcellulose suspension in distilled water) was used than when vehicle C was used. Aceclofenac C_{max}/D as well as AUC_{all}/D with vehicle B was also lower than those in other vehicles. The C_{max}/D of aceclofenac was the highest in vehicle C compared to all other vehicles. However, the AUC_{∞}/D of aceclofenac was comparable across all tested vehicles.

Table 2. Non-compartmental pharmacokinetic parameters of aceclofenac and diclofenac obtained after oral administration of vehicle A, B, C, and D containing aceclofenac (20 mg/kg for A, B, and C and 200 mg/kg for D) and esomeprazole (4 mg/kg for A, B, and C and 20 mg/kg for D) to rats.

Compound	Parameters	Vehicle A ($n = 5$)	Vehicle B ($n = 4$)	Vehicle C ($n = 6$)	Vehicle D ($n = 6$)
Aceclofenac	$t_{1/2}$ (h) [a]	2.13 ± 0.30	6.47 ± 5.59	0.94 ± 0.70	1.89 ± 1.65
	T_{max} (h)	0.57 ± 0.80	0.60 ± 0.93	0.17 ± 0.07	0.27 ± 0.21
	C_{max} (μg/mL)	2.53 ± 0.57	0.69 ± 0.33	5.12 ± 1.66	21.69 ± 6.48
	C_{max} (μg/mL)/D (mg/kg) [b]	0.13 ± 0.03	0.03 ± 0.02	0.26 ± 0.08	0.11 ± 0.03
	AUC_{all} (μg·h/mL)	3.35 ± 1.72	0.88 ± 0.82	2.54 ± 0.51	34.75 ± 9.82
	AUC_{all} (μg·h/mL)/D (mg/kg) [c]	0.37 ± 0.07	0.07 ± 0.06	0.47 ± 0.05	0.63 ± 0.23
	AUC_{∞} (μg·h/mL)	3.53 ± 1.89	1.42 ± 1.14	2.57 ± 0.51	38.16 ± 9.00
	AUC_{∞} (μg·h/mL)/D (mg/kg)	0.18 ± 0.09	0.07 ± 0.06	0.13 ± 0.03	0.19 ± 0.05
	CL/F (mL/min/kg)	116.07 ± 51.38	446.08 ± 358.98	134.77 ± 32.32	91.01 ± 23.36
Diclofenac	$t_{1/2}$ (h) [d]	1.97 ± 0.35	3.04 ± 1.42	3.82 ± 1.65	5.57 ± 3.21
	T_{max} (h)	0.60 ± 0.78	0.69 ± 0.88	0.28 ± 0.11	1.33 ± 1.67
	C_{max} (μg/mL)	5.98 ± 3.06	0.63 ± 0.28	10.76 ± 2.74	43.69 ± 14.61
	AUC_{all} (μg·h/mL)	7.41 ± 1.35	1.46 ± 1.30	9.44 ± 1.10	125.81 ± 46.49
	AUC_{∞} (μg·h/mL)	7.51 ± 1.38	1.58 ± 1.44	10.1 ± 1.35	129.86 ± 44.66
	AUC_{DIC}/AUC_{ACE} [a]	3.04 ± 1.06	2.03 ± 0.24	4.64 ± 1.32	4.33 ± 0.85
Esomeprazole	$t_{1/2}$ (h)	1.69 ± 0.75	5.14 ± 5.30	3.87 ± 2.21	3.72 ± 0.38
	T_{max} (h)	1.80 ± 3.47	0.21 ± 0.08	0.15 ± 0.14	0.21 ± 0.08
	C_{max} (ng/mL)	15.43 ± 3.36	13.54 ± 4.08	57.14 ± 25.94	319 ± 136.81
	C_{max} (ng/mL)/D (mg/kg) [e]	3.86 ± 0.84	3.39 ± 1.02	14.28 ± 6.49	15.95 ± 6.84
	AUC_{all} (ng·h/mL)	33.83 ± 10.1	27.28 ± 6.43	27.68 ± 13.39	143.85 ± 48.71
	AUC_{all} (ng·h/mL)/D (mg/kg)	8.46 ± 2.53	6.82 ± 1.61	6.92 ± 3.35	7.19 ± 2.44
	AUC_{∞} (ng·h/mL)	42.09 ± 19.27	37.03 ± 11.85	30.91 ± 12.76	151.35 ± 51.65
	AUC_{∞} (ng·h/mL)/D (mg/kg)	10.52 ± 4.82	9.26 ± 2.96	7.73 ± 3.19	7.57 ± 2.58
	CL/F (mL/min/kg)	1786.9 ± 670.64	1910.9 ± 518.68	2442.37 ± 884.54	2356.49 ± 602.56

[a] ANOVA ($p < 0.05$, post hoc: Tukey, B vs. C); [b] ANOVA ($p < 0.05$, post hoc: Tukey, C vs. A, B, D); [c] ANOVA ($p < 0.05$, post hoc: Tukey, B vs. A, C, D); [d] ANOVA ($p < 0.05$, post hoc: Tukey, A vs. D); [e] ANOVA ($p < 0.05$, post hoc: Tukey, A, B vs. C, D); * Statistical significance was only presented for dose-independent parameters.

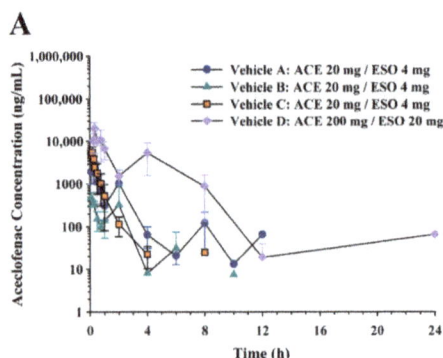

Figure 3. *Cont.*

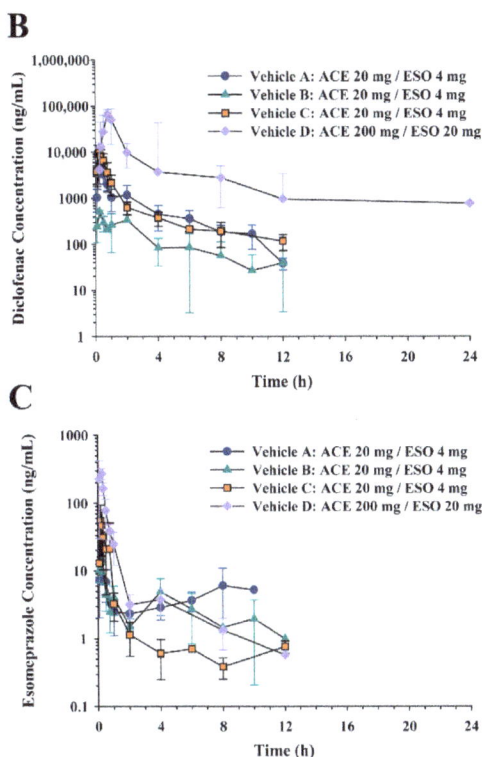

Figure 3. Average plasma concentration-time profiles of (**A**) aceclofenac, (**B**) diclofenac, and (**C**) esomeprazole following oral administration of vehicle A, B, C, and D containing aceclofenac (20 mg/kg for A, B, and C and 200 mg/kg for D) and esomeprazole (4 mg/kg for A, B, and C and 20 mg/kg for D) in rats.

Most pharmacokinetic parameters of diclofenac except $t_{1/2}$ were similar regardless of the dosing vehicle. The fraction metabolized, i.e., AUC_{DIC}/AUC_{ACE}, after aceclofenac administration was higher in vehicle C compared to that in vehicle B.

Most pharmacokinetic parameters of esomeprazole were not changed by different dosing vehicles, except C_{max}/D. The C_{max}/D values were similar between vehicles C and D, which were over 3.7-fold higher than those in vehicles A and B (Table 2).

3.4. Food Effects on the Pharmacokinetics of Aceclofenac and Esomeprazole

To evaluate food effects on aceclofenac and esomeprazole pharmacokinetics, aceclofenac (20 mg/kg) and esomeprazole (4 mg/kg) prepared in vehicle A were orally administered in fasting and fed conditions. Plasma concentration vs. time profiles of aceclofenac, diclofenac, and esomeprazole are shown in Figure 4. Non-compartmental pharmacokinetic parameters of aceclofenac, diclofenac, and esomeprazole in fasting and fed conditions are summarized in Table 3. Although overall plasma concentration vs. time profiles of aceclofenac and diclofenac were similar between fasting and fed conditions (Figure 4A,B), a longer $t_{1/2}$ was observed in fasting conditions for aceclofenac. In contrast, there was no significant difference between the $t_{1/2}$ in the fasting and fed conditions for diclofenac (Table 3). Conversely, overall esomeprazole plasma concentrations were lower in the fed condition than in the fasting condition (Figure 4C). The $t_{1/2}$ was longer and C_{max} and AUC_{all} were significantly lower for esomeprazole in the fed condition (Table 3).

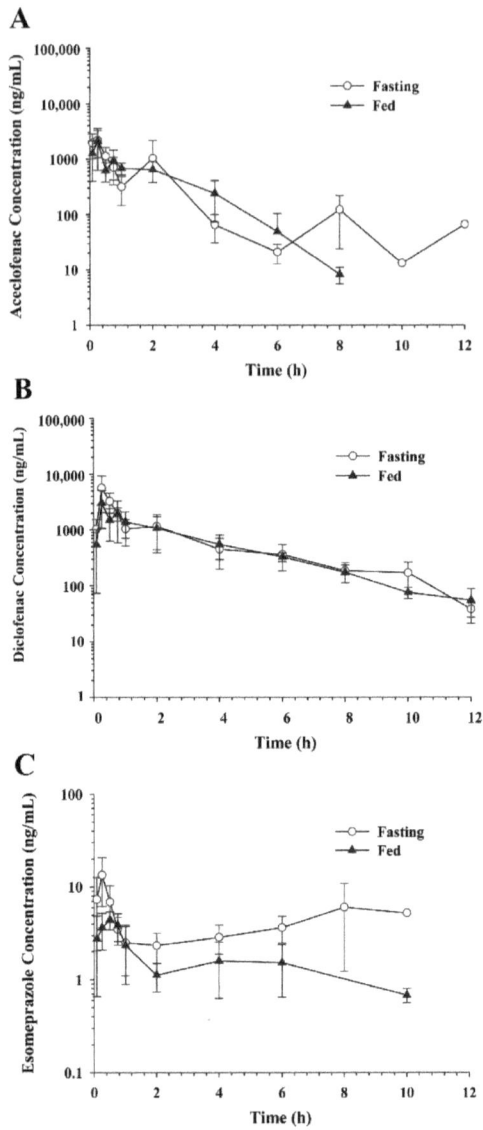

Figure 4. Average plasma concentration-time profiles of (**A**) aceclofenac, (**B**) diclofenac, and (**C**) esomeprazole following oral administration of aceclofenac (20 mg/kg) in combination with esomeprazole (4 mg/kg) in rats with fasting vs. fed conditions. Data represent mean ± SD (*n* = 4–5).

Table 3. Non-compartmental pharmacokinetic parameters of aceclofenac, diclofenac, and esomeprazole obtained after oral administration of aceclofenac (20 mg/kg) and esomeprazole (4 mg/kg) to rats under fasted and fed state.

Compound	Parameters	Fasted (*n* = 5)	Fed (*n* = 4)
Aceclofenac	$t_{1/2}$ (h) *	2.13 ± 0.30	0.81 ± 0.21
	T_{max} (h)	0.57 ± 0.80	0.65 ± 0.91
	C_{max} (µg/mL)	2.53 ± 0.57	2.27 ± 1.38
	AUC_{all} (µg·h/mL)	3.35 ± 1.72	2.95 ± 0.41
	AUC_{∞} (µg·h/mL)	3.53 ± 1.89	2.97 ± 0.41
	CL/F (mL/min/kg)	116.07 ± 51.38	114.1 ± 17.25
Diclofenac	$t_{1/2}$ (h)	1.97 ± 0.35	2.22 ± 0.59
	T_{max} (h)	0.60 ± 0.78	0.69 ± 0.88
	C_{max} (µg/mL)	5.98 ± 3.06	3.12 ± 1.91
	AUC_{all} (µg·h/mL)	7.41 ± 1.35	6.36 ± 1.27
	AUC_{∞} (µg·h/mL)	7.51 ± 1.38	6.56 ± 1.31
	AUC_{DIC}/AUC_{ACE}	3.04 ± 1.06	2.57 ± 0.27
Esomeprazole	$t_{1/2}$ (h) *	1.69 ± 0.75	3.18 ± 1.02
	T_{max} (h)	1.80 ± 3.47	0.40 ± 0.29
	C_{max} (ng/mL) *	15.43 ± 3.36	4.84 ± 0.94
	AUC_{all} (ng·h/mL) *	33.83 ± 10.10	13.96 ± 4.82
	AUC_{∞} (ng·h/mL)	42.09 ± 19.27	17.26 ± 4.42
	CL/F (mL/min/kg)	1786.9 ± 670.64	4061.35 ± 1041.26

* *t*-test ($p < 0.05$, Fasted vs. Fed).

4. Discussion

This study demonstrated no significant pharmacokinetic interactions between aceclofenac and esomeprazole in rats. Metabolic formation of diclofenac from aceclofenac was fast and extensive, which was consistent with previous reports [6,7]. Aceclofenac metabolism to diclofenac was also largely unaffected by concurrent administration of esomeprazole. Although diclofenac may be present at lower levels in humans than in rats, it significantly inhibits enzymatic activity of COX enzymes and contributes to the pharmacological action of aceclofenac in both humans and rats. Moreover, consistent with results in humans [22,23,25], our results indicate that esomeprazole may suppress gastric mucosal damage induced by aceclofenac in rats.

Substantial lesions were observed in the gastric mucosa following single dose oral administration of aceclofenac at 200 mg/kg in rats compared to that following vehicle administration (Figure 1). Co-administration of esomeprazole significantly suppressed gastric mucosal damage. Similarly, esomeprazole has demonstrated efficacy in the prevention and treatment of NSAIDs-induced gastric ulcers in humans [22,23,25] and experimental animals [30]. However, esomeprazole prevention of gastric ulcers was not dose-dependent in our study (Figure 1). While gastric ulceration induced by aceclofenac was almost entirely prevented by co-administration with esomeprazole at 10 and 20 mg/kg, no additional benefit was seen at the higher esomeprazole dose (40 mg/kg).

The gastro-protective effects of esomeprazole in combination with NSAIDs are potentially attributed to multiple mechanisms. Both acid-dependent and acid-independent mechanisms were proposed. Esomeprazole significantly inhibited gastric acid secretion in parallel with a significant reduction in mucosal damage in rats treated with indomethacin for 2 weeks [30]. In addition, esomeprazole restored proliferating cell nuclear antigen (PCNA) and Ki-67 expression and decreased malondialdehyde (MDA) levels and caspase-3 expression [30]. Reduction of oxidative tissue damage may also contribute to the gastroprotective actions of esomeprazole [31,32]. Digestive effects of esomeprazole may also confer gastroprotection [31]. Although the present study mainly focused on apparent gastric injury, we also analyzed the biomarkers that may contribute to gastric injury in mucosal samples. However, measured levels of MDA and protein expression of NF-κB, PCNA, and caspase-3 were variable and not dependent on aceclofenac administration. Minor changes in these biomarkers were observed with esomeprazole co-administration. It is possible that mucosal samples may be damaged during macroscopic examination in the present experimental setting. In addition, experimental conditions (i.e., a single dose administration of aceclofenac and esomeprazole) are different from studies that examined the effects of repeated exposures of indomethacin for two weeks followed by one week of esomeprazole co-administration [30]. The mechanism of gastroprotective effects of esomeprazole in combination with aceclofenac should be evaluated in further studies.

When pharmacokinetics of aceclofenac and esomeprazole were compared in fed vs. fasted conditions, the $t_{1/2}$ of aceclofenac was longer in fasting conditions. Multiple peaks were observed in the plasma concentration vs. time profiles and were more prominent in the fasting conditions (Figure 4A). These results agree with those of previous studies in which multiple peaks were present [6]. The multiple-peak phenomenon may result from the presence of either enterohepatic recirculation or a complicated absorption process [33,34], which may be favorable in fasting conditions [6]. The pharmacokinetics of the metabolite diclofenac were not altered by the presence of food. However, a significant reduction in systemic exposure to esomeprazole was observed in the fed versus fasting condition (Table 3). This is consistent with previous reports that the mean exposure after administration of a single dose of esomeprazole was decreased by 43–53% after food intake compared to fasting conditions resulting in the recommendation for esomeprazole to be taken at least one hour before meals [35].

During the present study, we also found that both aceclofenac and esomeprazole pharmacokinetics were significantly dependent on dosing vehicles. Among four different dosing vehicles, vehicle C (citric urea buffer solution) allowed for the most rapid absorption of aceclofenac, as evidenced by the highest C_{max}/D with a short T_{max} (Table 2). A previous study reported that a mixture of urea and sodium citrate similar to vehicle C markedly increased aceclofenac water solubility [6]. Increased water solubility may have contributed to the increased rate of aceclofenac absorption. On the contrary, vehicle B (0.5% methylcellulose suspension in distilled water) induced lower C_{max}/D and AUC_{all}/D with a longer $t_{1/2}$ compared to the solution vehicle, which may be due to slower absorption of the suspension. However, the overall extent of absorption and AUC_{∞} of aceclofenac were comparable across suspension and solution vehicles. For esomeprazole, a significantly higher C_{max} was observed when esomeprazole was dosed in vehicles C and D than in vehicles A and B (Table 2). Esomeprazole stability is pH-dependent, and it degrades rapidly in an acidic environment [35]. Vehicles C and D contained neutral buffers, which may have prevented acid-catalyzed degradation of esomeprazole in the stomach leading to a higher C_{max}. When omeprazole was given in combination with sodium bicarbonate, bioavailability was reported to increase by 2-fold [36].

5. Conclusions

Potential interactions between aceclofenac and esomeprazole were evaluated with regard to pharmacokinetics and GI adverse effects. While metabolism and pharmacokinetic profiles of aceclofenac were mostly unaltered, gastric ulceration associated with aceclofenac was significantly inhibited by concurrent administration of esomeprazole. The clinical benefits, as well as the optimal dose of the combination of aceclofenac and esomeprazole, should be evaluated in further studies. Since both aceclofenac and esomeprazole absorption was affected by dosing vehicles, design of optimal formulations may provide further advantages with regard to pharmacokinetics and efficacy.

Author Contributions: Conceptualization, T.H.K., S.S., and B.S.S.; Methodology, T.H.K., S.K.T., Y.-W.C., S.-M.C., K.-Y.N., W.-H.K., S.S., and B.S.S.; Investigation, T.H.K., S.K.T., D.Y.L., S.E.C., J.Y.L., H.M.J., C.H.S., and B.S.S.; Formal analysis, T.H.K., S.K.T., S.S., and B.S.S.; Resources, S.S. and B.S.S.; Writing-Original Draft Preparation, T.H.K., S.S., and B.S.S.; Writing-Review and Editing, T.H.K., S.S., and B.S.S. Supervision, B.S.S.; Funding Acquisition, S.S., Y.-W.C., W.-H.K., and B.S.S.

Funding: This research was supported by the Small and Medium Business Administration of Korea Grant No. S2318312, Ministry of Food and Drug Safety (MFDS) Grant No. 16173MFDS542 in 2018, and the National Research Foundation (NRF) of Korea Grant No. 2015R1D1A1A09059248.

Conflicts of Interest: The authors declare no conflict of interest. Y.-W.C., S.-M.C., K.-Y.N., and W.-H.K. are full-time employees of Korea United Pharm. Inc. The funders had no role in the design of the study; in the collection, analyses, or interpretation of data; in the writing of the manuscript, and in the decision to publish the results.

References

1. Ward, D.E.; Veys, E.M.; Bowdler, J.M.; Roma, J. Comparison of aceclofenac with diclofenac in the treatment of osteoarthritis. *Clin. Rheumatol.* **1995**, *14*, 656–662. [CrossRef] [PubMed]
2. Martin-Mola, E.; Gijon-Banos, J.; Ansoleaga, J.J. Aceclofenac in comparison to ketoprofen in the treatment of rheumatoid arthritis. *Rheumatol. Int.* **1995**, *15*, 111–116. [CrossRef] [PubMed]
3. Batlle-Gualda, E.; Figueroa, M.; Ivorra, J.; Raber, A. The efficacy and tolerability of aceclofenac in the treatment of patients with ankylosing spondylitis: A multicenter controlled clinical trial. Aceclofenac indomethacin study group. *J. Rheumatol.* **1996**, *23*, 1200–1206. [PubMed]
4. Schattenkirchner, M.; Milachowski, K.A. A double-blind, multicentre, randomised clinical trial comparing the efficacy and tolerability of aceclofenac with diclofenac resinate in patients with acute low back pain. *Clin. Rheumatol.* **2003**, *22*, 127–135. [CrossRef] [PubMed]
5. Movilia, P.G. Evaluation of the analgesic activity and tolerability of aceclofenac in the treatment of post-episiotomy pain. *Drugs Exp. Clin. Res.* **1989**, *15*, 47–51. [PubMed]
6. Noh, K.; Shin, B.S.; Kwon, K.I.; Yun, H.Y.; Kim, E.; Jeong, T.C.; Kang, W. Absolute bioavailability and metabolism of aceclofenac in rats. *Arch. Pharm. Res.* **2015**, *38*, 68–72. [CrossRef] [PubMed]
7. Bort, R.; Ponsoda, X.; Carrasco, E.; Gomez-Lechon, M.J.; Castell, J.V. Comparative metabolism of the nonsteroidal antiinflammatory drug, aceclofenac, in the rat, monkey, and human. *Drug Metab. Dispos.* **1996**, *24*, 969–975. [PubMed]
8. Henrotin, Y.; de Leval, X.; Mathy-Hartet, M.; Mouithys-Mickalad, A.; Deby-Dupont, G.; Dogne, J.M.; Delarge, J.; Reginster, J.Y. In vitro effects of aceclofenac and its metabolites on the production by chondrocytes of inflammatory mediators. *Inflamm. Res.* **2001**, *50*, 391–399. [CrossRef] [PubMed]
9. Scheiman, J.M. Nsaids, gastrointestinal injury, and cytoprotection. *Gastroenterol. Clin. North Am.* **1996**, *25*, 279–298. [CrossRef]
10. Dooley, M.; Spencer, C.M.; Dunn, C.J. Aceclofenac: A reappraisal of its use in the management of pain and rheumatic disease. *Drugs* **2001**, *61*, 1351–1378. [CrossRef] [PubMed]
11. Perez-Ruiz, F.; Alonso-Ruiz, A.; Ansoleaga, J.J. Comparative study of the efficacy and safety of aceclofenac and tenoxicam in rheumatoid arthritis. *Clin. Rheumatol.* **1996**, *15*, 473–477. [CrossRef] [PubMed]
12. Diaz, C.; Rodriguez de la Serna, A.; Geli, C.; Gras, X. Efficacy and tolerability of aceclofenac versus diclofenac in the treatment of knee osteoarthritis: A multicentre study. *Eur. J. Rheumatol. Inflamm.* **1996**, *16*, 17–22.
13. Pasero, G.; Marcolongo, R.; Serni, U.; Parnham, M.J.; Ferrer, F. A multi-centre, double-blind comparative study of the efficacy and safety of aceclofenac and diclofenac in the treatment of rheumatoid arthritis. *Curr. Med. Res. Opin.* **1995**, *13*, 305–315. [CrossRef] [PubMed]
14. Torri, G.; Vignati, C.; Agrifoglio, E.; Benvenuti, M.; Ceciliani, L.; Raschella, B.F.; Letizia, G.; Martorana, U.; Tessari, L.; Thovez, G.; et al. Aceclofenac versus piroxicam in the management of osteoarthritis of the knee: A double-blind controlled study. *Curr. Ther. Res.* **1994**, *55*, 576–583. [CrossRef]
15. Pasero, G.; Ruju, G.; Marcolongo, R.; Senesi, M.; Seni, U.; Mannoni, A.; Accardo, S.; Seriolo, B.; Colombo, B.; Ligniere, G.C.; et al. Aceclofenac versus naproxen in the treatment of ankylosing spondylitis: A double-blind, controlled study. *Curr. Ther. Res.* **1994**, *55*, 833–842. [CrossRef]
16. Perez Busquier, M.; Calero, E.; Rodriguez, M.; Castellon Arce, P.; Bermudez, A.; Linares, L.F.; Mesa, J.; Ffernandez Crisostomos, C.; Garcia, C.; Garcia Lopez, A.; et al. Comparison of aceclofenac with piroxicam in the treatment of osteoarthritis. *Clin. Rheumatol.* **1997**, *16*, 154–159. [CrossRef] [PubMed]
17. Kornasoff, D.; Frerick, H.; Bowdler, J.; Montull, E. Aceclofenac is a well-tolerated alternative to naproxen in the treatment of osteoarthritis. *Clin. Rheumatol.* **1997**, *16*, 32–38. [CrossRef] [PubMed]
18. Kornasoff, D.; Maisenbacher, J.; Bowdler, J.; Raber, A. The efficacy and tolerability of aceclofenac compared to indomethacin in patients with rheumatoid arthritis. *Rheumatol. Int.* **1996**, *15*, 225–230. [CrossRef] [PubMed]
19. Villa Alcazar, L.F.; de Buergo, M.; Rico Lenza, H.; Montull Fruitos, E. Aceclofenac is as safe and effective as tenoxicam in the treatment of ankylosing spondylitis: A 3 month multicenter comparative trial. Spanish study group on aceclofenac in ankylosing spondylitis. *J. Rheumatol.* **1996**, *23*, 1194–1199. [PubMed]

20. Lanza, F.L.; Chan, F.K.; Quigley, E.M. Practice Parameters Committee of the American College of, G. Guidelines for prevention of nsaid-related ulcer complications. *Am. J. Gastroenterol.* **2009**, *104*, 728–738. [CrossRef] [PubMed]

21. Agrawal, N.M.; Campbell, D.R.; Safdi, M.A.; Lukasik, N.L.; Huang, B.; Haber, M.M. Superiority of lansoprazole vs ranitidine in healing nonsteroidal anti-inflammatory drug-associated gastric ulcers: Results of a double-blind, randomized, multicenter study. Nsaid-associated gastric ulcer study group. *Arch. Intern. Med.* **2000**, *160*, 1455–1461. [CrossRef] [PubMed]

22. Goldstein, J.L.; Johanson, J.F.; Suchower, L.J.; Brown, K.A. Healing of gastric ulcers with esomeprazole versus ranitidine in patients who continued to receive nsaid therapy: A randomized trial. *Am. J. Gastroenterol.* **2005**, *100*, 2650–2657. [CrossRef] [PubMed]

23. Hawkey, C.; Talley, N.J.; Yeomans, N.D.; Jones, R.; Sung, J.J.; Langstrom, G.; Naesdal, J.; Scheiman, J.M.; Group, N.S.S. Improvements with esomeprazole in patients with upper gastrointestinal symptoms taking non-steroidal antiinflammatory drugs, including selective cox-2 inhibitors. *Am. J. Gastroenterol.* **2005**, *100*, 1028–1036. [CrossRef] [PubMed]

24. Morgner, A.; Miehlke, S.; Labenz, J. Esomeprazole: Prevention and treatment of nsaid-induced symptoms and ulcers. *Expert Opin. Pharmacother.* **2007**, *8*, 975–988. [CrossRef] [PubMed]

25. Scheiman, J.M.; Yeomans, N.D.; Talley, N.J.; Vakil, N.; Chan, F.K.; Tulassay, Z.; Rainoldi, J.L.; Szczepanski, L.; Ung, K.A.; Kleczkowski, D.; et al. Prevention of ulcers by esomeprazole in at-risk patients using non-selective nsaids and cox-2 inhibitors. *Am. J. Gastroenterol.* **2006**, *101*, 701–710. [CrossRef] [PubMed]

26. Lanas, A.; Polo-Tomas, M.; Roncales, P.; Gonzalez, M.A.; Zapardiel, J. Prescription of and adherence to non-steroidal anti-inflammatory drugs and gastroprotective agents in at-risk gastrointestinal patients. *Am. J. Gastroenterol.* **2012**, *107*, 707–714. [CrossRef] [PubMed]

27. Dries, A.M.; Richardson, P.; Cavazos, J.; Abraham, N.S. Therapeutic intent of proton pump inhibitor prescription among elderly nonsteroidal anti-inflammatory drug users. *Aliment. Pharmacol. Ther.* **2009**, *30*, 652–661. [CrossRef] [PubMed]

28. Andrade, S.F.; Antoniolli, D.; Comunello, E.; Cardoso, L.G.V.; Carvalho, J.C.T.; Bastos, J.K. Antiulcerogenic activity of crude extract, fractions and populnoic acid isolated from austroplenckia populnea (celastraceae). *Z. Naturforsch. C* **2006**, *61*, 329–333. [CrossRef] [PubMed]

29. Adinortey, M.B.; Ansah, C.; Galyuon, I.; Nyarko, A. In vivo models used for evaluation of potential antigastroduodenal ulcer agents. *Ulcers* **2013**, *2013*, 12. [CrossRef]

30. Fornai, M.; Colucci, R.; Antonioli, L.; Awwad, O.; Ugolini, C.; Tuccori, M.; Fulceri, F.; Natale, G.; Basolo, F.; Blandizzi, C. Effects of esomeprazole on healing of nonsteroidal anti-inflammatory drug (nsaid)-induced gastric ulcers in the presence of a continued nsaid treatment: Characterization of molecular mechanisms. *Pharmacol. Res.* **2011**, *63*, 59–67. [CrossRef] [PubMed]

31. Suzuki, H.; Hibi, T. Novel effects other than antisecretory action and off-label use of proton pump inhibitors. *Expert Opin. Pharmacother.* **2005**, *6*, 59–67. [CrossRef] [PubMed]

32. Pastoris, O.; Verri, M.; Boschi, F.; Kastsiuchenka, O.; Balestra, B.; Pace, F.; Tonini, M.; Natale, G. Effects of esomeprazole on glutathione levels and mitochondrial oxidative phosphorylation in the gastric mucosa of rats treated with indomethacin. *Naunyn Schmiedebergs Arch. Pharmacol.* **2008**, *378*, 421–429. [CrossRef] [PubMed]

33. Metsugi, Y.; Miyaji, Y.; Ogawara, K.; Higaki, K.; Kimura, T. Appearance of double peaks in plasma concentration-time profile after oral administration depends on gastric emptying profile and weight function. *Pharm. Res.* **2008**, *25*, 886–895. [CrossRef] [PubMed]

34. Kim, T.H.; Shin, S.; Landersdorfer, C.B.; Chi, Y.H.; Paik, S.H.; Myung, J.; Yadav, R.; Horkovics-Kovats, S.; Bulitta, J.B.; Shin, B.S. Population pharmacokinetic modeling of the enterohepatic recirculation of fimasartan in rats, dogs, and humans. *AAPS J.* **2015**, *17*, 1210–1223. [CrossRef] [PubMed]

35. U.S. FDA, NDA 21-153/S-022: Nexium (esomeprazole magnesium) delayed-release capsules. 2001. Available online: http://www.accessdata.fda.gov/drugsatfda_docs/label/2006/021153s022lbl.pdf (accessed on 31 July 2018).

36. Pilbrant, A.; Cederberg, C. Development of an oral formulation of omeprazole. *Scand. J. Gastroenterol. Suppl.* **1985**, *108*, 113–120. [CrossRef] [PubMed]

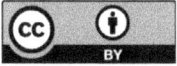

pharmaceutics

MDPI

Article

Simultaneous Determination of Chlorogenic Acid Isomers and Metabolites in Rat Plasma Using LC-MS/MS and Its Application to A Pharmacokinetic Study Following Oral Administration of *Stauntonia Hexaphylla* Leaf Extract (YRA-1909) to Rats

Won-Gu Choi [1,†], Ju-Hyun Kim [1,2,†], Dong Kyun Kim [1], Yongnam Lee [3], Ji Seok Yoo [3], Dae Hee Shin [3] and Hye Suk Lee [1,*]

[1] BK21 PLUS Team for Creative Leader Program for Pharmacomics-based Future Pharmacy and Drug Metabolism and Bioanalysis Laboratory, College of Pharmacy, The Catholic University of Korea, Bucheon 420-743, Korea; cwg0222@catholic.ac.kr (W.-G.C.); noraekajoa@gmail.com (J.-H.K.); kdk3124@catholic.ac.kr (D.K.K.)
[2] College of Pharmacy, Yeungnam University, Gyeongsan 38541, Korea
[3] Central R&D Institute, YUNGJIN PHARM. CO., LTD., Suwon 16229, Korea; nami0209@yungjin.co.kr (Y.L.); jsyoo@yungjin.co.kr (J.S.Y.); sdh580509@gmail.com (D.H.S.)
* Correspondence: sianalee@catholic.ac.kr; Tel.: +82-2-2164-4061
† These authors contributed equally to this work.

Received: 9 August 2018; Accepted: 28 August 2018; Published: 2 September 2018

Abstract: *Stauntonia hexaphylla* leaf extract (YRA-1909), which is widely used for the antirheumatic properties, has been under phase 2 clinical trials in patients with rheumatoid arthritis since April 2017. Liquid chromatography-tandem mass spectrometric method while using liquid–liquid extraction with ethyl acetate was validated for the simultaneous determination of the major active components of YRA-1909, including chlorogenic acid (CGA), neochlorogenic acid (NCGA), cryptochlorogenic acid (CCGA), and their metabolites (i.e., caffeic acid (CA), caffeic acid 3-*O*-glucuronide (CA-3-G), caffeic acid 4-*O*-glucuronide (CA-4-G), and ferulic acid (FA)) in rat plasma and applied to a pharmacokinetic study of YRA-1909 in rats. Seven analytes were separated on Halo C18 while using gradient elution of formic acid and methanol, and then quantified in selected reaction monitoring mode while using negative electrospray ionization. Following oral administration of YRA-1909 at doses of 25, 50, and 100 mg/kg to male Sprague-Dawley rats, CGA, NCGA, and CCGA were rapidly absorbed and metabolized to CA, CA-3-G, and CA-4-G. The area under the plasma concentration-time curve (AUC_{last}) of CGA, NCGA, CCGA, and three metabolites linearly increased as the YRA-1909 dose increased. Other pharmacokinetic parameters were comparable among three doses studied. AUC_{last} values for CA, CA-3-G, and CA-4-G exceeded those for CGA, NCGA, and CCGA.

Keywords: *Stauntonia hexaphylla* leaf extract; YRA-1909; pharmacokinetics; chlorogenic acid; neochlorogenic acid; cryptochlorogenic acid; caffeic acid; caffeic acid *O*-glucuronides; LC-MS/MS

1. Introduction

Stauntonia hexaphylla (Lardizabalaceae) is widely distributed throughout Korea, Japan, and China, and is a popular herbal supplement in Korean and Chinese folk medicine due to its analgesic, sedative, and diuretic properties [1,2]. It exhibits anti-osteoporosis [3], antidiabetic activity [4], and anti-inflammatory effects in carrageenan-induced paw edema rats [5]. *Stauntonia hexaphylla* leaf extract, YRA-1909, is associated with the antirheumatic activity [6] and has been undergoing in phase 2 clinical trials in the Republic of Korea since April 2017 to evaluate its safety and efficacy for treating patients suffering from rheumatoid arthritis (ClinicalTrials.gov identifier NCT03275025) [7]. Chlorogenic acid (CGA), neochlorogenic acid (NCGA), and cryptochlorogenic acid (CCGA) have been identified as the active ingredients in *Stauntonia hexaphylla* [4,5] and YRA-1909. CGA and NCGA are associated with various pharmacological properties, including antioxidant [8], anti-cancer [9], anti-virus [10], anti-coagulant, and anti-thrombotic properties [11]. CGA, NCGA, and CCGA are metabolized to caffeic acid (CA) and quinic acid by esterase [12–15]. CA is further metabolized to caffeic acid 3-*O*-glucuronide (CA-3-G) and caffeic acid 4-*O*-glucuronide (CA-4-G) by uridine-5′-diphosphate-glucuronosyltransferase (UGT) 1A1 and 1A9 enzymes, caffeic acid 3- and 4-*O*-sulfate by sulfotransferase (SULT) 1A1 and 1E1 enzymes, and ferulic acid (FA) and isoferulic acid by catechol-*O*-methyltransferase (COMT), which are metabolized to FA 4-*O*-glucuronide, FA 4-*O*-sulfate, and isoferulic acid 3-*O*-sulfate (Figure 1) [12–16]. CA and FA are active metabolites that are associated with various biological activities, including antioxidant [17], anti-mutagenic [18], and anti-cancer [19,20] effects.

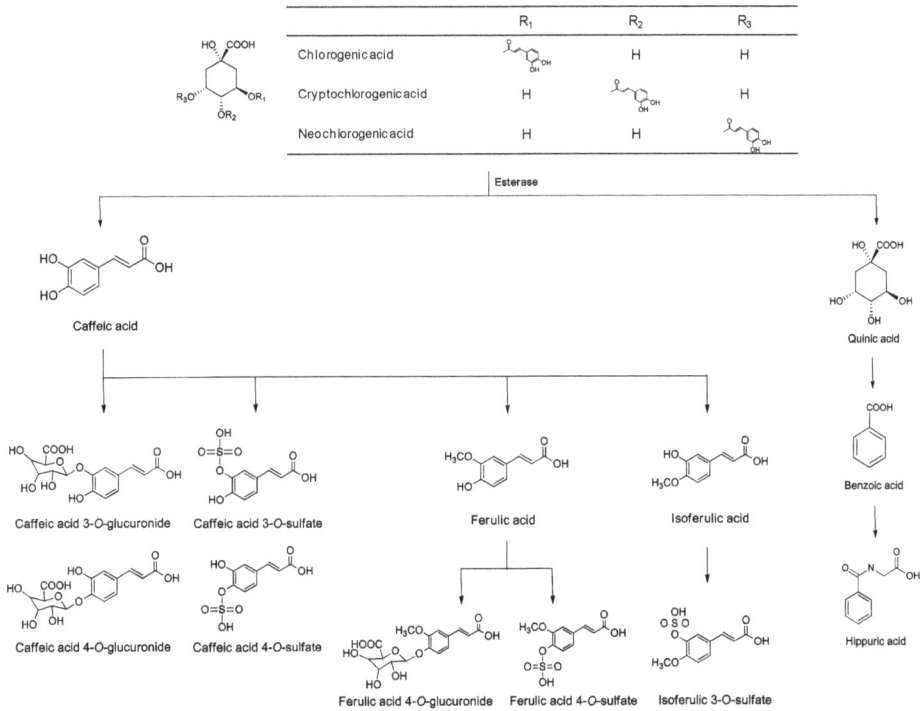

Figure 1. Metabolic pathways of chlorogenic acid, neochlorogenic acid, and cryptochlorogenic acid in rats and humans.

Pharmacokinetic evaluation of herbal drugs is helpful for determining dosage regimens and interpreting the pharmacological effects under clinical conditions. However, typical pharmacokinetic studies can be difficult to apply to herbal drugs that consist of multiple constituents, with frequently unidentified pharmacologically active components. As such, simultaneous determination of the various potential active constituents, major constituents, and/or their metabolites is recommended for the satisfactory pharmacokinetic evaluation of herbal drugs [21–23].

Several studies have applied liquid chromatography-mass spectrometry (LC-MS) or tandem mass spectrometry (LC-MS/MS) methods for the simultaneous determination of CGA, NCGA, CCGA, CA, or FA in human and rat plasma (50–500 µL) while using liquid–liquid extraction [24–27], or solid phase extraction [28], protein precipitation [29], or protein precipitation with disperse solid phase extraction [30]. The LC-MS has also been used in pharmacokinetic studies of these acids following the administration of herbal drugs to rats and humans. For example, one such study used the LC-MS/MS method to simultaneously determine phenolic acids and their metabolites in human plasma following the ingestion of instant coffee containing various chlorogenic and phenolic acids; the study used protein precipitation to prepare samples [31]. The negative [24,26,28–31] and positive [25,27] electrospray ionization (ESI) modes were used for the ionization of phenolic acids in mass spectrometry.

There are currently no reports on the pharmacokinetics of YRA-1909. In this study, we developed a sensitive and selective LC-MS/MS method for evaluating the pharmacokinetics of the active constituents of YRA-1909 (i.e., CGA, NCGA, and CCGA) and their active metabolites (i.e., CA, CA-3-G, CA-4-G, and FA) after the oral administration of YRA-1909 at doses of 25, 50, and 100 mg/kg to the rats.

2. Materials and Methods

2.1. Materials

CGA (purity, 98.1%) was obtained from Hunan Yuanhang Biology Technology Co., Ltd (Changsha, China). CCGA (purity, 99.7%) was obtained from Dailan Meilun Biotech Co., Ltd (Dailan, China). NCGA (purity, 98.0%), CA (purity, 98.0%), FA (purity, 99.0%), dimethyl sulfoxide, and formic acid were purchased from Sigma Aldrich Co. (St. Louis, MO, USA). CA-3-G (purity, 98.1%), CA-4-G (purity, 98.0%), and ferulic acid-d3 (FA-d3)(purity, 98.0%; used as an internal standard) were obtained from Toronto Research Chemicals Inc. (Toronto, Canada). Water and methanol (LC-MS grade) were supplied from Burdick and Jackson Inc. (Muskegon, MI, USA). All the other chemicals used were of the highest quality available.

Stauntonia hexaphylla leaves were collected from cultivated fields, in accordance with Good Agricultural Practice guidelines, in Jangheung (Jeonnam, Korea). YRA-1909 was prepared by extracting *Stauntonia hexalphylla* leaves with distilled water, followed by purification using column chromatography. YRA-1909 was produced by KGCYebon (Chungju, Korea) according to the protocol recommended by the International Conference on Harmonization and Good Manufacturing Practice. The contents of CGA, NCGA, and CCGA in YRA-1909 (batch no.: YR-1001) were 4.74, 1.10, and 3.49 mg/g, respectively, as quantified while using high-performance liquid chromatographic method for quality control developed by YUNGJIN PHARM CO., LTD (Suwon, Korea). CA and FA were not detected in YRA-1909.

2.2. Preparation of Clibration Standards and Quality Control Samples

Each standard stock solution was prepared separately by dissolving CGA, NCGA, CCGA, and their four metabolites (1 mg each) in 1 mL dimethyl sulfoxide. A mixed standard stock solution was prepared by mixing each stock solution to final concentrations of 10 µg/mL for CGA and NCGA, 50 µg/mL for CCGA, CA, CA-3-G, and CA-4-G, and 250 µg/mL for FA. Working standard solutions of the seven analytes were prepared by diluting a mixed standard stock solution with methanol. The internal standard working solution (FA-d3, 20 µg/mL) was prepared by diluting an aliquot of stock solution with methanol. All such standard solutions were stored at 4 °C in darkness for four weeks.

Rat plasma calibration standards were prepared at eight concentration levels by adding 2 µL working standard solution to 50 µL of drug-free rat plasma: 0.5, 1.0, 2.0, 5.0, 10.0, 25.0, 50,0, 100, and 200 ng/mL for CGA and NCGA, 2.5, 5.0, 10.0, 25.0, 50,0, 250, 500, and 1000 ng/mL for CCGA, CA, CA-3-G, and CA-4-G, and 12.5, 25.0, 50.0, 125, 250, 1250, 3750, and 5000 ng/mL for FA, respectively.

5 μL of 5% formic acid was added and vortex-mixed to improve the plasma stability of CGA, CCGA, and NCGA [24,32]. Quality control (QC) samples were prepared at the concentrations of 1.5, 25, and 160 ng/mL for CGA and NCGA, 7.5, 125, and 800 ng/mL for CCGA, CA, CA-3-G, and CA-4-G, and 37.5, 625, and 4000 ng/mL for FA in drug-free rat plasma and then stored at −80 °C until analysis.

2.3. Sample Preparation

50 μL aliquot of blank rat plasma, calibration standards, and QC samples stored on ice were vortex-mixed with 5 μL FA-d$_3$ in methanol (20 μg/mL), 100 μL 1 M hydrochloric acid, and 600 μL ethyl acetate for 2 min. Following centrifugation at 13000 rpm for 8 min, 475 μL the supernatant was transferred into a new polypropylene tube. The aqueous layer was extracted once more with 600 μL ethyl acetate, and the supernatants were transferred after centrifugation. The organic layer was evaporated to dryness at 35 °C for 20 min while using a vacuum evaporator. The residues were dissolved in 50 μL 10% methanol and centrifuged. An aliquot (3 μL) was injected onto the LC-MS/MS system for analyses.

2.4. LC-MS/MS Analysis

An ultra-performance liquid chromatograph, Agilent 1290, coupled with Agilent 6495 tandem mass spectrometer (Agilent Technologies, Wilmington, DE, USA) was used. Chromatographic separation was performed on a Halo C$_{18}$ column (2.7 μm, 2.1 mm i.d. × 100 mm, Advanced Material Technology, Wilmington, DE, USA) while using a gradient elution of 0.1% formic acid in water (mobile phase A) and 0.1% formic acid in methanol (mobile phase B) at a flow rate of 0.3 mL/min, as follows: 10% mobile phase B for 0.5 min, 10% to 25% mobile phase B for 5.5 min, 25% to 37% mobile phase B for 1 min, 37% mobile phase B for 2 min, 37% to 10% mobile phase B for 0.1 min, and 10% mobile phase B for 2.4 min. The column and autosampler tray were maintained at 35 °C and 4 °C, respectively. The ESI source settings for the ionization of the analytes in negative mode were as follows: gas temperature, 230 °C; gas flow, 19 L/min; Nebulizer, 45 psi; sheath gas temperature, 400 °C; sheath gas flow, 10 L/min; capillary voltage, 3000 V; nozzle voltage, 1000 V. Fragmentation of analytes was performed at collision energy of 14 eV for CGA, NCGA, and CCGA, 8 eV for CA, 20 eV for CA-3-G and CA-4-G, 12 eV for FA, and 10 eV for FA-d$_3$, respectively, while using nitrogen gas as a collision gas at a pressure of 2 bar on the instrument. Selected reaction monitoring (SRM) mode was employed for the quantification: *m/z* 352.8 → 191.0 for CGA, NCGA, and CCGA; *m/z* 179.1 → 135.0 for CA; *m/z* 355.0 → 178.9 for CA-3-G and CA-4-G; *m/z* 192.9 → 133.9 for FA; *m/z* 196.1 → 134.0 for FA-d$_3$. Mass Hunter software (Agilent Technologies) was used for LC-MS/MS system control and data processing.

2.5. Method Validation

Method validation was performed according to the FDA Guidance on Bioanalytical Method Validation. For the evaluation of intra-and inter-day precision and accuracy, we analyzed batches of calibration standards and QC samples in five replicates on three different days, as follows: 0.5, 1.5, 25, and 160 ng/mL for CGA and NCGA, 2.5, 7.5, 125, and 800 ng/mL for CCGA, CA, CA-3-G, and CA-4-G, and 12.5, 37.5, 625, and 4000 ng/mL for FA were analyzed. Accuracy was defined as relative error (RE, %) of the measured mean value deviated from the nominal value, and precision was defined as the coefficient of variation (CV, %) of the measured concentration.

The stability of each of the seven analytes in rat plasma was evaluated by analyzing low and high QC samples in triplicate: post-preparation sample stability in the autosampler at 4 °C for 24 h, short-term storage stability following storage of plasma samples on ice for 2 h, long-term storage stability following the storage of plasma samples at −80 °C for 28 days, and three freeze-thaw cycles.

The matrix effect for each analyte was assessed by comparing the mean peak areas of the analytes that were spiked after extraction into blank plasma extracts originating from six different rats to mean peak areas for neat solutions of the analytes at 1.5, 25, and 160 ng/mL for CGA and NCGA, 7.5, 125, and 800 ng/mL for CCGA, CA, CA-3-G, and CA-4-G, and 37.5, 625, and 4000 ng/mL for FA.

The recoveries of each analyte were determined by comparing the mean peak areas of the extract of analyte-spiked plasma with those of the analytes spiked post-extraction into six different blank plasma extracts at three concentration levels.

2.6. Pharmacokinetic Study of YRA-1909 in Rats

This validated method was applied to the pharmacokinetic study of CGA, NCGA, CCGA, and their metabolites, such as CA, CA-3-G, CA-4-G, and FA after a single oral administration of YRA-1909 at doses of 25 (n = 6), 50 (n = 12), and 100 mg/kg (n = 6) and repeated oral administration of 50 mg/kg YRA-1909 for seven days (n = 6) to male Sprague-Dawley (SD) rats (body weight, 220–260 g, Samtako Co., Osan, Korea). The effective oral doses of YRA-1909 on preclinical pharmacology studies were 25–100 mg/kg in rats (internal reports of YUNGJIN PHARM CO., LTD). The study protocol was approved by the Institutional Animal Care and Use Committee of The Catholic University of Korea (Approval No. 2015–015). The animals were kept in plastic cages with unlimited access to standard rat diet (Samtako Co.) and water before the experiment. Animals were maintained at a temperature of 23 ± 2 °C with a 12 h light/dark cycle and relative humidity of $50 \pm 10\%$. The rats were anesthetized while using isoflurane and they were cannulated with polyethylene tubing (PE-50, Nastsume Co., Tokyo, Japan) in the jugular vein for blood sampling. Each rat was housed individually in a metabolic cage and permitted a recovery time of one day following anesthesia prior to the study's commencement. During the recovery period, rats were fasted but let free access to water and were not restrained at any time. To prevent blood clotting, each catheter was flushed with heparin in a physiological saline solution (10 U/mL). YRA-1909 was dissolved in purified water and administered to the rats at doses of 25, 50, and 100 mg/kg (equivalent to 1.2, 2.4, and 4.8 mg/kg CGA; 0.275, 0.55, and 1.10 mg/kg NCGA; 0.87, 1.74, and 3.48 mg/kg CCGA). Blood samples (approximately 200 µL) were collected before (control) and 0.083, 0.25, 0.5, 1, 1.5, 2, 3, 4, 6, 8, and 24 h after drug administration. Plasma samples were harvested by centrifugation at 3000 g for 5 min at 4 °C and 50 µL plasma samples were immediately collected and vortex-mixed with 5 µL 5% formic acid. The samples were stored at −80 °C until analyses.

Pharmacokinetic parameters were analyzed while using noncompartment analysis (WinNonlin, Pharsight, Mountain View, CA, USA), including the area under the plasma concentration-time curve during the period of observation (AUC_{last}), the terminal half-life ($t_{1/2}$), and mean residence time (MRT). The peak plasma concentration (C_{max}) and the time to reach C_{max} (T_{max}) were directly obtained from the experimental data. All data are expressed as the means $\pm$ standard deviations (S.D.).

3. Results

3.1. LC-MS/MS Analysis

For the simultaneous quantification of CGA, NCGA, CCGA, CA, CA-3-G, CA-4-G, and FA, MS/MS parameters for all analytes were optimized by the flow-injection method to achieve maximum sensitivity, and SRM transitions of the precursor ion ($[M - H]^-$) to the intense product ion were used for data acquisition owing to the high selectivity and sensitivity (Figure 2) [24,28–31].

The retention and base-line separation data are shown in Figure 3B. Analysis of blank plasma samples that were obtained from 30 different rats revealed no significant interference peaks in the retention times across all analytes, which indicates the selectivity of the present method (Figure 3A). Figure 3C illustrates representative SRM chromatograms of a plasma sample obtained 5 min after oral administration of YRA-1909 at a 100 mg/kg dosage in a male SD rat.

3.2. Method Validation

Calibration curves were linear at concentration ranges of 0.5–200 ng/mL for CGA and NCGA, 12.5–5000 ng/mL for FA, and 2.5–1000 ng/mL for CCGA, CA, CA-3-G, and CA-4-G in rat plasma with coefficients of determination ≥ 0.9959 using linear regression analysis with a weighting of

1/concentration (Table 1). The RE and CV values of the calculated concentrations were less than ±15% and 15%, respectively, for all eight calibration points. The low CV values (≤12.2%) for the regression line slopes of the seven analytes indicated the repeatability of the method.

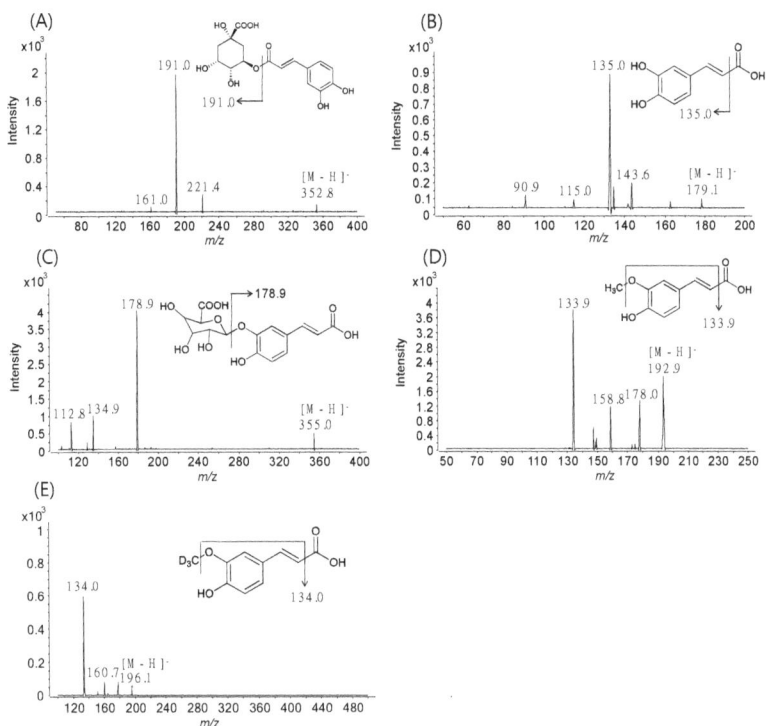

Figure 2. Product ion spectra of (**A**) chlorogenic acid (CGA), (**B**) caffeic acid (CA), (**C**) CA-3-G, (**D**) ferulic acid (FA), and (**E**) FA-d₃ (IS).

The lower limits of quantification (LLOQ), the lowest amounts of the analytes in rat plasma sample that can be quantified with S/N ratio >5 as well as both CV and RE within 20% of nominal concentration, were 0.5 ng/mL for CGA and NCGA, 12.5 ng/mL for FA, and 2.5 ng/mL for CCGA, CA, CA-3-G, and CA-4-G in rat plasma (Table 1).

The intra-day and inter-day precision and accuracy values for QC samples are presented in Table 1. The CV values of the seven analytes ranged from 2.4% to 12.5% at low, medium, and high QC levels and from 4.1% to 18.1% at LLOQ QC levels. The RE values ranged from −10.0% to 10.4% at low, medium, and high QC levels and from −8.8% to 16.0% at LLOQ QC levels. These results confirm the method's acceptable accuracy and precision levels.

A protein precipitation technique while using acetonitrile and methanol was examined as the sample preparation procedure for rat plasma but it was inadequate due to severe matrix effects. The recovery and matrix effects of all analytes in rat plasma were evaluated by extracting acidified rat plasma with ethyl acetate [25], ethyl acetate/ether [24], ethyl acetate/hexane [26], and methyl *ter*-butyl ether. Liquid–liquid extraction using ethyl acetate as the extraction solvent resulted in a higher degree of recovery and fewer matrix effects for all analytes (Table 2): the matrix effects and CV values were 86.5–98.0% and ≤11.8%, respectively. The recovery levels using liquid–liquid extraction at low, medium, and high QC levels are shown in Table 2. Based on the results, liquid–liquid extraction using ethyl acetate after acidification of rat plasma is deemed to be acceptable for the sample preparation procedure.

The processing (freeze-thaw, long-term storage at −80°C, and short-term storage on ice) and post-preparation stabilities of each analyte were evaluated; such processes had negligible effects on the stability of samples (Table 3).

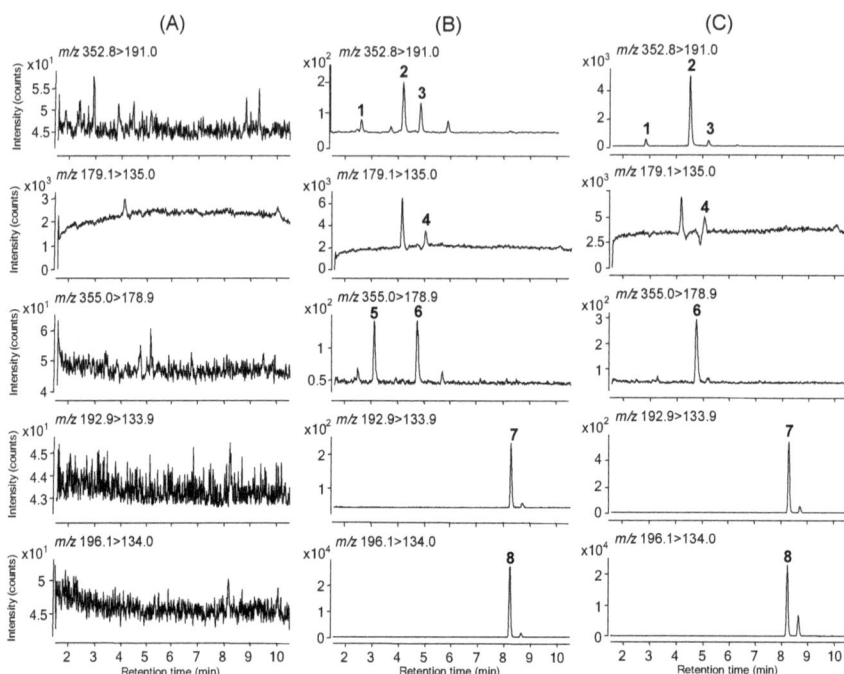

Figure 3. Selected reaction monitoring chromatograms of (**A**) rat blank plasma, (**B**) rat plasma spiked with CGA (0.5 ng/mL), NCGA (0.5 ng/mL), CCGA (2.5 ng/mL), CA (2.5 ng/mL), CA-3-G (2.5 ng/mL), CA-4-G (2.5 ng/mL), and FA (12.5 ng/mL) at lower limits of quantification (LLOQ) level, and (**C**) rat plasma obtained 5 min after oral administration of YRA-1909 at a dose of 100 mg/kg to a male SD rat. 1, NCGA; 2, CGA; 3, CCGA; 4, CA; 5, CA-4-G; 6, CA-3-G; 7, FA; 8, FA-d3.

Table 1. Linearity, LLOQ, intra-day and inter-day accuracy (RE, %) and precision (CV, %) of CGA, NCGA, CCGA, CA, CA-3-G, CA-4-G, and FA in rat plasma quality control (QC) samples.

Analytes	Concentration Range (ng/mL), Linear Equation [a], Linearity (r^2) [b], LLOQ (ng/mL)	QC Concentration (ng/mL)	Intra-day ($n = 5$)		Inter-day ($n = 15$)	
			RE (%)	CV (%)	RE (%)	CV (%)
CGA	0.5–200 $y = 0.01110x − 0.00054$ 0.9981 0.5	0.5	12.0	8.9	2.0	11.8
		1.5	−6.7	6.4	−4.7	11.2
		25	2.0	3.7	−1.9	10.5
		160	10.2	2.4	0.1	11.8
NCGA	0.5–200 $y = 0.00330x − 0.00039$ 0.9983 0.5	0.5	−2.0	4.1	−2.0	8.2
		1.5	−10.0	3.0	−1.3	10.1
		25	0.7	3.1	2.8	8.0
		160	10.4	2.0	2.0	12.5

Table 1. *Cont.*

Analytes	Concentration Range (ng/mL), Linear Equation [a], Linearity (r^2) [b], LLOQ (ng/mL)	QC Concentration (ng/mL)	Intra-day ($n = 5$)		Inter-day ($n = 15$)	
			RE (%)	CV (%)	RE (%)	CV (%)
CCGA	2.5–1000 $y = 0.00149x - 0.00068$ 0.9974 2.5	2.5 7.5 125 800	16.0 -6.3 3.0 -4.4	7.2 4.8 4.2 3.2	3.6 -3.9 2.8 -1.9	11.6 6.7 5.6 8.3
CA	2.5–1000 $y = 0.03784x - 0.00235$ 0.9959 2.5	2.5 7.5 125 800	-8.8 -3.9 6.5 4.1	7.9 8.3 5.0 5.8	-2.8 -2.8 6.5 0.9	18.1 8.6 6.2 9.2
CA-3-G	2.5–1000 $y = 0.00174x + 0.00022$ 0.9981 2.5	2.5 7.5 125 800	0.8 -8.3 4.3 8.8	7.1 4.2 2.4 5.1	-0.4 -5.9 2.4 0.9	8.0 9.6 6.2 10.4
CA-4-G	2.5–1000 $y = 0.00140x + 0.00031$ 0.9977 2.5	2.5 7.5 125 800	-6.8 -7.2 10.0 7.7	10.7 7.0 3.5 4.7	-5.2 0.3 6.7 1.2	9.3 11.6 6.4 9.6
FA	12.5–5000 $y = 0.00628x - 0.02194$ 0.9969 12.5	12.5 37.5 625 4000	12.6 -3.2 -3.0 4.8	8.5 7.2 3.8 3.9	9.0 -6.5 -7.4 -0.1	7.7 7.7 6.0 9.6

[a] y: peak area ratio, x: concentration; [b] r^2: coefficients of determination.

Table 2. Matrix effects and recoveries of CGA, NCGA, CCGA, CA, CA-3-G, CA-4-G, FA, and FA-d3 (IS) using six different rat plasma ($n = 6$).

Compounds	Nominal Concentration (ng/mL)	Matrix Effect [a] (%)		Recovery [b] (Mean ± SD, %)
		Mean	CV (%)	
CGA	1.5 25 160	91.6 92.0 87.1	7.6 11.0 5.4	63.0 ± 6.3 71.7 ± 6.9 71.9 ± 9.4
NCGA	1.5 25 160	96.1 90.8 89.0	3.6 3.2 7.1	41.4 ± 4.0 43.4 ± 3.7 41.8 ± 1.4
CCGA	7.5 125 800	98.0 92.4 89.3	6.6 2.2 6.2	61.5 ± 5.2 63.0 ± 7.8 65.2 ± 5.7
CA	7.5 125 800	87.7 93.0 88.6	7.2 11.8 6.2	94.0 ± 9.9 86.1 ± 10.4 91.2 ± 6.3
CA-3-G	7.5 125 800	95.9 95.8 88.5	2.0 7.4 8.5	46.5 ± 4.3 51.2 ± 3.4 52.8 ± 4.2
CA-4-G	7.5 125 800	92.7 95.6 86.5	1.7 5.3 9.7	51.3 ± 6.0 53.0 ± 3.4 55.8 ± 4.2
FA	37.5 625 4000	96.8 87.5 97.5	2.2 8.4 8.6	93.3 ± 8.7 96.9 ± 8.7 97.4 ± 4.2
FA-d3	20	96.0	5.4	100.1 ± 2.0

[a] Matrix effect expressed as the ratio of the mean peak area of an analyte spiked post-extraction to the mean peak area of same analyte standards multiplied by 100. [b] Recovery calculated as the ratio of the mean peak area of an analyte–spiked plasma prior to liquid–liquid extraction to the mean peak of an analyte spiked after liquid-liquid extraction of blank plasma multiplied by 100.

Table 3. Post-preparation, short-term, long-term and freeze-thaw stabilities of CGA, NCGA, CCGA, CA, CA-3-G, CA-4-G, and FA in rat plasma quality control samples (*n* = 3).

Analytes and Nominal Concentration (ng/mL)	Post-Preparative (24 h at 4 °C)		Short-Term (2 h on ice)		Long-Term (28 days at −80 °C)		Freeze-Thaw 3 Cycles (−80 °C to room temp.)	
	CV, %	RE, %	CV, %	RE, %	CV, %	RE, %	CV, %	RE, %
CGA								
1.5	8.8	−9.3	2.3	−12.0	7.0	−14.0	6.2	−14.0
160	2.1	9.4	2.5	−5.4	4.1	−12.3	3.2	−10.0
NCGA								
1.5	14.4	−2.7	2.3	−12.0	3.7	−9.3	10.1	−14.0
160	2.7	11.2	4.2	−5.9	5.6	−6.3	5.9	−5.3
CCGA								
7.5	5.1	−3.2	3.7	−14.3	5.9	−8.9	7.6	−11.9
800	1.3	5.5	2.9	−4.6	4.4	−14.4	3.0	−9.4
CA								
7.5	4.1	−0.1	9.0	−12.4	7.3	−6.3	8.3	−7.2
800	0.9	10.6	2.1	−7.7	7.6	−12.7	2.1	−11.0
CA-3-G								
7.5	9.9	−10.0	6.1	−14.6	7.3	−7.1	9.1	−10.5
800	1.1	9.1	2.8	−1.5	2.2	−14.8	4.4	−11.9
CA-4-G								
7.5	6.2	−9.6	8.1	−9.3	7.9	1.6	4.7	−3.6
800	1.0	10.9	3.2	−0.4	2.1	−13.9	4.7	−9.4
FA								
37.5	3.2	−7.0	5.4	−11.2	5.9	−11.0	5.6	−7.7
4000	4.6	−8.6	2.7	−4.8	6.1	−8.8	3.9	−8.4

3.3. Pharmacokinetics of YRA-1909 in Male SD Rats

Mean plasma concentration-time profiles of CGA, NCGA, CCGA, CA, CA-3-G, and CA-4-G following a single oral administration of YRA-1909 at doses of 25, 50, and 100 mg/kg to male SD rats are shown in Figure 4. Plasma concentrations of CGA, NCGA, CA, CA-3-G, and CA-4-G were below LLOQ 6, 4, 4, 4, and 4 h after oral administration of YRA-1909 at a dosage of 100 mg/kg. Plasma concentrations of CCGA were under LLOQ (2.5 ng/mL) following 25 mg/kg dose (equivalent to 0.87 mg/kg CCGA), and 1 and 3 h after administration of 50 and 100 mg/kg doses of YRA-1909, respectively. Plasma concentrations of FA, which is a metabolite, were under LLOQ (12.5 ng/mL), except in samples taken 0.083 and/or 0.25 h after oral administration of 50 and 100 mg/kg YRA-1909. Therefore, the pharmacokinetic parameters of FA were not calculated. The relevant pharmacokinetic parameters of all other analytes are shown in Table 4.

No significant differences were observed among plasma concentrations and pharmacokinetic parameters of CGA, NCGA, CCGA, CA, CA-3-G, and CA-4-G between single and seven-day repeated administration of 50 mg/kg YRA-1909 (Figure 4, Table 4).

Table 4. Pharmacokinetic parameters of CGA, CCGA, NCGA, CA, CA-3-G, and CA-4-G after a single oral administration of YRA-1909 at doses of 25, 50, and 100 mg/kg (equivalent to 1.2, 2.4, and 4.8 mg/kg CGA; 0.275, 0.55, and 1.10 mg/kg NCGA; 0.87, 1.74 and 3.48 mg/kg CCGA) and repeated administration of 50 mg/kg YRA-1909 for seven days to male rats (mean ± SD).

| Compounds | PK Parameters | Dose of YRA-1909 (mg/kg) | | | |
| | | Single Oral Dosing | | | 7-Day Repeated Oral Dosing |
		25 (n = 6)	50 (n = 12)	100 (n = 6)	50 (n = 6)
CGA	C_{max} (ng/mL)	3.11 ± 0.96	5.59 ± 1.61	8.73 ± 2.83	4.85 ± 1.25
	T_{max} [1] (h)	0.25 (0.083–0.25)	0.25 (0.083–0.5)	0.25	0.25 (0.083–0.5)
	AUC_{last} (ng·h/mL)	4.29 ± 1.92	8.16 ± 3.65	14.38 ± 5.06	7.54 ± 1.86
	$t_{1/2}$ (h)	NC	NC	1.52 ± 0.79	NC
	MRT (h)	1.19 ± 0.22	1.48 ± 0.50	1.67 ± 0.63	1.48 ± 0.18
CCGA	C_{max} (ng/mL)	NC	4.01 ± 0.82	5.64 ± 1.45	3.81 ± 0.72
	T_{max} [1] (h)	NC	0.25 (0.083–0.5)	0.25 (0.083–0.25)	0.25 (0.083–0.5)
	AUC_{last} (ng·h/mL)	NC	4.15 ± 4.10	6.26 ± 4.70	3.35 ± 3.42
	MRT (h)	NC	0.61 ± 0.55	0.84 ± 0.65	0.56 ± 0.57
NCGA	C_{max} (ng/mL)	0.70 ± 0.12	1.18 ± 0.26	1.69 ± 0.43	1.08 ± 0.28
	T_{max} [1] (h)	0.17 (0.083–0.5)	0.25 (0.083–0.5)	0.25 (0.083–0.25)	0.25 (0.083–0.25)
	AUC_{last} (ng·h/mL)	0.81 ± 0.22	1.61 ± 0.90	3.40 ± 1.97	1.60 ± 0.79
	MRT (h)	0.68 ± 0.30	1.00 ± 0.58	1.66 ± 0.91	1.09 ± 0.55
CA	C_{max} (ng/mL)	3.92 ± 1.47	7.31 ± 2.12	16.72 ± 5.45	6.07 ± 0.94
	T_{max} [1] (h)	1.25 (1.0–1.5)	0.25 (0.083–1.0)	0.25 (0.25–2.0)	0.17 (0.083–2.0)
	AUC_{last} (ng·h/mL)	5.60 ± 1.30	12.40 ± 4.03	29.73 ± 15.24	11.75 ± 3.31
	MRT (h)	0.90 ± 0.11	1.29 ± 0.31	1.74 ± 0.87	1.26 ± 0.33
CA-3-G	C_{max} (ng/mL)	69.09 ± 25.06	129.05 ± 30.41	238.55 ± 97.46	132.18 ± 26.70
	T_{max} [1] (h)	0.38 (0.25–1.0)	0.38 (0.25–1.0)	0.25 (0.25–1.0)	0.38 (0.25–1.0)
	AUC_{last} (ng·h/mL)	111.15 ± 37.32	208.77 ± 80.46	405.33 ± 188.56	216.38 ± 25.06
	$t_{1/2}$ (h)	1.05 ± 0.38	0.93 ± 0.23	0.82 ± 0.23	0.88 ± 0.19
	MRT (h)	1.49 ± 0.52	1.33 ± 0.24	1.68 ± 0.69	1.33 ± 0.12
CA-4-G	C_{max} (ng/mL)	3.86 ± 0.94	6.97 ± 1.91	9.38 ± 2.56	7.77 ± 1.85
	T_{max} [1] (h)	1.0 (1.0–1.5)	0.75 (0.25–2.0)	1.0 (0.5–2.0)	1.5 (1.0–2.0)
	AUC_{last} (ng·h/mL)	6.04 ± 0.77	14.95 ± 4.03	25.59 ± 10.84	18.95 ± 3.30
	MRT (h)	1.01 ± 0.18	1.48 ± 0.27	1.77 ± 0.46	± 0.23

[1] T_{max} presented median value with the range in parentheses. NC: Not calculable.

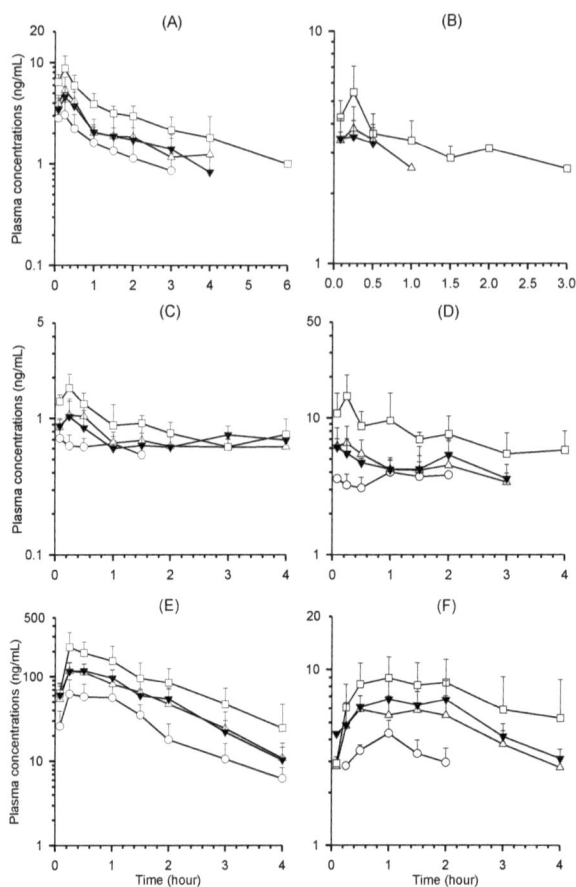

Figure 4. Mean plasma concentration-time profiles of (**A**) CGA, (**B**) CCGA, (**C**) neochlorogenic acid (NCGA), (**D**) CA, (**E**) CA-3-G, and (**F**) CA-4-G after a single oral administration of YRA-1909 at the doses of 25 ($\bigcirc$, n = 6), 50 ($\triangle$, n = 12), and 100 ($\square$, n = 6) mg/kg (equivalent to 1.2, 2.4, and 4.8 mg/kg CGA; 0.275, 0.55, and 1.10 mg/kg NCGA; 0.87, 1.74 and 3.48 mg/kg CCGA) and repeated administration of 50 mg/kg YRA-1909 once/day for seven days ($\blacktriangledown$, n = 6) in male rats. Each point represents mean ± SD.

4. Discussion

We developed a LC-MS/MS method for the simultaneous determination of CGA, NCGA, CCGA, and their metabolites, such as CA, CA-3-G, CA-4-G, and FA in rat plasma. A gradient elution of formic acid and methanol, as the mobile phase, resulted in less peak tailing and an increase in the ionization efficiency of the seven analytes, when compared to previously reported gradient elution of acetic acid-acetonitrile used as the mobile phase for the analyses of phenolic acids, sulfates, and glucuronides [31]. For sample preparation, liquid–liquid extraction using ethyl acetate at acidic pH resulted in smaller sample volume (50 vs. 100 μL), superior sensitivity (0.5 vs. 1.77 ng/mL for CGA and NCGA), and reduced matrix effects compared to the protein precipitation technique [31]. We successfully applied the present method to study pharmacokinetics of CGA, NCGA, CCGA, and their metabolites after oral administration of YRA-1909 (Figure 4, Table 4).

CGA, NCGA, and CCGA were rapidly absorbed after oral administration of YRA-1909 at doses of 25, 50, and 100 mg/kg; each was detected at the first blood sampling time point (5 min) with rapid T_{max},

0.17–0.25 h for all three doses (Table 4). The AUC_{last} values for CGA and NCGA increased linearly as the oral dose increased. The dose-normalized (based on 25 mg/kg YRA-1909) AUC_{last} of CGA and NCGA were comparable among the doses studied: 4.29 ± 1.92, 4.08 ± 1.82, and 3.60 ± 1.27 ng·h/mL for CGA, respectively, and 0.81 ± 0.22, 0.81 ± 0.45, and 0.85 ± 0.49 ng·h/mL for NCGA in 25, 50, and 100 mg/kg YRA-1909, respectively. Moreover, the slopes between the log AUC_{last} and log dose of CGA and NCGA were close to 1. Plasma concentrations of CCGA were less than LLOQ (2.5 ng/mL) in the group that was administered a 25 mg/kg dose of YRA-1909, but the dose-normalized (based on 50 mg/kg YRA-1909) AUC_{last} values of CCGA were also comparable: 4.15 ± 4.10 and 3.13 ± 2.35 ng·h/mL for 50 and 100 mg/kg YRA-1909, respectively.

CGA, NCGA, and CCGA were absorbed by passive diffusion and hydrolyzed to CA by gastric esterase, and then, CA was metabolized to ferulic acid by COMT [13]. The bioavailability and urinary recovery of CGA or CA were very low after oral administration of CGA or CA in rats due to extensive metabolism [14,15,31]. After oral administration of YRA-1909 at doses of 25, 50, and 100 mg/kg, CA, CA-3-G, CA-4-G, and FA, which were reported as the major metabolites of CGA, CCGA, and NCGA (Figure 1) [12–15], were determined in plasma that was obtained after oral administration of YRA-1909 (Figure 3, Table 4). AUC_{last} and C_{max} values of CA, CA-3-G, and CA-4-G linearly increased with an increase in YRA-1909 dose (Figure 4, Table 4). For CA, dose-normalized (based on 25 mg/kg YRA-1909) AUC_{last} values were 5.60 ± 1.30, 6.20 ± 2.01, and 7.43 ± 3.81 ng·h/mL for 25, 50, and 100 mg/kg YRA-1909, respectively. CA-3-G and CA-4-G were formed from CA, as shown in Figure 1 [12–16] and their dose-normalized (based on 25 mg/kg YRA-1909) AUC_{last} values were 111.15 ± 37.32, 104.39 ± 40.23, and 101.33 ± 47.14 ng·h/mL for CA-3-G and 6.04 ± 0.77, 7.47 ± 2.02, and 6.40 ± 2.71 ng·h/mL for CA-4-G, respectively. AUC_{last} and C_{max} values of CA-3-G were higher than those for CA and CA-4-G, which suggests that CA-3-G may be a major metabolite after oral administration of YRA-1909. FA, which was formed via methylation of CA [12–15], was detected 0.083 or 0.25 h after oral administration of YRA-1909. After oral administration of YRA-1909, the AUC_{last} values of the metabolites, CA, CA-3-G, and CA-4-G were higher than those of CGA, CCGA, and NCGA due to extensive metabolism, which were similar to the metabolism of CGA, CCGA, and NCGA in humans and rats [12,14,15].

Repeated administration of YRA-1909 at 50 mg/kg for seven days to male SD rats did not affect the plasma concentrations and pharmacokinetic parameters of any compounds when compared to those that received single administrations (Figure 4, Table 4).

5. Conclusions

A selective and sensitive LC-MS/MS method using liquid–liquid extraction as sample clean-up procedure was developed and validated for the simultaneous determination of CGA, CCGA, NCGA, and their metabolites, such as CA, CA-3-G, CA-4-G, and FA in rat plasma. The method was successfully applied to characterize the pharmacokinetics of CGA, CCGA, NCGA, CA, CA-3-G, CA-4-G, and FA after oral administration of YRA-1909 at 25, 50, and 100 mg/kg doses to male SD rats. These results constitute useful information for the development of YRA-1909 as a new herbal medicine for the treatment of rheumatoid arthritis, based on the evaluation of the pharmacokinetic properties of its main components (i.e., CGA, CCGA, and NCGA) and their active metabolites (CA, CA-3-G, and CA-4-G).

Author Contributions: Conceptualization, H.S.L. Y.L., J.S.Y, and D.H.S.; Methodology, W.G.C., J.H.K., K.D.K., and H.S.L.; Validation, W.G.C., J.H.K Y.L., and J.S.Y.; Formal Analysis, W.G.C., J.H.K., D.K.K., and H.S.L.; Investigation, W.G.C., J.H.K. and H.S.L.; Resources, W.G.C., J.H.K, Y.L., and J.S.Y.; Data Curation, W.G.C., J.H.K. and H.S.L.; Writing-Original Draft Preparation, W.G.C., J.H.K., and D.K.K.; Writing-Review & Editing, H.S.L. Y.L., J.S.Y., and D.H.S.; Visualization, W.G.C., J.H.K. and H.S.L; Supervision, H.S.L.; Project Administration, H.S.L.; Funding Acquisition, H.S.L.

Funding: This research was supported by the Technology Innovation Program (10051145) funded by the Ministry of Trade, Industry & Energy (MOTIE, Korea).

Conflicts of Interest: The authors declare no conflict of interest.

References

1. Wang, H.-B.; Mayer, R.; Rücker, G.; Yang, J.-J.; Matteson, D.S. A phenolic glycoside and triterpenoids from *Stauntonia hexaphylla*. *Phytochemistry* **1998**, *47*, 467–470. [CrossRef]
2. Park, Y.J.; Park, Y.S.; Towantakavanit, K.; Park, J.O.; Kim, Y.M.; Jung, K.J.; Cho, J.Y.; Lee, K.D.; Heo, B.G. Chemical components and biological activity of *Stauntonia hexaphylla*. *Korean J. Plant. Resour.* **2009**, *22*, 403–411.
3. Cheon, Y.H.; Baek, J.M.; Park, S.H.; Ahn, S.J.; Lee, M.S.; Oh, J.; Kim, J.Y. *Stauntonia hexaphylla* (Lardizabalaceae) leaf methanol extract inhibits osteoclastogenesis and bone resorption activity via proteasome-mediated degradation of c-Fos protein and suppression of NFATc1 expression. *BMC Complement. Altern. Med.* **2015**, *15*, 280. [CrossRef] [PubMed]
4. Hwang, S.H.; Kwon, S.H.; Kim, S.B.; Lim, S.S. Inhibitory activities of *Stauntonia hexaphylla* leaf constituents on rat lens aldose reductase and formation of advanced glycation end products and antioxidant. *Biomed. Res. Int.* **2017**, *2017*, 4273257. [CrossRef] [PubMed]
5. Kim, J.; Kim, H.; Choi, H.; Jo, A.; Kang, H.; Yun, H.; Im, S.; Choi, C. Anti-inflammatory effects of a *Stauntonia hexaphylla* Fruit Extract in lipopolysaccharide-activated RAW-264.7 macrophages and rats by carrageenan-induced hind paw swelling. *Nutrients* **2018**, *10*, E110. [CrossRef] [PubMed]
6. Yoo, H.J.; Kim, J.Y.; Kang, S.E.; Yoo, J.S.; Lee, Y.; Lee, D.G.; Park, J.S.; Lee, E.B.; Lee, E.Y.; Song, Y.W. YRA-1909 suppresses production of pro-inflammatory mediators and MMPs through downregulating Akt, p38, JNK and NF-κb activation in rheumatoid arthritis fibroblast-like synoviocytes. In Proceedings of the 81st American College of Rheumatology and the 52nd Association of Rheumatology Health Professionals Annual Scientific Meeting, San Diego, CA, USA, 6 November 2017; Abstract Number, 1412.
7. A Phase 2 Study to Evaluate the Safety and Efficacy of YRA-1909 in Patients with Rheumatoid Arthritis. Available online: https://clinicaltrials.gov/ct2/archive/NCT03275025 (accessed on 7 November 2017).
8. Sato, Y.; Itagaki, S.; Kurokawa, T.; Ogura, J.; Kobayashi, M.; Hirano, T.; Sugawara, M.; Lseki, K. In vitro and in vivo antioxidant properties of chlorogenic acid and caffeic acid. *Int. J. Pharm.* **2011**, *403*, 136–138. [CrossRef] [PubMed]
9. Kurata, R.; Adachi, M.; Yamakawa, O.; Yoshimoto, M. Growth suppression of human cancer cells by polyphenolics from sweetpotato (*Ipomoea batatas* L.) leaves. *J. Agric. Food Chem.* **2007**, *55*, 185–190. [CrossRef] [PubMed]
10. Ooi, L.S.; Wang, H.; He, Z.; Ooi, V.E. Antiviral activities of purified compounds from *Youngia japonica* (L.) DC (Asteraceae, Compositae). *J. Ethnopharmacol.* **2006**, *106*, 187–191. [CrossRef] [PubMed]
11. Choi, J.H.; Kim, S. Investigation of the anticoagulant and antithrombotic effects of chlorogenic acid. *J. Biochem. Mol. Toxicol.* **2017**, *31*, e21865. [CrossRef] [PubMed]
12. Del Rio, D.; Stalmach, A.; Calani, L.; Crozier, A. Bioavailability of coffee chlorogenic acids and green tea flavan-3-ols. *Nutrients* **2010**, *2*, 820–833. [CrossRef] [PubMed]
13. Farrell, T.L.; Dew, T.P.; Poquet, L.; Hanson, P.; Williamson, G. Absorption and metabolism of chlorogenic acids in cultured gastric epithelial monolayers. *Drug Metab. Dispos.* **2011**, *39*, 2338–2346. [CrossRef] [PubMed]
14. Omar, M.H.; Mullen, W.; Stalmach, A.; Auger, C.; Rouanet, J.M.; Teissedre, P.L.; Caldwell, S.T.; Hartley, R.C.; Crozier, A. Absorption, disposition, metabolism, and excretion of [3-(14)C] caffeic acid in rats. *J. Agric. Food Chem.* **2012**, *60*, 5205–5214. [CrossRef] [PubMed]
15. Azuma, K.; Ippoushi, K.; Nakayama, M.; Ito, H.; Higashio, H.; Terao, J. Absorption of chlorogenic acid and caffeic acid in rats after oral administration. *J. Agric. Food Chem.* **2000**, *48*, 5496–5500. [CrossRef] [PubMed]
16. Wong, C.C.; Meinl, W.; Glatt, H.R.; Barron, D.; Stalmach, A.; Steiling, H.; Crozier, A.; Williamson, G. In vitro and in vivo conjugation of dietary hydroxycinnamic acids by UDP-glucuronosyltransferases and sulfotransferases in humans. *J. Nutr. Biochem.* **2010**, *21*, 1060–1068. [CrossRef] [PubMed]
17. Piazzon, A.; Vrhovsek, U.; Masuero, D.; Mattivi, F.; Mandoj, F.; Nardini, M. Antioxidant activity of phenolic acids and their metabolites: synthesis and antioxidant properties of the sulfate derivatives of ferulic and caffeic acids and of the acyl glucuronide of ferulic acid. *J. Agric. Food Chem.* **2012**, *60*, 12312–12323. [CrossRef] [PubMed]
18. Yamada, J.; Tomita, Y. Antimutagenic activity of caffeic acid and related compounds. *Biosci. Biotech. Biochem.* **1996**, *60*, 328–329. [CrossRef] [PubMed]

19. Guo, D.; Dou, D.; Ge, L.; Huang, Z.; Wang, L.; Gu, N. A caffeic acid mediated facile synthesis of silver nanoparticles with powerful anti-cancer activity. *Colloids Surf. B Biointerfaces* **2015**, *134*, 229–234. [CrossRef] [PubMed]

20. Yang, G.W.; Jiang, J.S.; Lu, W.Q. Ferulic acid exerts anti-angiogenic and anti-tumor activity by targeting fibroblast growth factor receptor 1-mediated angiogenesis. *Int. J. Mol. Sci.* **2015**, *16*, 24011–24031. [CrossRef] [PubMed]

21. Shi, P.; Lin, X.; Yao, H. A comprehensive review of recent studies on pharmacokinetics of traditional Chinese medicines (2014–2017) and perspectives. *Drug Metab. Rev.* **2018**, *50*, 161–192. [CrossRef] [PubMed]

22. Li, Y.; Wang, Y.; Tai, W.; Yang, L.; Chen, Y.; Chen, C.; Liu, C. Challenges and solutions of pharmacokinetics for efficacy and safety of traditional chinese medicine. *Curr. Drug Metab.* **2015**, *16*, 765–776. [CrossRef] [PubMed]

23. Jeong, J.H.; Kim, D.K.; Ji, H.Y.; Oh, S.R.; Lee, H.K.; Lee, H.S. Liquid chromatography-atmospheric pressure chemical ionization tandem mass spectrometry for the simultaneous determination of dimethoxyaschantin, dimethylliroresinol, dimethylpinoresinol, epimagnolin A, fargesin and magnolin in rat plasma. *Biomed. Chromatogr.* **2011**, *25*, 879–889. [CrossRef] [PubMed]

24. Wang, X.; Ma, X.; Li, W.; Chu, Y.; Guo, J.; Li, S.; Wang, J.; Zhang, H.; Zhou, S.; Zhu, Y. Simultaneous determination of five phenolic components and paeoniflorin in rat plasma by liquid chromatography-tandem mass spectrometry and pharmacokinetic study after oral administration of Cerebralcare granule. *J. Pharm. Biomed. Anal.* **2013**, *86*, 82–91. [CrossRef] [PubMed]

25. Zhou, W.; Liu, S.; Ju, W.; Shan, J.; Meng, M.; Cai, B.; Di, L. Simultaneous determination of phenolic acids by UPLC-MS/MS in rat plasma and its application in pharmacokinetic study after oral administration of Flos Lonicerae preparations. *J. Pharm. Biomed. Anal.* **2013**, *86*, 189–197. [CrossRef] [PubMed]

26. De Oliveira, D.M.; Pinto, C.B.; Sampaio, G.R.; Yonekura, L.; Catharino, R.R.; Bastos, D.H. Development and validation of methods for the extraction of phenolic acids from plasma, urine, and liver and analysis by UPLC-MS. *J. Agric. Food Chem.* **2013**, *61*, 6113–6121. [CrossRef] [PubMed]

27. Zhou, W.; Shan, J.; Wang, S.; Ju, W.; Meng, M.; Cai, B.; Di, L. Simultaneous determination of caffeic acid derivatives by UPLC-MS/MS in rat plasma and its application in pharmacokinetic study after oral administration of Flos Lonicerae-Fructus Forsythiae herb combination. *J. Chromatogr. B* **2014**, *949–950*, 7–15. [CrossRef] [PubMed]

28. Zeng, L.; Wang, M.; Yuan, Y.; Guo, B.; Zhou, J.; Tan, Z.; Ye, M.; Ding, L.; Chen, B. Simultaneous multi-component quantitation of Chinese herbal injection Yin-zhi-huang in rat plasma by using a single-tube extraction procedure for mass spectrometry-based pharmacokinetic measurement. *J. Chromatogr B* **2014**, *967*, 245–254. [CrossRef] [PubMed]

29. Marmet, C.; Actis-Goretta, L.; Renouf, M.; Giuffrida, F. Quantification of phenolic acids and their methylates, glucuronides, sulfates and lactones metabolites in human plasma by LC-MS/MS after oral ingestion of soluble coffee. *J. Pharm. Biomed. Anal.* **2014**, *88*, 617–625. [CrossRef] [PubMed]

30. Wang, X.; Li, W.; Ma, X.; Chu, Y.; Li, S.; Guo, J.; Jia, Y.; Zhou, S.; Zhu, Y.; Liu, C. Simultaneous determination of caffeic acid and its major pharmacologically active metabolites in rat plasma by LC-MS/MS and its application in pharmacokinetic study. *Biomed. Chromatogr.* **2015**, *29*, 552–559. [CrossRef] [PubMed]

31. Chang, Y.X.; Ge, A.H.; Yu, X.A.; Jiao, X.C.; Li, J.; He, J.; Tian, J.; Liu, W.; Azietaku, J.T.; Zhang, B.L.; et al. Simultaneous determination of four phenolic acids and seven alkaloids in rat plasma after oral administration of traditional Chinese medicinal preparation Jinqi Jiangtang Tablet by LC-ESI-MS/MS. *J. Pharm. Biomed. Anal.* **2016**, *117*, 1–10. [CrossRef] [PubMed]

32. Jung, J.W.; Kim, J.M.; Jeong, J.S.; Son, M.; Lee, H.S.; Lee, M.G.; Kang, H.E. Pharmacokinetics of chlorogenic acid and corydaline in DA-9701, a new botanical gastroprokinetic agent, in rats. *Xenobiotica* **2014**, *44*, 635–643. [CrossRef] [PubMed]

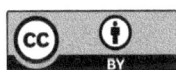

pharmaceutics

MDPI

Article

Characterization of CYPs and UGTs Involved in Human Liver Microsomal Metabolism of Osthenol

Pil Joung Cho [1], Sanjita Paudel [1], Doohyun Lee [1], Yun Ji Jin [1], GeunHyung Jo [1], Tae Cheon Jeong [2], Sangkyu Lee [1,*] and Taeho Lee [1,*]

[1] BK21 Plus KNU Multi-Omics-based Creative Drug Research Team, College of Pharmacy, Research Institute of Pharmaceutical Sciences, Kyungpook National University, Daegu 41566, Korea; whvlfwjd@naver.com (P.J.C.); sanjitapdl99@gmail.com (S.P.); newkiy@hanmail.net (D.L.); yundzzang@naver.com (Y.J.J.); cgh0605@naver.com (G.J.)

[2] College of Pharmacy, Yeungnam University, Gyeongsan 38541, Korea; taecheon@ynu.ac.kr

* Correspondence: sangkyu@knu.ac.kr (S.L.); tlee@knu.ac.kr (T.L.); Tel.: +82-53-950-8571 (S.L.); +82-53-950-8573 (T.L.); Fax: +82-53-950-8557 (S.L. & T.L.)

Received: 11 July 2018; Accepted: 27 August 2018; Published: 30 August 2018

Abstract: Osthenol is a prenylated coumarin isolated from the root of *Angelica koreana* and *Angelica dahurica*, and is an *O*-demethylated metabolite of osthole in vivo. Its various pharmacological effects have been reported previously. The metabolic pathway of osthenol was partially confirmed in rat osthole studies, and 11 metabolic products were identified in rat urine. However, the metabolic pathway of osthenol in human liver microsomes (HLM) has not been reported. In this study, we elucidated the structure of generated metabolites using a high-resolution quadrupole-orbitrap mass spectrometer (HR-MS/MS) and characterized the major human cytochrome P450 (CYP) and uridine 5′-diphospho-glucuronosyltransferase (UGT) isozymes involved in osthenol metabolism in human liver microsomes (HLMs). We identified seven metabolites (M1-M7) in HLMs after incubation in the presence of nicotinamide adenine dinucleotide phosphate (NADPH) and uridine 5′-diphosphoglucuronic acid (UDPGA). As a result, we demonstrated that osthenol is metabolized to five mono-hydroxyl metabolites (M1-M5) by CYP2D6, 1A2, and 3A4, respectively, a 7-*O*-glucuronide conjugate (M6) by UGT1A9, and a hydroxyl-glucuronide (M7) from M5 by UGT1A3 in HLMs. We also found that glucuronidation is the dominant metabolic pathway of osthenol in HLMs.

Keywords: Osthenol; CYP; UGT; human liver microsomes; glucuronidation

1. Introduction

Osthenol (7-hydroxy-8-(3-methyl-2-butenyl)-2H-1-benzopyran-2-one, Figure 1a) is a prenylated coumarin isolated from the root of *Angelica koreana* and *Angelica dahurica* [1,2]. Its intermediate is a C8-prenylated derivative of umbelliferone, which is converted to an angelicin by angelicin and columbianetin synthase in the furanocoumarin biosynthetic pathway [3]. In previous studies, osthenol has shown anti-tumor, anti-fungal, anti-bacterial, and anti-inflammatory pharmacological effects. Osthenol showed the most potent inhibitory activity with only weak cytotoxicity on Raji cells, and mouse skin tumor promotion [4]. In addition, osthenol has strong antibacterial and antifungal activities against Gram-positive bacteria, as well as *Candida albicans* and *Aspergillus fumigatus* [5,6]. For anti-inflammatory effects, osthenol was shown to inhibit 5-lipoxygenase and cyclooxygenase in vitro [7].

The diverse pharmacological effects of osthenol have been reported, and it was assumed that osthenol, as the major metabolite of osthole (osthol, 7-methoxy-8-(3-methyl-2-butenyl)-2H-1-benzopyran-2-one, Figure 1b) in vivo, was involved in physiological effects of osthole, a natural coumarin found in the traditional herb Cnidii Fructus [8,9]. Osthole can convert to osthenol by

O-demethylation, which was identified as phase I and phase II metabolites in rat urine after 40 mg/kg of osthole oral administration [10]. Nevertheless, the metabolic pathway of osthenol in humans still remains unclear. The aim of the present study was to investigate the metabolism of osthenol in human liver microsomes. We elucidated the structure of the generated metabolites using a high-resolution quadrupole-orbitrap mass spectrometer (HR-MS/MS) and characterized the major human cytochrome P450 (CYP) and UDP-glucuronosyltransferase (UGT) isozymes involved in osthenol metabolism.

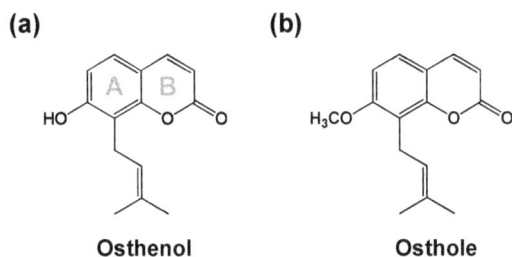

Figure 1. Chemical structures of osthenol (a) and osthole (b).

2. Materials and Methods

2.1. Materials

Osthenol (purity > 99%) was synthesized from 8-allyl-7-hydroxy-2H-chromen-2-one [11]. Pooled human liver microsomes (HLMs, UltraPool^{TM} HLM 50$^{®}$), human recombinant cDNA-expressed CYP isoforms, and cDNA-expressed UDP-glucuronosyltransferase (UGT, Supersomes^{TM}) were obtained from Corning Gentest (Woburn, MA, USA). Glucose 6-phosphate, glucose 6-phosphate dehydrogenase, uridine 5′-diphosphoglucuronic acid (UDPGA), β-glucuronidase, alamethicin, and 1,4-saccharolactone were purchased from Sigma-Aldrich (St. Louis, MO, USA). β-Nicotinamide adenine dinucleotide phosphate reduced form (β-NADPH) was purchased from Oriental Yeast Co. (Tokyo, Japan). All other chemicals were of analytical grade and used as received.

2.2. Identification of Osthenol Metabolites in Human Liver Microsomes

For Phase I metabolism, 20 μM osthenol was combined with 1 mg/mL pooled HLMs at 37 °C for 60 min with reduced nicotinamide adenine dinucleotide phosphate (β-NADPH)-regenerating system (NGS) in a 200 μL reaction volume in the presence of 0.1 M potassium phosphate buffer (Kpi, pH 7.4). To identify Phase II metabolites, 1 mg/mL HLM was treated with 0.5 mg/mL alamethicin and kept on ice for 15 min to activate the enzymes; then, 20 μM osthenol along with 0.1 M Kpi buffer (pH 7.4) was added to the mixture and incubated at 37 °C for 5 min. The reaction was initiated by the addition of 10 mM UDPGA and NGS solution and incubated for 60 min at 37 °C. The reaction was terminated by the addition of 400 μL 100% acetonitrile (ACN) mixed thoroughly and centrifuged at 13,000 rpm for 10 min. A 550 μL aliquot of the supernatant was transferred to a new tube and dried using vacuum concentrator. The dried sample was dissolved in 100 μL 20% MeOH containing 0.1% formic acid, and 10 μL of this mixture was injected onto a C18 column for liquid chromatograph tandem-mass spectrometer (LC-MS/MS) analysis.

2.3. Metabolism of Osthenol in Human Recombinant cDNA-Expressed CYP and UGT Isoforms

The reaction mixture consisted of 5 pmoles of human recombinant cDNA-expressed CYP isoforms (CYP1A2, 2B6, 2C8, 2C9, 2C19, 2D6, 2E1, 3A4, and 3A5) and 20 μM osthenol with NGS system in a 200 μL reaction volume in the presence of 0.1 M Kpi buffer (pH 7.4). Human recombinant UGT isoforms (UGT1A1, 1A3, 1A4, 1A6, 1A9, and 2B7, 50 μg/mL) were used for the analysis of the metabolites of UGT isoforms instead of human liver microsomes. Osthenol (10 μM) was pre-incubated in a 200 µL reaction mixture containing 0.1 mg/mL human recombinant UGT isoforms and 0.5 mg/mL alamethicin at 37 °C for 5 min, then and kept on ice for 15 min to activate the enzymes. Then, 0.1 M Kpi buffer (pH 7.4) was added to the mixture and incubated at 37 °C for 5 min. The reaction was initiated by the addition of 10 mM UDPGA and NGS solution and incubated for 60 min at 37 °C. The reaction was terminated by the addition of 400 µL 100% ACN, and mixed thoroughly. After incubation, the mixtures were centrifuged at 13,000 rpm for 10 min, and then 550 µL of supernatant was transferred to a new tube. The solvent was completely evaporated using a vacuum concentrator. The residue was dissolved in 100 µL 20% MeOH containing 0.1% formic acid. The analysis of osthenol metabolites was as described in the above section.

2.4. Reaction Phenotyping for M7

Aliquots of 50, 100, and 250 U of β-glucuronidase in 150 mM sodium acetate were added to the Phase II reaction sample and incubated at 37 °C for 20 h. The reaction was terminated by the addition of 300 µL 100% ACN, mixed thoroughly and centrifuged at 13,000 rpm for 10 min. A 100 µL aliquot of the supernatant was collected, and 10 µL was injected onto a C18 column for LC-MS/MS analysis. To investigate the UGT isoform associated with glucuronidation from the hydroxylated osthenol, 10 µM osthenol was combined with 5 pmoles human recombinant CYP 1A1 and 1A2 in 0.1 M Kpi buffer (pH 7.4). The reaction was initiated by the addition of NGS solution and incubated for 30 min at 37 °C. Then, 50 µg/mL human recombinant UGT isoforms and 10 mM UDPGA were added and incubated at 37 °C for 30 min. The reaction was terminated by the addition of 400 µL 100% ACN.

2.5. Instruments

The LC-MS/MS system consisted of a Thermo Scientific UHPLC system (Thermo Fisher Scientific, Waltham, MA, USA) equipped with a HPG-3400RS Standard binary pump, WPS 3000 TRS analytical autosampler, and TCC-3000 SD Column compartment. The LC system was coupled with a high-resolution mass spectrometer (Q Exactive™ Focus quadrupole-Orbitrap MS; Thermo Fisher Scientific, Bremen, Germany). A heated electrospray ionization source II (HESI-II) probe was used as an ion generator with nitrogen used as the auxiliary, sheath and sweep gas. The mass spectrometry was operated in negative ion mode, with sheath gas, and the auxiliary gas was set to 45 and 10 aux units, respectively. The other parameters were set as follows: spray voltage to 2.5 KV, capillary temperature to 250 °C, S-lens RF level to 50, and Aux gas heater temperature to 400 °C. The LC method consisted of water (mobile phase A) and ACN (mobile phase B), both of which contained 0.1% formic acid, at a flow rate of 0.24 mL/min at 45 °C. For metabolic profiling, the gradient conditions were as follows: 15–57% of B at 0–21 min, 57–95% of B at 21–23 min, 5% of B at 23–25 min, 95–15% of B at 25–25.1 min, 15% of B at 25.1–30 min. The analytes were separated with a Kinetex® C18 column (150 mm × 2.1 mm, 2.6 µm, Phenomenex, Torrance, CA, USA).

3. Results

3.1. Identification of Phase I and Phase II Metabolites of Osthenol in HLMs

Representative extracted ion chromatograms (EICs) following the incubation of pooled human liver microsomes with osthenol are shown in Figure 2. Osthenol was detected at *m/z* 229 at 13.7 min in negative mode, which showed a stronger intensity compared to the positive mode. After 60 min incubation in the presence of NGS and UDPGA, seven metabolites were generated, and protonated ions in negative ion mode were observed at *m/z* 245 (M1–M5) at 6.6–11.8 min, *m/z* 407 (M6) at 7.0 min and *m/z* 421 (M7) at 8.0 min corresponding to monohydroxylation, *O*-glucuronide conjugate and hydroxyl-glucuronide conjugate, in pooled human liver microsomes, respectively (Table 1). The mass signal of the generated metabolites (M1–M5) in negative ion mode was stronger than in positive ion mode, and M6 and M7 were only detected in negative ion mode. The experiment was carried out through in negative ion mode.

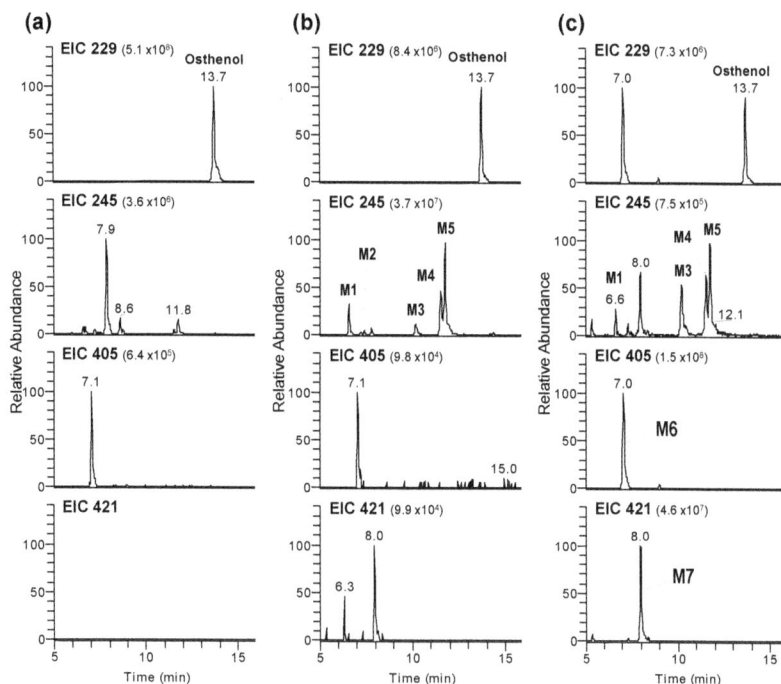

Figure 2. LC-MS/MS analysis of osthenol and its metabolites. Extracted ion chromatograms for osthenol (20 μM) and its metabolites (M1–M7) after 60 min of incubation with 1 mg/mL pooled human liver microsomes in the absence (**a**) and the presence (**b**) of a reduced nicotinamide adenine dinucleotide phosphate (β-NADPH)-regenerating system (NGS), and in the presence NGS with 5 mM uridine 5′-diphosphoglucuronic acid (**c**).

Table 1. Elemental composition of key product ions of osthenol and its metabolites in human liver microsomes using high-resolution quadrupole-orbitrap mass spectrometry.

Compound	Precursor Ions (m/z)			HCD (eV)	Product Ion (m/z)	Elemental Comp. (exp.)	Error (ppm)	Mass Shift (Da)
	MS^2	Elemental Comp. (exp.)	Error (ppm)					
Osthenol	229.0864	$C_{14}H_{13}O_3$	−0.5	25	206.0214	Unknown	NA	
				25	174.0315	$C_{10}H_6O_3$	−1.1	
				25	145.0285	$C_9H_5O_2$	−3.2	
				25	130.0416	C_9H_6O	−1.8	
				25	108.0206	$C_6H_4O_2$	−5.0	
M1	245.0816	$C_{14}H_{13}O_4$	1.0	25	227.0708	$C_{14}H_{11}O_3$	−0.1	-H_2O
				25	215.0708	$C_{13}H_{11}O_3$	−0.1	-CH_2O
				25	206.0214	Unknown	NA	
				25	183.0807	$C_{13}H_{11}O$	−1.4	
				25	174.0315	$C_{10}H_6O_3$	−1.3	
				25	145.0285	$C_9H_5O_2$	−2.9	
				25	108.0207	$C_6H_4O_2$	−4.2	
M2	245.0816	$C_{14}H_{13}O_4$	2.9	25	227.0708	$C_{14}H_{11}O_3$	2.7	-H_2O
				25	215.0707	$C_{13}H_{11}O_3$	2.2	
				25	206.0214	Unknown	NA	
				25	183.0808	$C_{13}H_{11}O$	1.9	
				25	174.0314	$C_{10}H_6O_3$	1.5	
				25	145.0285	$C_9H_5O_2$	0.9	

Table 1. *Cont.*

| Compound | Precursor Ions (m/z) | | | HCD (eV) | Product Ion (m/z) | Elemental Comp. (exp.) | Error (ppm) | Mass Shift (Da) |
	MS^2	Elemental Comp. (exp.)	Error (ppm)					
M3	245.0816	$C_{14}H_{13}O_4$	3.2	15	217.0865	$C_{13}H_{13}O_3$	2.7	
				15	201.0914	$C_{13}H_{13}O_2$	2.0	
				15	133.0285	$C_8H_5O_2$	0.5	
M4	245.0817	$C_{14}H_{13}O_4$	3.4	25	229.0501	$C_{13}H_9O_4$	2.5	
				25	222.0164	$C_{10}H_6O_6$	2.3	206 + 16
				25	201.0914	$C_{13}H_{13}O_2$	1.9	
				25	190.0264	$C_{10}H_6O_4$	1.8	174 + 16
				25	173.0965	$C_{12}H_{13}O$	2.4	
				25	162.0314	$C_9H_6O_3$	1.4	
				25	132.0207	$C_8H_4O_2$	0.9	
M5	245.0816	$C_{14}H_{13}O_4$	1.0	25	229.0501	$C_{13}H_9O_4$	0.2	213 + 16
				25	222.0163	$C_{10}H_6O_6$	−0.4	206 + 16
				25	217.0865	$C_{13}H_{13}O_3$	0.4	
				25	190.0264	$C_{10}H_6O_4$	−1.4	174 + 16
				25	174.0314	$C_{10}H_6O_3$	−1.6	
				25	166.0262	$C_8H_6O_4$	−2.3	
				25	162.0314	$C_9H_6O_3$	−1.5	
				25	161.0235	$C_9H_5O_3$	−2.6	145 + 16
				25	132.0206	$C_8H_4O_2$	−3.7	
M6	405.1186	$C_{20}H_{21}O_9$	1.5	15	229.0865	$C_{14}H_{13}O_3$	2.7	
				15	175.0239	$C_6H_7O_6$	1.3	
				15	113.0233	$C_5H_5O_3$	−0.1	
M7	421.1137	$C_{20}H_{21}O_{10}$	1.8	15	245.0816	$C_{14}H_{13}O_4$	3.1	
				15	217.0863	$C_{13}H_{13}O_3$	1.8	
				15	175.0239	$C_6H_7O_6$	1.3	
				15	113.2333	$C_5H_5O_3$	−0.2	

3.2. Elucidation of Metabolite Structure

To elucidate the chemical structure of osthenol metabolites, the HR-MS/MS of osthenol and M1–M7 were characterized using HR-MS/MS. The product ions and fragments were matched to their elemental composition with less than 5 ppm error (Table 1). The product ion spectrum of protonated osthenol is depicted in Figure 3a. The precursor ion spectra of protonated osthenol were observed at [M-H]$^-$ 229.0864 ($C_{14}H_{13}O_3$) in negative mode and the dominant fragment ions of MS^2 were at *m/z* 174.0315 ($C_{10}H_6O_3$) and 145.0285 ($C_9H_5O_2$), indicating the loss of a methylpropene, and methylbutene with hydroxyl group moiety, respectively. Another dominant fragment ion at *m/z* 206.0214 ($C_{10}H_6O_5$, loss of 23 Da) was detected, although we could not trace the exact fragment mechanism; it was assumed to indicate 2H-chromen-2-one (coumarin), which would be the key ion to determine the hydroxylation position of metabolites.

(a) Osthenol

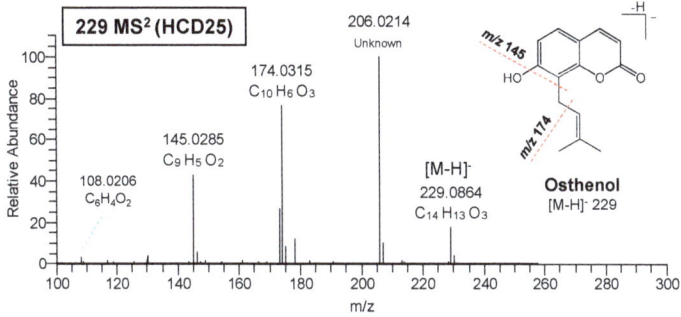

(b) M1

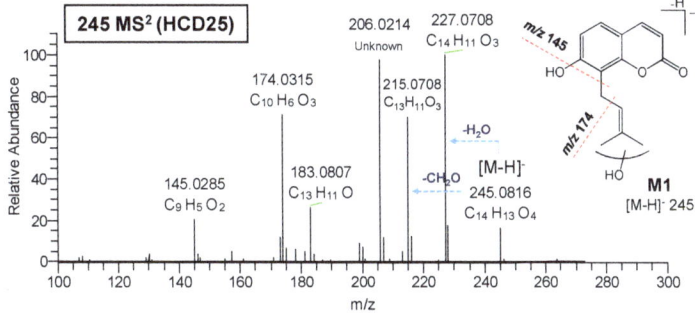

(c) M3

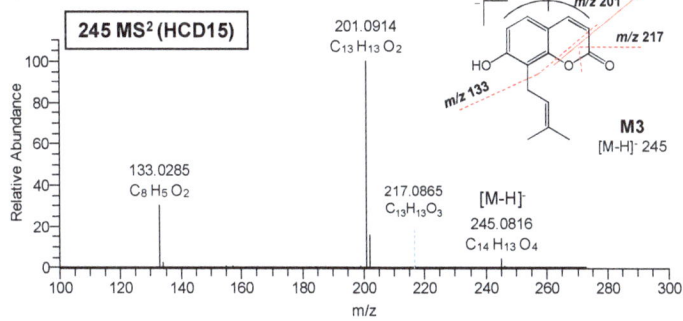

Figure 3. *Cont.*

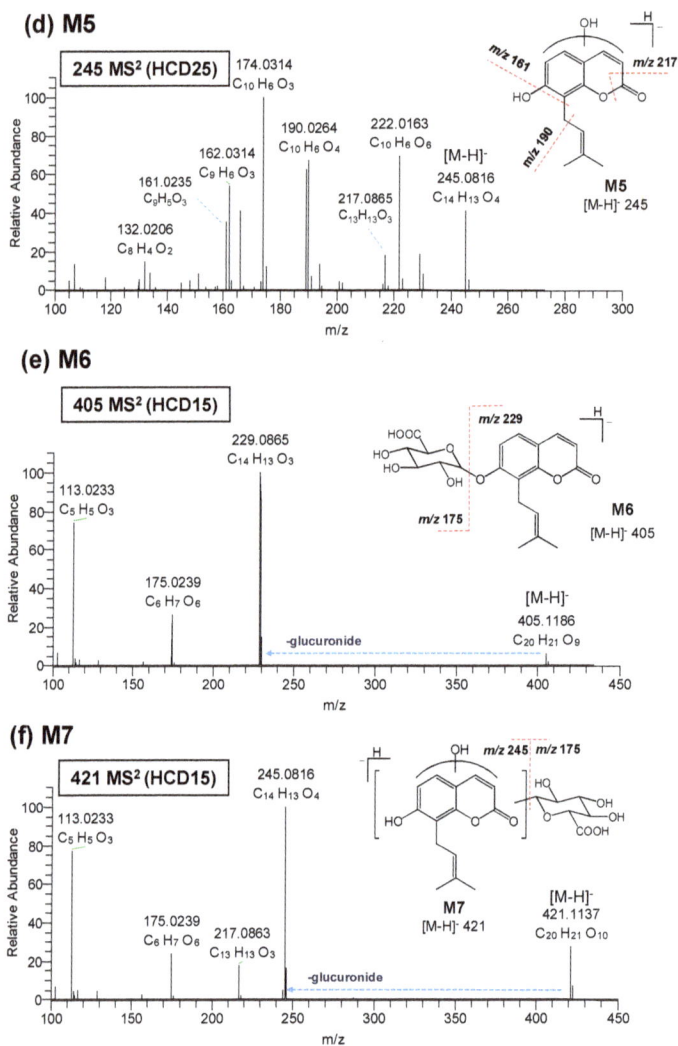

Figure 3. MS/MS spectra of protonated osthenol (**a**), 5 hydroxylated osthenol (M1–M5, (**b**)–(**d**)), osthenol-glucuronide (M6, (**e**)), and hydroxyl glucuronide osthenol (M7, (**f**)) using high-resolution/high-accuracy tandem mass spectrometry.

The M1 was observed at m/z 245.0816 ($C_{14}H_{13}O_4$) as monohydroxylated metabolites in HLMs. The MS^2 spectrum of M1 shows major product ions at 227.0708, 215.0708, 206.0214, 174.0351, and 145.0285 (Figure 3a). At first, two major product ions at m/z 227.0708 ($C_{14}H_{11}O_3$) and 215.0708 ($C_{13}H_{11}O_3$) indicated the loss of H_2O (18 Da) and CH_2O (30 Da), respectively. Another three characteristic ions at m/z 206.0214 ($C_{10}H_6O_5$), 174.0315 ($C_{10}H_6O_3$), and 145.0285 ($C_9H_5O_2$) were the same as those observed in the MS^2 spectrum of osthenol. Based on these results, these metabolites were proposed to be monohydroxylated on the methyl group in the pentane moiety. The M2 showed the same higher-energy collisional dissociation (HCD) spectra as M1 (Table 1), and was also proposed as a monohydroxylated osthenol in the pentane moiety.

As depicted in Figure 3c, the MS^2 spectrum of M3 at m/z 245.0816 ($C_{14}H_{13}O_4$) showed a different pattern compared to osthenol and other metabolites. The three product ions detected at m/z 217.0865 ($C_{13}H_{13}O_3$), 201.0914 ($C_{13}H_{13}O_2$), and 133.0285 ($C_8H_5O_2$) indicate the fragmentation in the 2H-chromen-2-one moiety (Table 1). The ion at m/z 217 corresponds to loss of -CH_2O in 5,6-dihydro-2H-pyran-2-one moiety (B ring), and the ion at m/z 201 was also the result of being connected to the ion at m/z 217. The ion at m/z 133 indicates the loss of a pentane moiety from the ion at m/z 201. However, these fragment ions do not indicate the exact position of monohydroxylation. As a result, M3 is postulated as monohydroxyl osthenol in the 2H-chromen-2-one moiety.

The M4 (m/z 245.0817, $C_{14}H_{13}O_4$) and M5 (m/z 245.0816, $C_{14}H_{13}O_4$) showed similar MS^2 fragment patterns (Table 1). The ions at m/z 190.0264 ($C_{10}H_6O_4$) and 161.0235 ($C_9H_5O_3$) were observed as newly generated fragment ions compared to osthenol (Figure 3d) and were >16 Da than the corresponding osthenol ions at m/z 174 and 145, indicating monohydroxylation in the 2H-chromen-2-one moiety. Although the MS^2 fragment patterns of M4 and M5 show different patterns compared to M3, they were tentatively assigned as monohydroxyl derivatives at the 2H-chromen-2-one (coumarin moiety).

In addition, the hydroxylation position of M1–M5 was confirmed by MS/MS fragment in positive ion mode (data not shown). Osthenol showed the specific fragment ion as m/z 175 for the loss of 56 Da, which could assume the existence of hydroxylation in the methyl propane moiety. The MS^2 fragment of M1 and M2 (m/z 247.0961) showed the m/z 175.0387 ($C_{10}H_7O_2$), indicating the loss of hydroxyl methyl propane moiety (72 Da). On the contrary, the MS^2 fragment of M3-M5 (m/z 247.0960) showed the m/z 191.0335 ($C_{10}H_7O_4$), indicating the loss of the methyl propane moiety (56 Da). Therefore, the structure of the metabolites can be estimated once more through this result.

The precursor ion spectra of the protonated monoglucuronide metabolite M6 of osthenol was observed at m/z 405.1186 ($C_{20}H_{21}O_9$) in negative mode (Figure 3e). The fragment ions are listed in Table 1. We confirmed that m/z 229.0865 ($C_{14}H_{13}O_3$) indicates the loss of glucuronide moiety from osthenol. The two fragment ions at m/z 175.0239 ($C_6H_7O_6$) and 111.0233 ($C_5H_5O_3$) indicate the glucuronide moiety. Based on the osthenol structure, M6 is the osthenol-7-O-β-D-glucuronide formed in HLMs.

The precursor ion spectra of the protonated monohydroxyl glucuronide metabolite M7 of osthenol was observed at m/z 421.1137 ($C_{20}H_{21}O_{10}$) in negative mode (Figure 3e). We also confirmed that m/z 245.0816 ($C_{14}H_{13}O_4$) indicates the loss of the glucuronide moiety from hydroxyl osthenol. The ion at m/z 217.0863 ($C_{14}H_{13}O_4$) was newly detected, indicating the loss of -CH_2O in 5,6-dihydro-2H-pyran-2-one moiety (B ring). The two fragment ions at m/z 175.0239 ($C_6H_7O_6$) and 113.0233 ($C_9H_7O_2$) were the same as detected in M6. Based on the signature ion at m/z 217, M7 was determined to be derived from M3, M4, or M5, which are monohydroxylated osthenol metabolites at the 2H-chromen-2-one (coumarin moiety).

3.3. Reaction Phenotyping of Osthenol Metabolism Using cDNA-Expressed Recombinant CYP and UGT Isoforms

For identification of the osthenol metabolic enzymes in HLMs, we incubated osthenol with nine human recombinant CYP (10 pmoles) or six UGT (10 pmoles) isoforms in the presence of NGS or UDPGA, respectively (Figure 4). There are three different groups of CYP isoforms to selectively metabolize to hydroxyl-osthenol. At the first, CYP2D6 mainly generated the formation of M1, monohydroxyl osthenol, in the pentane moiety. While M3 is generated highly by CYP3A4, and another mono-hydroxylated metabolite, 2H-chromen-2-one, M4 and M5 are mainly metabolized by CYP1A1 and 1A2. In addition, CYP2C19 and 2D6 were also partially involved in the formation of M5. Although the structures of M3, M4 and M5 are predicted to be hydroxylation on the 2H-chromen-2-one moiety, their hydroxyl position was presumed to be different because the related enzymes were different, as CYP3A4/3A5 generated M3, and CYP1A1/1A2 contributed to the formation of M4 and M5. M6, the monoglucuronide conjugate, showed the highest formation in incubation with human recombinant UGT1A9, while UGT1A6 was also slightly involved in the formation of M6.

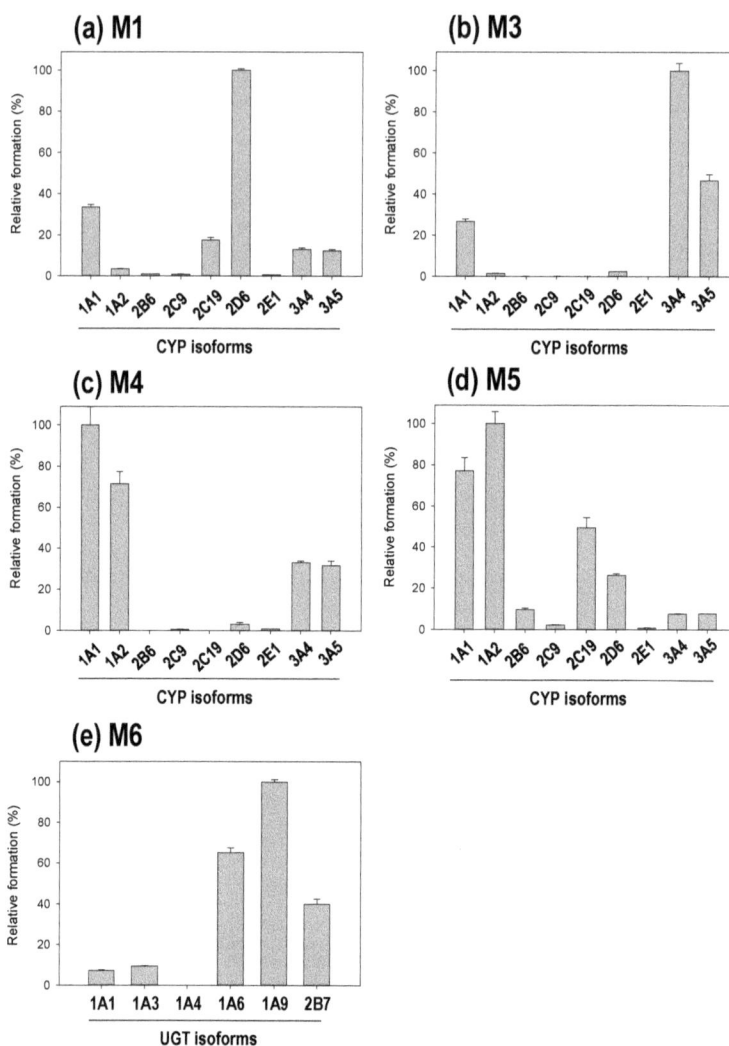

Figure 4. The formation of osthenol metabolites in human recombinant cDNA-expressed cytochrome P450 (CYP) isoforms (**a–d**) or cDNA-expressed uridine 5′-diphospho-glucuronosyltransferase (UGT) isoforms (**e**). Osthenol (20 μM) was incubated with each enzyme (5 pmole) for 60 min at 37 °C in the presence of a NADPH-regenerating system and 5 mM uridine 5′-diphosphoglucuronic acid. Data are expressed as the means ± SE of three independent determinations.

M7 is assigned as the hydroxyl-glucuronide conjugate of osthenol by the interpretation of MS^2 analysis (Figure 3f), which is a product of the two step metabolic pathways. In Figure 3f, the M7 is assumed to be derived from the M4 or M5 by the signature ion at m/z 217. Moreover, to confirm the enzyme reaction phenotyping for M7, we additionally treated with β-glucuronidase to remove glucuronide from M7 after the osthenol was incubated in presence of NGS and UDPGA in HLMs (Figure 5a). After the β-glucuronidase treatment, M5 increased greatly compared to without β-glucuronidase treatment, which means that M5 is the intermediate for M7 generation. Moreover, to identify the UGT isoform related to M7 conjugation from M5, we incubated it with the human recombinant UGT isoforms UGT1A1, 1A3, 1A4, 1A6, 1A9, and 2B7, after the incubation of osthenol with human recombinant CYP 1A2 (Figure 5b). M7 was mainly generated by UGT1A3, and UGT 1A1 and 1A6 slightly contributed to the formation of M7 from M5.

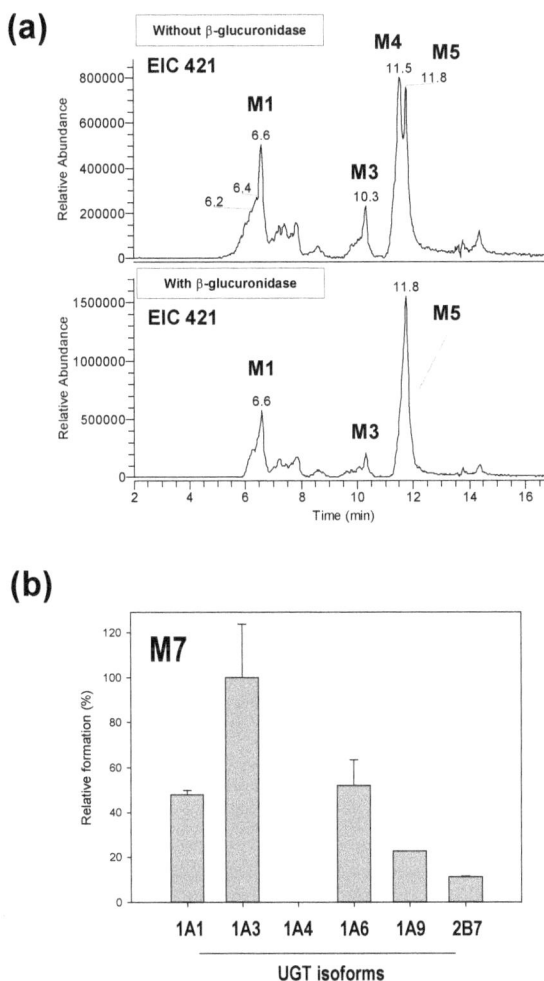

Figure 5. The formation of M7 in human liver microsomes (HLMs). Extracted ion chromatograms for M7 after incubation for 60 min with 1 mg/mL HLMs in the absence and the presence of β-glucuronidase (**a**) and the formation of M7 from M5 in human recombinant cDNA-expressed uridine 5′-diphospho-glucuronosyltransferase (UGT) isoforms (**b**) after treatment with β-glucuronidase.

4. Discussion

Osthenol is a prenylated coumarin, and is known to be a major metabolite of osthole, desmethyl-osthole [9,10]. Although osthole is known to be the major component of the bioactive reaction of Cnidii Fructus [8], osthenol also shows bioactivation, such as the inhibition of skin tumor promotion [4], strong antibacterial and antifungal activities [5,6] and anti-inflammatory effects [7]. To date, the metabolite directly generated from osthenol has not been identified, and the metabolic enzymes involved in osthenol metabolism remain unknown. Here, we investigated the metabolic pathway of osthenol in HLMs and identified five hydroxylated metabolites by CYPs, and two glucuronide conjugates of osthenol by UGTs (Figure 6).

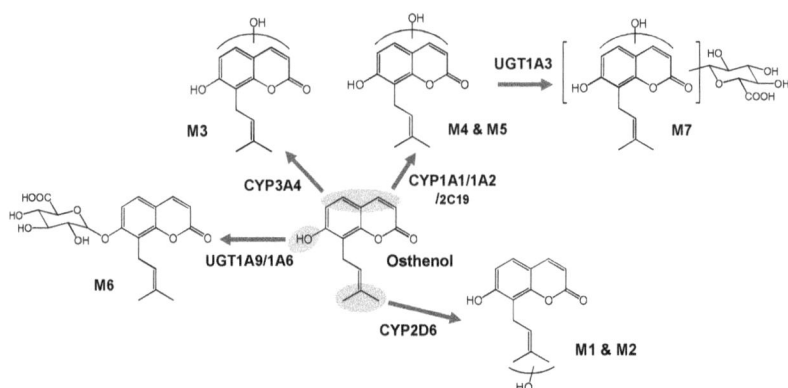

Figure 6. Postulated metabolic pathways of osthenol in human liver microsomes.

Previously, the metabolic pathway of osthenol was partially identified in a study of osthole in rats. In 2013, the metabolites of osthole, 7-*O*-methyl-osthenol, were isolated from rat urine, and the structures of 10 phase I and three phase II metabolites were identified using the 2D-NMR technique [10]. Among these metabolites, osthenol-related metabolites were identified, including 5′-hydroxyl-osthenol, 4′-hydroxyl-2′, 3′-dihydro-osthenol, 4′-hydroxyl-osthenol for phase I, and osthenol-7-*O*-β-D-glucuronide for phase II. In addition, Li et al. studied the metabolism of osthole in rat urine by UPLC-QTOF/MS in 2013 [12]. They identified a total of 11 metabolites by 7-demethylation, 8-dehydrogenation, hydroxylation on coumarin, 3,4-epoxide, and sulfate conjugation.

Based on these studies, we expected that the metabolic pathway of osthenol would show it to be monohydroxylated at the 4′C or 5′C position, and between 3C to 6C in 2H-chromen-2-one, with dehydrogenation at 2′-3′C for phase I, and 7-*O*-glucuronidation and 7-*O*-sulfation for phase II. First, we identified five monohydroxylated metabolites that could be distinguished by three distinct features (Figure 6). M1 and M2 are monohydroxylated metabolites at 4′C or 5′C and are metabolized by CYP2D6. The typical substrate of CYP2D6 usually consists of lipophilic bases with a planar hydrophobic aromatic ring and a nitrogen atom, however CYP2D6 can also react with several atypical substrates that do not contain a basic nitrogen atom [13]. M3 is produced by monohydroxylation on a 2H-chromen-2-one moiety by CYP3A4 and CYP3A5, which prefer relatively large, structurally diverse molecules [14]. M4 and M5 are also monohydroxylated metabolites of a 2H-chromen-2-one moiety; the hydroxylation positions of M4 and M5 are expected to be different from those of M3. Although M5 was generated by CYP2C19 and 2D6, CYP1A1 and 1A2 are the main isoforms that generate M4 and M5 in HLMs. Planar molecules, neutral or basic in character, are typical substrates of CYP1A2 [14]. Although the dehydrogenated metabolite of osthenol was reported in rat urine and microsomal enzymes can mediate dehydrogenation, this metabolite was not detected in the present study.

In natural phenolic phytochemicals, glucuronidation is linked to significant physiological properties, such as its solubility, bioactivity, bioavailability, and inter- and intracellular transport [15]. Moreover, extensive glucuronidation can be a barrier to oral bioavailability as the first-pass glucuronidation of orally administered agents usually results in poor oral bioavailability and a lack of efficacy [16]. In the present study, osthenol and hydroxyl-osthenol (M5) were strongly glucuronidated by UGT in HLMs, and M6, 7-*O*-glucuronide-osthenol, was produced 200-fold more than hydroxyl osthenol in the presence of NGS and UDPGA (Figure 2c). The hydroxylated metabolite (M5) of osthenol

Pharmaceutics **2018**, *10*, 141

was also strongly converted to glucuronide conjugate (M7), and the concentration of hydroxylated metabolites decreased, indicating that the glucuronidation of osthenol is major metabolic pathway and controls the pharmacokinetic parameters of osthenol in vivo. Here UGT1A6 and 1A9 mainly contributed to the 7-*O*-glucuronidation of osthenol, which is consistent with previous studies of the glucuronidation of coumarins. For example, 4-methylumbelliferone is metabolized by human UGT1A6, 1A7, and 1A10 [17]. Human UGT1A6 and 1A9 were shown to be major isoforms involved in daphnetin glucuronidation in human intestine and liver microsomes [18]. Scopoletin is rapidly metabolized by UGT1A3, 1A6, and 1A9 [19]. In addition, UGT1A3 is dominantly associated with M7 generation from M5, where coumarin moiety is glucuronidated.

In conclusion, we demonstrated that osthenol is metabolized to five monohydroxyl metabolites (M1–M5) by CYP2C19, 2D6, 1A2, and 3A4, respectively, and a 7-*O*-glucuronide conjugate (M6) by UGT1A9 and a hydroxyl-glucuronide (M7) by UGT1A3 in HLMs. We also found that glucuronidation is a dominant metabolic pathway of osthenol in HLMs. The structures of the metabolites were proposed using high-resolution/high-accuracy tandem mass spectrometry, and the possible metabolic fate of osthenol in HLMs is summarized in Figure 6.

Author Contributions: Conceptualization, S.L. and T.L.; Data Curation, P.J.C. and S.L.; Formal Analysis, P.J.C.; Funding Acquisition, T.L.; Methodology, P.J.C. and S.P.; Resources, D.L., Y.J.J., G.J. and T.L.; Writing—Original Draft Preparation, P.J.C.; Writing—Review & Editing, T.C.J., S.L. and T.L.

Funding: This research was funded by the National Research Foundation of Korea (NRF) grant funded by the Korean Government, grant number NRF-2017R1A1A1A05001129.

References

1. Seo, E.K.; Kim, K.H.; Kim, M.K.; Cho, M.H.; Choi, E.; Kim, K.; Mar, W. Inhibitors of 5alpha -reductase type I in LNCaP cells from the roots of Angelica koreana. *Planta Med.* **2002**, *68*, 162–163. [CrossRef] [PubMed]
2. Chen, Y.; Fan, G.; Chen, B.; Xie, Y.; Wu, H.; Wu, Y.; Yan, C.; Wang, J. Separation and quantitative analysis of coumarin compounds from Angelica dahurica (Fisch. ex Hoffm) Benth. et Hook. f by pressurized capillary electrochromatography. *J. Pharm. Biomed. Anal.* **2006**, *41*, 105–116. [CrossRef] [PubMed]
3. Karamat, F.; Olry, A.; Munakata, R.; Koeduka, T.; Sugiyama, A.; Paris, C.; Hehn, A.; Bourgaud, F.; Yazaki, K. A coumarin-specific prenyltransferase catalyzes the crucial biosynthetic reaction for furanocoumarin formation in parsley. *Plant J.* **2014**, *77*, 627–638. [CrossRef] [PubMed]
4. Ito, C.; Itoigawa, M.; Ju-ichi, M.; Sakamoto, N.; Tokuda, H.; Nishino, H.; Furukawa, H. Antitumor-promoting activity of coumarins from citrus plants. *Planta Med.* **2005**, *71*, 84–87. [CrossRef] [PubMed]
5. Montagner, C.; de Souza, S.M.; Groposoa, C.; Delle Monache, F.; Smania, E.F.; Smania, A., Jr. Antifungal activity of coumarins. *Z. Naturforsch. C* **2008**, *63*, 21–28. [CrossRef] [PubMed]
6. de Souza, S.M.; Delle Monache, F.; Smania, A., Jr. Antibacterial activity of coumarins. *Z. Naturforsch. C* **2005**, *60*, 693–700. [CrossRef] [PubMed]
7. Liu, J.H.; Zschocke, S.; Reininger, E.; Bauer, R. Inhibitory effects of Angelica pubescens f. biserrata on 5-lipoxygenase and cyclooxygenase. *Planta Med.* **1998**, *64*, 525–529. [CrossRef] [PubMed]
8. Zhang, Z.R.; Leung, W.N.; Cheung, H.Y.; Chan, C.W. Osthole: A review on its bioactivities, pharmacological properties, and potential as alternative medicine. *Evid. Based Complement. Altern. Med.* **2015**, *2015*, 919616. [CrossRef] [PubMed]
9. Yuan, Z.; Xu, H.; Wang, K.; Zhao, Z.; Hu, M. Determination of osthol and its metabolites in a phase I reaction system and the Caco-2 cell model by HPLC-UV and LC-MS/MS. *J. Pharm. Biomed. Anal.* **2009**, *49*, 1226–1232. [CrossRef] [PubMed]
10. Lv, X.; Wang, C.Y.; Hou, J.; Zhang, B.J.; Deng, S.; Tian, Y.; Huang, S.S.; Zhang, H.L.; Shu, X.H.; Zhen, Y.H.; et al. Isolation and identification of metabolites of osthole in rats. *Xenobiotica* **2012**, *42*, 1120–1127. [CrossRef] [PubMed]
11. Cho, P.J.; Nam, W.; Lee, D.; Lee, T.; Lee, S. Selective inhibitory effect of osthenol on human cytochrome 2C8. *Bull. Korean Chem. Soc.* **2018**, *39*, 801–805. [CrossRef]

12. Li, J.; Chan, W. Investigation of the biotransformation of osthole by liquid chromatography/tandem mass spectrometry. *J. Pharm. Biomed. Anal.* **2013**, *74*, 156–161. [CrossRef] [PubMed]

13. Zhou, S.F.; Liu, J.P.; Lai, X.S. Substrate specificity, inhibitors and regulation of human cytochrome P450 2D6 and implications in drug development. *Curr. Med. Chem.* **2009**, *16*, 2661–2805. [CrossRef] [PubMed]

14. Lewis, D.F.; Dickins, M. Substrate SARs in human P450s. *Drug Discov. Today* **2002**, *7*, 918–925. [CrossRef]

15. Docampo, M.; Olubu, A.; Wang, X.; Pasinetti, G.; Dixon, R.A. Glucuronidated flavonoids in neurological protection: Structural analysis and approaches for chemical and biological synthesis. *J. Agric. Food Chem.* **2017**, *65*, 7607–7623. [CrossRef] [PubMed]

16. Wu, B.; Kulkarni, K.; Basu, S.; Zhang, S.; Hu, M. First-pass metabolism via UDP-glucuronosyltransferase: A barrier to oral bioavailability of phenolics. *J. Pharm. Sci.* **2011**, *100*, 3655–3681. [CrossRef] [PubMed]

17. Uchaipichat, V.; Mackenzie, P.I.; Guo, X.H.; Gardner-Stephen, D.; Galetin, A.; Houston, J.B.; Miners, J.O. Human udp-glucuronosyltransferases: Isoform selectivity and kinetics of 4-methylumbelliferone and 1-naphthol glucuronidation, effects of organic solvents, and inhibition by diclofenac and probenecid. *Drug Metab. Dispos.* **2004**, *32*, 413–423. [CrossRef] [PubMed]

18. Liang, S.C.; Ge, G.B.; Liu, H.X.; Zhang, Y.Y.; Wang, L.M.; Zhang, J.W.; Yin, L.; Li, W.; Fang, Z.Z.; Wu, J.J.; et al. Identification and characterization of human UDP-glucuronosyltransferases responsible for the in vitro glucuronidation of daphnetin. *Drug Metab. Dispos.* **2010**, *38*, 973–980. [CrossRef] [PubMed]

19. Luukkanen, L.; Taskinen, J.; Kurkela, M.; Kostiainen, R.; Hirvonen, J.; Finel, M. Kinetic characterization of the 1A subfamily of recombinant human UDP-glucuronosyltransferases. *Drug Metab. Dispos.* **2005**, *33*, 1017–1026. [CrossRef] [PubMed]

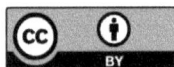

pharmaceutics

MDPI

Article

Pharmacokinetics and Brain Distribution of the Active Components of DA-9805, Saikosaponin A, Paeonol and Imperatorin in Rats

Mi Hye Kwon [1], Jin Seok Jeong [2], Jayoung Ryu [2], Young Woong Cho [2] and Hee Eun Kang [1,*]

[1] College of Pharmacy and Integrated Research Institute of Pharmaceutical Sciences, The Catholic University of Korea, 43 Jibong-ro, Wonmi-gu, Bucheon 14662, Korea; mihye8699@hanmail.net
[2] Research Center, Dong-A ST Co., Ltd., 21 Geumhwa-ro, 105beon-gil, Giheung-gu, Yongin 17073, Korea; treadwheel@donga.co.kr (J.S.J.); jyryu@donga.co.kr (J.R.); herojoe@donga.co.kr (Y.W.C.)
* Correspondence: kanghe@catholic.ac.kr; Tel.: +82-2-2164-4055

Received: 25 July 2018; Accepted: 18 August 2018; Published: 20 August 2018

Abstract: DA-9805 is a botanical anti-Parkinson's drug candidate formulated from ethanol extracts of the root of *Bupleurum falcatum*, the root cortex of *Paeonia suffruticosa*, and the root of *Angelica dahurica*. The pharmacokinetics (PKs) and brain distribution of active/representative ingredients of DA-9805, Saikosaponin a (SSa; 1.1–4.6 mg/kg), Paeonol (PA; 14.8–59.2 mg/kg), and Imperatorin (IMP; 1.4–11.5 mg/kg) were evaluated following the intravenous or oral administration of each pure component and the equivalent dose of DA-9805 in rats. All three components had greater dose-normalized areas under the plasma concentration-time curve (AUC) and slower clearance with higher doses, following intravenous administration. By contrast, dose-proportional AUC values of SSa, PA, and IMP were observed following the oral administration of each pure component (with the exception of IMP at the highest dose) or DA-9805. Compared to oral administration of each pure compound, DA-9805 administration showed an increase in the AUC of SSa (by 96.1–163%) and PA (by 155–164%), possibly due to inhibition of their metabolism by IMP or other component(s) in DA-9805. A delay in the absorption of PA and IMP was observed when they were administered as DA-9805. All three components of DA-9805 showed greater binding values in brain homogenates than in plasma, possibly explaining why the brain-to-plasma ratios were greater than unity following multiple oral administrations of DA-9805. By contrast, their levels in cerebrospinal fluid were negligible. Our results further our understanding of the comprehensive PK characteristics of SSa, PA, and IMP in rats and the comparative PKs between each pure component and DA-9805.

Keywords: DA-9805; saikosaponin a; paeonol; imperatorin; pharmacokinetics; brain distribution

1. Introduction

Recently, the potential role of herbal products in the treatment of Parkinson's disease has emerged [1]. Neuroprotective or neurorestorative agents for the treatment of this disease by either inhibiting primary neurodegenerative events or boosting compensatory and regenerative mechanisms in the brain remain an unmet medical need [2]. DA-9805, a novel botanical neuroprotective anti-Parkinson's drug candidate, was formulated from ethanol extracts of the mixture (1:1:1, $w/w/w$) of three herbal drugs, the root of *Bupleurum falcatum* L. (Apiaceae), the root cortex of *Paeonia suffruticosa* Andrews (Paeoniaceae), and the root of *Angelica dahurica* Benth et Hook (Umbelliferae). An investigational new drug application for DA-9805 for a phase II clinical study was recently submitted to the U.S. Food and Drug Administration. The neuroprotective effects of each of the three herbal constituents in DA-9805 have been reported in various in vitro and animal models. Ethanol extracts of the root of *B. falcatum* have been shown to inhibit neuroinflammation in murine microglial cells [3], improve behavioral defects after spinal-cord injury [4], and alleviate stress-induced memory impairment [5]. Extracts from the root cortex of *P. suffruticosa* have been found to have neuroprotective effects in an 1-methyl-4-phenyl-1,2,3,6-tetrahydropyridine (MPTP)-induced Parkinson's disease model [6]. Extracts from *A. dahurica* reduce apoptotic cell death and improve functional recovery after spinal cord injury [7].

Saikosaponin a (SSa, [3β,4α,16β]-13,28-epoxy-16,23-dihydroxyolean-11-en-3-yl-6-deoxy-3-O-β-D-glucopyranosyl-β-D-galactopyranoside; Figure 1A), originated from the root of *B. falcatum*, is a representative component of DA-9805, for which it is used as a quality control (QC) ingredient (at >0.297%). The quantity of SSa is listed in the Chinese Pharmacopeia for QC of a traditional Chinese medicine (TCM) prescribed with Radix Bupleuri [8]. Its pharmacological activity and structure are similar to those of steroids [9], and its antiepileptic [10] and neuroprotective effects [11] have recently been reported. However, its toxicity, including an ability to cause hemolysis and liver damage, has also been reported [12]. The pharmacokinetics (PKs) of SSa following intravenous administration of 15 mg/kg [8] and oral administration of the extract of the dried roots of *B. chinense* DC (equivalent to ~40 mg/kg SSa) [13] have been reported.

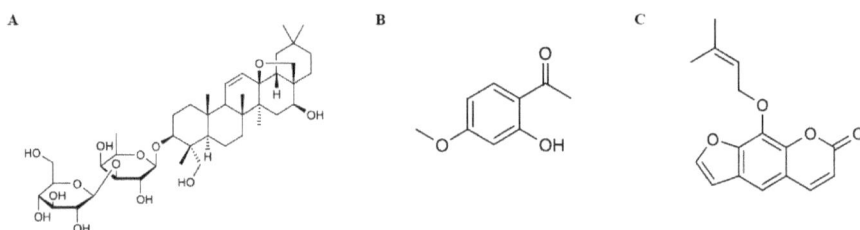

Figure 1. Chemical structures of three active/representative components in DA-9805: (**A**) saikosaponin a (SSa); (**B**) paeonol (PA); (**C**) imperatorin (IMP).

Paeonol (PA; 1-[2-hydroxy-4-methoxyphenyl]ethanone; Figure 1B), a marker component of the root cortex of *P. suffruticosa* [14], is the most abundant active compound in DA-9805 (at >2.802%). It has various pharmacological activities [15–17] and neuroprotective effects in various murine models [18–20]. Its PKs and/or tissue distribution have been reported after intravenous (2.5–10 mg/kg) [21] and oral administration (35–140 mg/kg) [14,22], as well as after oral administration of herbal products containing PA or TCM prescriptions (equivalent to 17.5–100 mg/kg PA) [23,24].

Imperatorin (IMP, 9-[3-methylbut-2-enoxy]-7-furo[3,2-g]chromenone; Figure 1C), an active ingredient in the root of *A. dahurica*, is another representative component of DA-9805 (at >0.512%). It has anti-inflammatory effects [25,26] and other favorable effects in the central nervous system (CNS) including neuroprotective, anticonvulsant, anxiolytic, and procognitive activities [27–29]. Its PKs following intravenous and oral administration (6.25–25 mg/kg or 80 mg/kg) in rats have been reported [30,31], as has its brain distribution after oral administration of 20 mg/kg of IMP [32] or ~26 mg/kg in an extract [33].

The efficacy and safety of herbal medicines remain major issues of concern. Up to now, a widely accepted approach for evaluating in vivo efficacy of an herbal medicine is that the efficacy of mixed herbal preparation can be correlated with pharmacokinetic behavior of one or several known active ingredients [34]. PKs studies of these three active/representative ingredients of DA-9805 are essential for botanical drug development to evaluate not only the efficacy of the drug but also its potential drug interactions and toxicity. Despite the promising neuroprotective activities of DA-9805 as an anti-Parkinson's agent, the PKs of its active/representative ingredients at relatively low doses have not been characterized comprehensively. Moreover, PKs of each active ingredient following DA-9805 administration may be altered by the multiple components in DA-9805.

In this study, the PKs of pure SSa, PA, and IMP and their dose dependency were evaluated following the intravenous and oral administration of each pure component. The PKs of each marker compound following the oral administration of DA-9805 were also compared to those following the respective equivalent dose of the pure marker components. Moreover, the distribution of the three active components in the brain, which is the site of action, was evaluated following multiple oral administrations of DA-9805.

2. Materials and Methods

2.1. Materials and Reagents

DA-9805 (Lot No. PD15702; containing 0.456% SSa, 5.919% PA, and 0.576% IMP, as determined by HPLC-UV) was obtained from Dong-A ST (Yongin, Korea). SSa (98.32% purity) and IMP (99.17% purity) were products from Letopharm, Ltd. (Shanghai, China), and PA (99.8% purity) was obtained from Sigma-Aldrich (St. Louis, MO, USA). Internal standard (IS) for SSa, PA, and IMP (dexamethasone, bumetanide, indomethacin, respectively), hydroxypropyl-methylcellulose (HPMC), dimethylsulfoxide (DMSO), Tween® 80, and Solutol® HS 15 were purchased from Sigma-Aldrich (St. Louis, MO, USA). Other chemicals were of reagent or HPLC grade.

2.2. Animals

Animal-study protocols were approved by the Department of Laboratory Animals, Institutional Animal Care and Use Committee on the Sungsim Campus of the Catholic University of Korea (Approval No. 2015-011; Bucheon, Korea). Male Sprague-Dawley rats, 7–8 weeks old and weighing 195–300 g, were purchased from Young Bio (Sungnam, Korea). The procedures used for the housing and handling of rats were similar to those previously described [35].

2.3. Intravenous Drug Administration

For intravenous administration, the carotid artery and jugular vein were cannulated using previously reported procedures [35]. Thereafter, each pure active component of DA-9805 was infused for 1 min via the jugular vein: SSa (dissolved in 2:1:7 [$v/v/v$] DMSO:Tween 80:distilled water (DW)) at doses of 2.3 and 4.6 mg (2 mL)/kg (n = 5 and 4, respectively); PA (dissolved in 2:2:6 [$v/v/v$] DMSO:Tween 80:20% Solutol in DW) at doses of 14.8, 29.6, and 59.2 mg (2 mL)/kg (n = 5, 5, and 6, respectively); and IMP (dissolved in 2:2:6 [$v/v/v$] DMSO:Tween 80: DW) at doses of 2.9, 5.8, and 11.5 mg (2 mL)/kg (n = 5, 6 and 5, respectively). A blood sample of ~200 μL was collected via the carotid artery at time 0 (prior to dosing), 1 (at the end of the infusion), and 5, 15, 30, 60, 90, 120, 180, 240, 360, and 480 min after the start of infusion. After centrifugation (13,000× g for 2 min), 100 μL aliquots of plasma were collected and stored at −20 °C until liquid chromatography-tandem mass spectrometry (LC-MS/MS) analyses. The preparation and handling of 24 h urine samples (Ae$_{0–24h}$) and gastrointestinal tract (GI) samples (including their contents at 24 h and feces during 0–24 h) at 24 h (GI$_{24h}$) were similar to a previously reported method [35].

2.4. Oral Drug Administration

DA-9805 (dissolved in 2:7.75, 2:7.5, and 2:7 [v/v] DMSO:DW with 2% HPMC, respectively) at doses of 250, 500, and 1000 mg (10 mL)/kg was administered orally using a gastric gavage tube (n = 5 each). Equivalent doses of each pure SSa, PA, and IMP (dissolved in 2:7.75:0.25, 2:7.5:0.5, and 2:7:1 [$v/v/v$] DMSO:DW with 2% HPMC:ethanol with dose elevation) were also administered orally (n = 4 or 5 each). Doses of 1.1, 2.3, and 4.6 mg (10 mL)/kg pure SSa; 14.8, 29.6, and 59.2 mg (10 mL)/kg pure PA; and 1.4, 2.9, and 5.8 mg (10 mL)/kg pure IMP were orally administered. A blood sample of ~200 μL was collected via the carotid artery at 0, 5, 15, 30, 45, 60, 90, 120, 180, 240, 360, 480, and 600 min after oral administration. Other procedures for the oral study were similar to those used for the intravenous study.

2.5. Brain Distribution of Saikosaponin A(SSa), Paeonol (PA), and Imperatorin (IMP) Following Multiple Oral Doses of DA-9805

DA-9805 (dissolved in 2:7 [v/v] DMSO:DW with 2% HPMC and diluted 2-fold with DW to a final concentration of 250 mg/5 mL) at a dose of 250 mg (5 mL)/kg/day was orally administered for 8 days. At 2 and 6 h after the final oral dose, the rats were euthanized (n = 3 at each time point) by carbon-dioxide asphyxiation, and cerebrospinal fluid (CSF) was collected from each rat. Blood samples were collected via cardiac puncture. Next, the mixed brain (whole of left hemisphere), frontal cortex, striatum, hippocampus, and cerebellum (from the right hemisphere) were excised and blotted on tissue paper. Each tissue sample was homogenized (Minilys®; Bertin Technologies, Montigny le Bretonneux, France) with 3 volumes (3 mL/g tissue) of methanol and centrifuged at 9000 g for 10 min. Two 100 µL aliquots of the supernatant and plasma samples were collected and stored at −70 °C until subsequent LC-MS/MS analyses.

2.6. Measurement of the Protein Binding of SSa, PA, and IMP in Rat Plasma and Brain Homogenates

The protein-binding abilities of SSa, PA, and IMP in fresh rat plasma and brain homogenates were measured using a single-use rapid equilibrium dialysis device (molecular weight cutoff of 8 kDa; Thermo Scientific, Rockford, IL, USA) in accordance with the manufacturer's instructions. For binding studies with rat plasma, SSa, PA, and IMP were spiked into each 1200 µL blank plasma sample (n = 6) to produce a final concentration of 0.5, 2, and 0.5 µg/mL, respectively. A triplicate of the above samples (each containing 300 µL) was placed into each sample chamber to minimize potential errors during sample processing, and was dialyzed against 500 µL isotonic phosphate buffer (pH 7.4) in each buffer chamber. After 4 h incubation in a water bath shaker (37 °C, 50 oscillations/min), the plasma and buffer samples were collected, and each 100 µL sample was used for LC-MS/MS analyses of SSa, PA, and IMP. For the binding study with rat brain (hippocampus, striatum, mixed brain) homogenates, each brain tissue sample was homogenized (Minilys®; Bertin Technologies, Montigny le Bretonneux, France) with 3 volumes (3 mL/g tissue) of isotonic phosphate buffer (pH 7.4). SSa, PA, and IMP were spiked into each blank brain homogenate to produce a final concentration of 0.2, 1, and 0.2 µg/mL, respectively. One (for the hippocampus and striatum) and a duplicate (for the mixed brain) of the above homogenate samples (each 200 µL) were transferred into each sample chamber and dialyzed against 350 µL isotonic phosphate buffer (pH 7.4) in each buffer chamber. Other procedures were the same as those used in the plasma protein-binding study. The unbound fraction (f_u) in plasma was calculated as follows:

$$f_u = 1 - (C_p - C_b)/C_p, \tag{1}$$

where C_p is the drug concentration in the protein-containing compartment and C_b is the drug concentration in the buffer compartment. Because the brain homogenates were diluted during the homogenization process, it was necessary to correct the f_u value measured in a diluted sample ($f_{u\ measured}$) to generate the undiluted f_u value ($f_{u\ brain}$) using the following equation (Kalvass and Maurer, 2002):

$$f_{u\ brain} = \frac{1/D}{\{(1/f_{u\ measured}) - 1\} + 1/D} \tag{2}$$

where D is the dilution factor (=4) of the brain homogenates.

2.7. LC-MS/MS Analyses of SSa, PA, and IMP

The LC-MS/MS system comprised the Agilent 1260 LC System and the Agilent 6460 Triple Quadrupole Tandem Mass Spectrometer (Agilent, Waldbronn, Germany). Instrument control and data acquisition were performed using the Agilent MassHunter Workstation software (Version B. 04. 01). The concentrations of SSa, PA, and IMP in the samples were determined according to the LC-MS/MS method recently published from our laboratory [36]. The calibration curves were linear in a concentration range of 0.5–1000 ng/mL for SSa, 20–10,000 ng/mL for PA, and 0.2–1000 ng/mL for

IMP. The mean intra- and interday coefficients of variation of the analyses on 5 consecutive days were below 15.0%, and the assay accuracies ranged from 95.8 to 113%.

2.8. Pharmacokinetic Analyses

The total area under the plasma concentration–time curve from time zero to infinity (AUC_{0-inf}) or up to the last measured time (t) in plasma (AUC_{0-t}) was calculated using the trapezoidal rule-extrapolation method [37]. Calculation of the following PK parameters was performed using non-compartmental analyses (WinNonlin®; Pharsight Corporation, Mountain View, CA, USA): the time-averaged total body, renal, and nonrenal clearances (CL, CL_R, and CL_{NR}, respectively), terminal half-life, mean residence time (MRT), and apparent volume of distribution at steady state (V_{ss}) [38]. The maximum plasma concentration (C_{max}) and time to reach C_{max} (T_{max}) were directly read from the experimental data. For comparison, the extent of absolute oral bioavailability (F) was calculated by dividing the AUC value after oral administration by the AUC value after intravenous administration of equivalent doses of the pure component.

2.9. Statistical Analyses

The Statistical Package for Social Sciences program (SPSS Inc., Chicago, IL, USA) was used for statistical analyses. To compare two means of unpaired data, the t-test was used. To compare 3 means of unpaired data, the data were compared using one-way analysis of variance (ANOVA) and the post hoc Tukey test (for a homogenous subset), or Dunnett's T3 multiple-comparison test (for a non-homogenous subset). For data that were not normally distributed, nonparametric analyses (Kruskal-Wallis test) were used. A p value < 0.05 was considered statistically significant. All of the data are expressed as the means ± standard deviations (SD), except the median (range) for T_{max}.

3. Results

3.1. PKs of SSa, PA, and IMP after Intravenous Administration of Each Pure Compound

The mean arterial plasma concentration-time profiles and relevant PK parameters of SSa, PA, and IMP following intravenous administration of each pure compound are shown in Figure 2 and Table 1, respectively. The dose-normalized AUC values of SSa, PA, and IMP following intravenous administration tended to increase with dose elevation because of slower CL (particularly CL_{NR}) of the drugs in the higher dose group(s). A significantly greater (by 77.9%) dose-normalized AUC value of SSa following intravenous administration of 4.6 mg/kg SSa was observed with significantly slower CL (by 43.2%), CL_R (by 81.2%), and CL_{NR} (by 40.3%) than those of the 2.3 mg/kg dose group. A significantly smaller V_{ss} (by 19.0%), longer MRT (by 42.9%), and smaller Ae_{0-24h} (by 68.0%) of SSa were observed in the higher dose group. PA showed significantly greater (by 38.0%) dose-normalized AUC with slower CL (by 27.0%) and CL_{NR} (by 27.5%) in the highest intravenous dose (59.2 mg/kg) group than in the lowest dose (14.8 mg/kg) group. IMP also showed significantly greater (by 124% and 98.5%) dose-normalized AUC following the highest intravenous dose (11.5 mg/kg) with slower CL (by 56.4% and 50.5%) and CL_{NR} (by 56.4% and 50.5%) than the lower dose (2.9 and 5.8 mg/kg) groups. A significantly longer MRT (by 96.6% and 60.2%) was observed in the highest dose (11.5 mg/kg) IMP group than in the lower dose (2.9 and 5.8 mg/kg) groups. The 24 h urinary excretion of IMP was almost negligible (<0.1% of the intravenous dose).

Table 1. Pharmacokinetic parameters of Saikosaponin a (SSa), paeonol (PA), and imperatorin (IMP) after intravenous administration of each drug to rats (mean ± standard deviations (SD)).

Parameters	SSa			PA		IMP		
	2.3 mg/kg (n = 5)	4.6 mg/kg (n = 4)	14.8 mg/kg (n = 5)	29.6 mg/kg (n = 5)	59.2 mg/kg (n = 6)	2.9 mg/kg (n = 5)	5.8 mg/kg (n = 6)	11.5 mg/kg (n = 5)
Body weight (g)	290 ± 7.91	288 ± 8.66	262 ± 7.58	263 ± 12.5	258 ± 7.58	274 ± 10.7	280 ± 10.5	289 ± 11.9
$AUC_{0\text{-}inf}$ (µg·min/mL) [a]	517 ± 64.3	1840 ± 349 [b]	511 ± 65.3	1250 ± 250	2820 ± 400 [f]	55.9 ± 12.4	126 ± 23.9	496 ± 66.5 [h]
CL (mL/min/kg)	4.51 ± 0.583	2.56 ± 0.418 [c]	29.3 ± 3.60	24.4 ± 4.03	21.4 ± 3.29 [g]	53.9 ± 11.9	47.5 ± 9.85	23.5 ± 3.07 [i]
CL_R (µL/min/kg)	321 ± 177	60.2 ± 34.2 [d]	587 ± 535	232 ± 110	556 ± 382	39.4 ± 9.33	42.5 ± 27.7	13.8 ± 4.35
CL_{NR} (mL/min/kg)	4.19 ± 0.492	2.50 ± 0.387 [c]	28.7 ± 3.75	24.2 ± 3.98	20.8 ± 3.16 [g]	53.9 ± 11.9	47.5 ± 9.87	23.5 ± 3.07 [i]
V_{ss} (mL/kg)	126 ± 11.1	102 ± 8.16 [e]	1130 ± 290	1290 ± 327	1100 ± 429	1760 ± 595	1600 ± 333	1470 ± 254
MRT (min)	28.2 ± 4.33	40.3 ± 4.73 [e]	38.5 ± 8.43	53.5 ± 14.0	51.4 ± 18.9	32.1 ± 5.46	39.4 ± 15.2	63.1 ± 12.1 [i]
Terminal half-life (min)	93.9 ± 18.7	91.5 ± 16.0	81.5 ± 17.4	157 ± 53.7	214 ± 111	77.8 ± 5.58	75.1 ± 18.2	77.7 ± 36.0
$Ae_{0\text{-}24h}$ (% of dose)	6.94 ± 3.67	2.22 ± 1.16 [d]	2.06 ± 1.87	0.941 ± 0.362	2.55 ± 1.78	0.0750 ± 0.0191	0.0986 ± 0.0785	0.0605 ± 0.0223
Gl_{24h} (% of dose)	0.701 ± 1.17	0.481 ± 0.219	0.182 ± 0.124	0.186 ± 0.223	0.153 ± 0.165	0.0105 ± 0.00709	0.0103 ± 0.00265	0.0153 ± 0.0106

[a] Dose-normalized values were compared when statistical analysis was performed. [b] Dose-normalized value was significantly different from 2.3 mg/kg group ($p < 0.01$, t-test). [c] The value was significantly different from 2.3 mg/kg group ($p < 0.001$, t-test). [d] The value was significantly different from 2.3 mg/kg group ($p < 0.05$, t-test). [e] The value was significantly different from 2.3 mg/kg group ($p < 0.01$, t-test). [f] Dose-normalized value was significantly different from 14.8 mg/kg group ($p < 0.05$, one-way analysis of variance (ANOVA) with post hoc Tukey test). [g] The value was significantly different from 14.8 mg/kg group ($p < 0.05$, one-way ANOVA with post hoc Tukey test). [h] Dose-normalized value was significantly different from 2.9 and 5.8 mg/kg groups ($p < 0.05$, one-way ANOVA with post hoc Tukey test). [i] The value was significantly different from 2.9 and 5.8 mg/kg groups ($p < 0.05$, one-way ANOVA with post hoc Tukey test).

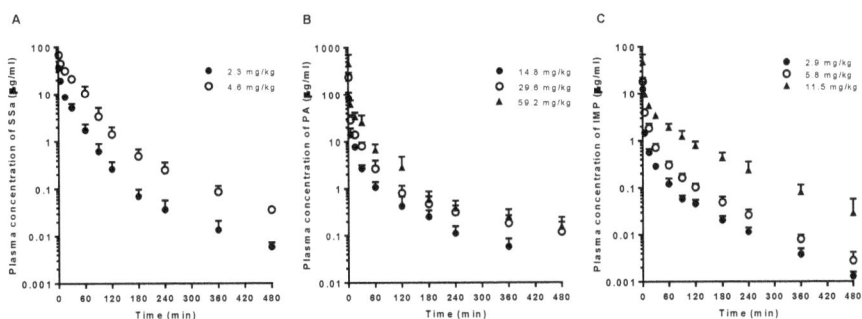

Figure 2. Mean arterial plasma concentration-time profiles of (**A**) SSa, (**B**) PA, and (**C**) IMP following 1-min intravenous administration of each pure compound at various doses (2.3 ($n = 5$) and 4.6 ($n = 4$) mg/kg of SSa; 14.8 ($n = 5$), 29.6 ($n = 5$), and 59.2 ($n = 6$) mg/kg of PA; and 2.9 ($n = 5$), 5.8 ($n = 6$), and 11.5 ($n = 5$) mg/kg of IMP) to rats. Vertical bars represent SD.

3.2. PKs of SSa after the Oral Administration of Pure SSa and DA-9805

The mean arterial plasma concentration-time profiles of SSa after oral administration in rats of pure SSa at doses of 2.3 and 4.6 mg/kg and DA-9805 at doses of 0.25, 0.5, and 1 g/kg (equivalent to 1.1, 2.3, and 4.6 mg/kg, respectively, as SSa) are shown in Figure 3. The relevant PK parameters are also listed in Table 2. Most of the plasma concentrations of SSa following oral administration of pure SSa at the lowest dose (1.1 mg/kg) were less than the lower limit of quantification (LLOQ; 0.5 ng/mL); thus, the data were excluded for PK analyses. The AUC and C_{max} values of SSa were dose-proportional following oral administration of pure SSa and DA-9805. Interestingly, the AUC_{0-8h} values of SSa following oral administration of DA-9805 were significantly greater (by 96.1% and 163%) than those following oral administration of each equivalent dose of pure SSa, whereas the C_{max} values were comparable between pure SSa and DA-9805. Therefore, the F values were greater (by 96.2% and 163%) following DA-9805 administration than after pure SSa administration. The F values of SSa following oral administration were extremely low (<0.1% of oral dose). Interestingly, the recovery from the GI tract ($GI_{24 h}$ values) was significantly higher (24.5- and 3.1-fold) in rats with DA-9805 administration than in rats with pure SSa administration.

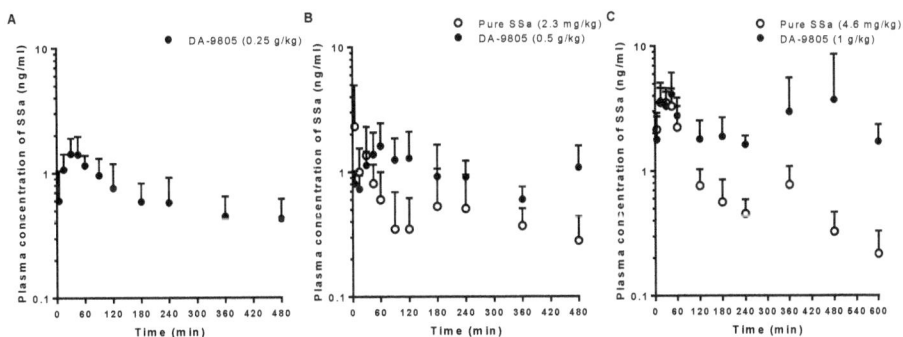

Figure 3. Mean arterial plasma concentration–time profiles of SSa following oral administration of DA-9805 (closed circle) at doses of 0.25 g/kg ((**A**); 1.1 mg/kg as SSa, $n = 5$), 0.5 g/kg ((**B**); 2.3 mg/kg as SSa, $n = 5$), and 1 g/kg ((**C**); 4.6 mg/kg as SSa, $n = 5$) and pure SSa (open circle) at doses of 2.3 mg/kg ((**B**); $n = 4$) and 4.6 mg/kg ((**C**); $n = 5$) to rats. Vertical bars represent SD.

Table 2. Pharmacokinetic parameters of SSa after oral administration of pure SSa or DA-9805 at doses equivalent to 1.1, 2.3, and 4.6 mg/kg of SSa to rats (mean ± SD).

Parameters	Oral Doses				
	1.1 mg/kg as SSa	2.3 mg/kg as SSa		4.6 mg/kg as SSa	
	DA-9805 0.25 g/kg (n = 5)	Pure SSa 2.3 mg/kg (n = 4)	DA-9805 0.5 g/kg (n = 5)	Pure SSa 4.6 mg/kg (n = 5)	DA-9805 1 g/kg (n = 5)
Body weight (g)	257 ± 5.70	249 ± 6.29	252 ± 6.71	204 ± 9.62	212 ± 5.70
AUC_{0-8h} (µg·min/mL) [a]	0.285 ± 0.0948	0.206 ± 0.129	0.404 ± 0.0839 *	0.460 ± 0.0451	1.21 ± 0.586 *
AUC_{0-10h} (µg·min/mL) [a]				0.490 ± 0.0521	1.49 ± 0.769 *
C_{max} (µg/mL) [a]	1.61 ± 0.248	3.00 ± 2.22	1.91 ± 0.808	4.67 ± 0.883	6.70 ± 3.46
T_{max} (min) [b]	45 (15–60)	17.5 (5–30)	60 (60–120)	30 (15–45)	45 (15–480)
GI_{24h} (% of dose)	2.19 ± 5.47	1.99 ± 1.49	26.5 ± 6.99 ***	14.2 ± 12.4	44.4 ± 7.17 ***
F (%)		0.0399	0.0783	0.0251	0.0659

[a] Dose-normalized values were compared when statistical analysis was performed. [b] T_{max} is expressed as median (range). * The value was significantly different from each same equivalent dose of pure SSa groups (* p < 0.05, *** p < 0.001; *t*-test).

3.3. PKs of PA after the Oral Administration of Pure PA and DA-9805

The mean arterial plasma concentration-time profiles of PA in rats after oral administration of pure PA at doses of 14.8, 29.6, and 59.2 mg/kg and equivalent doses of DA-9805 are shown in Figure 4. The relevant PK parameters are listed in Table 3. The AUC and C_{max} values of PA were proportional to PA doses following oral administration of pure PA and DA-9805. The AUC values of PA following oral administration of 0.5 and 1 g/kg of DA-9805 were significantly greater (by 164% and 155%) than those following the oral administration of each equivalent dose of pure PA, whereas the C_{max} values were comparable between pure PA and DA-9805 or even less than those in the pure PA group. Again, greater F values of PA were observed following DA-9805 administration than after pure PA administration (28.7–41.7% vs. 12.2–16.4%). Following the administration of DA-9805, slow absorption of PA supported by delayed T_{max} was observed compared to pure PA administration.

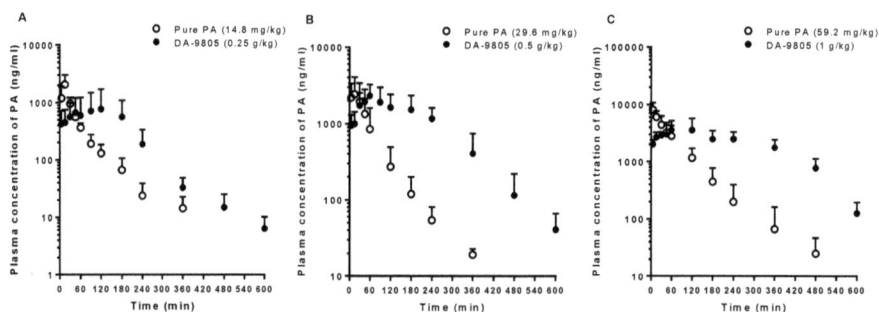

Figure 4. Mean arterial plasma concentration–time profiles of PA following oral administration of DA-9805 (closed circle) at doses of 0.25 g/kg (**A**; 14.8 mg/kg as PA, n = 5), 0.5 g/kg (**B**; 29.6 mg/kg as PA, n = 5), and 1 g/kg (**C**; 59.2 mg/kg as PA, n = 5) mg/kg and equivalent doses of pure PA (open circle; 14.8 mg/kg (**A**; n = 4), 29.6 mg/kg (**B**; n = 5), and 59.2 mg/kg (**C**; n = 4)) to rats. Vertical bars represent SD.

Table 3. Pharmacokinetic parameters of PA after oral administration of pure PA or DA-9805 at doses equivalent to 14.8, 29.6, and 59.2 mg/kg of PA to rats (mean $\pm$ SD).

Parameters	Oral Doses					
	14.8 mg/kg as PA		29.6 mg/kg as PA		59.2 mg/kg as PA	
	Pure PA 14.8 mg/kg ($n = 4$)	DA-9805 0.25 g/kg ($n = 5$)	Pure PA 29.6 mg/kg ($n = 5$)	DA-9805 0.5 g/kg ($n = 5$)	Pure PA 59.2 mg/kg ($n = 4$)	DA-9805 1 g/kg ($n = 5$)
Body weight (g)	251 $\pm$ 12.5	257 $\pm$ 5.70	247 $\pm$ 6.71	252 $\pm$ 6.71	204 $\pm$ 7.50	212 $\pm$ 5.70
AUC_{0-inf} ($\mu g \cdot min/mL$) [a]	82.4 $\pm$ 11.5	147 $\pm$ 129	153 $\pm$ 101	404 $\pm$ 83.9 *	462 $\pm$ 142	1180 $\pm$ 341 **
Terminal half-life (min)	79.1 $\pm$ 51.7	98.8 $\pm$ 56.1	70.5 $\pm$ 29.7	66.8 $\pm$ 15.6	50.5 $\pm$ 13.4	84.2 $\pm$ 55.4
C_{max} ($\mu g/mL$) [a]	2.05 $\pm$ 0.956	1.05 $\pm$ 0.855	2.78 $\pm$ 1.46	2.48 $\pm$ 0.853	8.20 $\pm$ 2.63	4.17 $\pm$ 1.53 *
T_{max} (min) [b]	15 (15)	30 (15–120)	15 (5–30)	60 (60–180)	5 (5–15)	120 (30–120)
GI_{24h} (% of dose)	0.406 $\pm$ 0.212	0.511 $\pm$ 1.01	0.0572 $\pm$ 0.0426	1.24 $\pm$ 1.39	0.119 $\pm$ 0.143	0.167 $\pm$ 0.128
F (%)	16.1	28.7	12.2	40.5	16.4	41.7

[a] Dose-normalized values were compared when statistical analysis was performed. [b] T_{max} is expressed as median (range). * The value was significantly different from each same equivalent dose of pure PA groups (* $p < 0.05$, ** $p < 0.01$; t-test).

3.4. PKs of IMP after the Oral Administration of Pure IMP and DA-9805

The mean arterial plasma concentration-time profiles of IMP after oral administration in rats of pure IMP at doses of 1.4, 2.9, and 5.8 mg/kg and equivalent doses of DA-9805 are shown in Figure 5. The relevant PK parameters are listed in Table 4. Following the oral administration of pure IMP, the dose-normalized AUC and C_{max} values of IMP at the highest level (5.8 mg/kg) were significantly greater (by 471% and 513%) than those in the lower dose groups (1.4 and 2.9 mg/kg). By contrast, DA-9805 showed dose-proportional AUC and C_{max} values of IMP in the equivalent oral dose range (0.25–1 g/kg; 1.4–5.8 mg/kg as IMP). Comparable AUC values of IMP were observed between the DA-9805 and pure IMP administration groups. Significantly delayed T_{max} values and/or lowered C_{max} values were observed following DA-9805 administration compared to those after each equivalent dose of pure IMP administration.

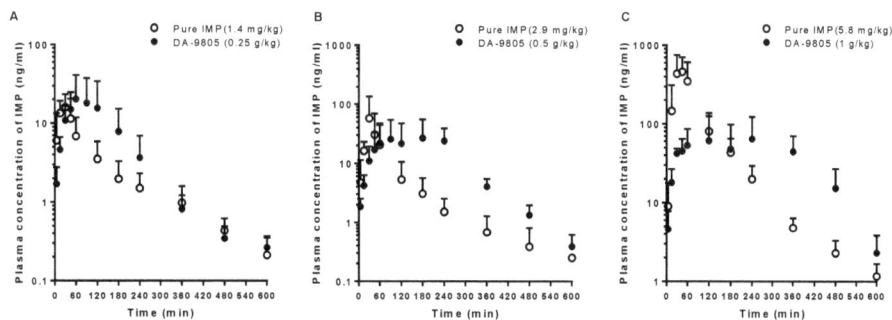

Figure 5. Mean arterial plasma concentration–time profiles of IMP following oral administration of DA-9805 (closed circle) at doses of 0.25 g/kg (**A**; 1.4 mg/kg as IMP, $n = 5$), 0.5 g/kg (**B**; 2.9 mg/kg as IMP, $n = 5$), and 1 g/kg (**C**; 5.8 mg/kg as IMP, $n = 5$) mg/kg and equivalent doses of pure IMP (open circle; 1.4 mg/kg (**A**; $n = 6$), 2.9 (**B**; $n = 6$), and 5.8 mg/kg (**C**; $n = 5$)) to rats. Vertical bars represent SD.

Table 4. Pharmacokinetic parameters of IMP after oral administration of pure IMP or DA-9805 at doses equivalent to 1.4, 2.9, and 5.8 mg/kg of DA-9805 to rats (mean $\pm$ SD).

Parameters	Oral Doses					
	1.4 mg/kg as IMP		2.9 mg/kg as IMP		5.8 mg/kg as IMP	
	Pure IMP 1.4 mg/kg ($n = 6$)	DA-9805 0.25 g/kg ($n = 5$)	Pure IMP 2.9 mg/kg ($n = 6$)	DA-9805 0.5 g/kg ($n = 5$)	Pure IMP 5.8 mg/kg ($n = 5$)	DA-9805 1 g/kg ($n = 5$)
Body weight (g)	258 ± 10.8	257 ± 5.70	253 ± 6.12	252 ± 6.71	204 ± 11.9	212 ± 5.70
AUC_{0-inf} (μg·min/mL) [a]	1.53 ± 0.851	3.02 ± 2.38	2.95 ± 3.13	6.74 ± 5.29	36.2 ± 18.1 [#]	22.5 ± 12.6
Terminal half-life (min)	121 ± 38.3	120 ± 51.1	99.9 ± 31.5	73.8 ± 24.7	101 ± 29.2	56.5 ± 7.26 [*]
C_{max} (μg/mL) [a]	17.7 ± 6.79	28.4 ± 20.8	58.6 ± 76.4	33.5 ± 25.7	568 ± 312 [#]	88.2 ± 46.2 [**]
T_{max} (min) [b]	22.5 (5–45)	60 (30–120)	30 (15–30)	240 (90–240)	30 (15–60)	240 (30–360)
GI_{24h} (% of dose)	0.0285 ± 0.0152	2.19 ± 5.47	0.153 ± 0.228	0.846 ± 0.854	1.37 ± 1.09	6.30 ± 2.89
F (%)			5.27	12.1	28.7	17.8

[a] Dose-normalized values were compared when statistical analysis was performed. [b] T_{max} is expressed as median (range). [#] The dose-normalized value was significantly different from lower dose groups ([#] $p < 0.05$; Kruskal-Wallis test). [*] The value was significantly different from each same equivalent dose of pure IMP group ([*] $p < 0.05$, [**] $p < 0.01$; *t*-test).

3.5. Protein Binding of SSa, PA, and IMP in Rat Plasma and Brain-Tissue Homogenates

The unbound fraction of SSa, PA, and IMP in rat plasma and brain-tissue homogenates are shown in Figure 6. The plasma protein-binding values of SSa, PA, and IMP were $97.3 \pm 0.516\%$ (free fraction of 2.7%), $28.5 \pm 15.4\%$ (free fraction of 71.5%), and $96.5 \pm 0.744\%$ (free fraction of 3.5%), respectively. Nonspecific binding of SSa, PA, and IMP to the equilibrium dialysis devices was negligible because their recovery after incubation was almost complete (>94.7%). The binding values of all three compounds were higher in brain homogenates than in plasma. The binding values of SSa in each brain tissue (striatum, hippocampus, and mixed brain) homogenate were $99.4 \pm 0.138\%$, $99.4 \pm 0.099\%$, and $99.3 \pm 0.124\%$ (free fraction of 0.618, 0.582, and 0.719%), respectively. The binding values of PA in the striatum, hippocampus, and mixed brain homogenates were $96.3 \pm 0.957\%$, $91.9 \pm 2.49\%$, and $90.5 \pm 0.996\%$ (free fraction of 3.75%, 8.10%, and 9.53%), respectively; and the corresponding IMP values were $99.0 \pm 0.10\%$, $98.9 \pm 0.037\%$, and $98.8 \pm 0.068\%$ (free fraction of 1.04%, 1.12%, and 1.22%), respectively.

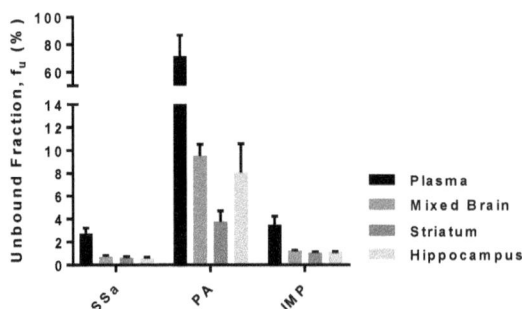

Figure 6. Mean unbound fraction (f_u, %) of SSa, PA, and IMP in rat plasma and brain (mixed brain, striatum, hippocampus) homogenates ($n = 6$ each). Vertical bars represent SD.

3.6. Brain and CSF Distribution of SSa, PA, and IMP after the Oral Administration of DA-9805

The mean plasma, brain regional (frontal cortex, striatum, hippocampus, and cerebellum), and CSF concentration–time profiles and tissue-to-plasma (T/P) ratios of SSa, PA, and IMP after multiple oral administration of DA-9805 (250 mg/kg/day for 8 days) are shown in Figure 7. The T/P ratios of SSa in each brain region were greater than unity (1.26–6.73) at 2 and 6 h, whereas the concentrations of

SSa in CSF were less than the LLOQ. For PA, the T/P ratios in each brain region were slightly greater than unity (1.13–1.98) at 2 h after the final DA-9805 oral dose, whereas the values, with the exception of those for the cerebellum, became smaller than unity at 6 h. The PA levels in the CSF were notably lower than those in the brain tissues and plasma. The T/P ratios of IMP in each brain region were greater than unity (1.24–3.04) at 2 h after the final dose, whereas the values became smaller than unity at 6 h. The concentrations of IMP in CSF were below the LLOQ.

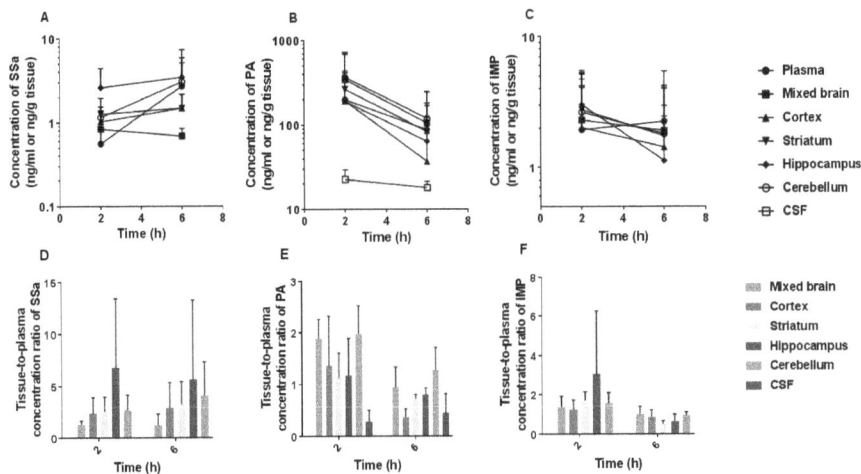

Figure 7. Mean plasma and brain regional concentration–time profiles of (**A**) SSa, (**B**) PA, and (**C**) IMP and their tissue-to-plasma (T/P) concentration ratios (**D**, **E**, and **F** for SSa, PA, and IMP, respectively) following multiple oral administration of DA-9805 (250 mg/kg/day for 8 days) at 2 h (*n* = 5) and 6 h (*n* = 4) after the final dose. Vertical bars represent SD.

4. Discussion

The effective oral dose of DA-9805 is 10–30 mg/kg/day in mice, and the planned dose regimen in the clinical study would be 30 mg or 60 mg three times a day (internal reports). However, the PKs of DA-9805 at this effective dose range could not be investigated due to the extremely low concentrations (<1%) of the two representative ingredients, SSa and IMP, in DA-9805. The doses of SSa (1.1–4.6 mg/kg), PA (14.8–59.2 mg/kg), and IMP (1.4–11.5 mg/kg) used in this study were determined based on the maximal tolerated dose of DA-9805, their concentrations in DA-9805, and assay sensitivity of each substance. Based on the relationship between the dose and PK parameters, the PKs of each component of DA-9805 in the effective dose range could be estimated.

The plasma concentrations of SSa after its intravenous administration at doses of 2.3 and 4.6 mg/kg decreased in a polyexponential fashion (Figure 2A). Based on the slower CL (primarily CL_{NR}) of SSa and greater dose-normalized AUC in the higher dose group, SSa was eliminated via a saturable process. The CL values of SSa were relatively slow compared to those of PA and IMP. Although the contribution of CL_R to CL was small (2.22–6.94%), renal excretion of SSa seemed to also be saturated in the higher dose group based on the slowed CL_R. The CL_R of SSa as the free (unbound to plasma proteins) fraction ($CL_{R,fu}$) was estimated based on the CL_R (Table 1) and free fraction of SSa in plasma. The estimated value was 2.23–11.9 mL/min/kg, similar to the reported glomerular filtration rate in rats at 5.24 mL/min/kg [39]. The V_{ss} values of SSa (102–126 mL/kg) were relatively small considering that the total body water in rats is 668 mL/kg [39]; hence, the distribution of SSa in tissues might be restricted due to its hydrophilicity, large molecular weight, and high binding affinity to plasma protein.

Interestingly, SSa showed linear PKs following the oral administration of pure SSa and DA-9805 based on the dose-proportional AUC and C_{max} values. This is because of the linear elimination of SSa at much lower plasma concentrations of SSa following oral administration in contrast to the saturation of SSa elimination following intravenous administration. The dose-normalized AUC of SSa following oral administration of 4.6 mg/kg of pure SSa is also similar to the dose-normalized value in previous reports with a much higher dose in TCM (~42 mg/kg as SSa) [13]. Note that the F values of SSa following oral administration were extremely low (<0.1%). Slow SSa CL (Table 1) suggested that its first-pass metabolism is not considerable. Therefore, the extremely low F value of SSa was most likely due to incomplete absorption. The low permeability of SSa because of its large molecular weight (>700 Da) and hydrophilicity may contribute to incomplete absorption. Considering the extremely low F values of SSa, its recovery from the GI tract ($GI_{24 h}$ values, Table 2) seems incomplete due to possible decomposition in the GI tract. SSa, which includes an unstable allyl oxide linkage, could be converted into diene saponin by gastric juice [40]. In addition, both the SSa and diene-transformed saikosaponins could be stripped of their sugar moieties by intestinal flora [40,41]. Therefore, the decomposition of SSa in the GI tract could also be one of the possible reasons for the incomplete absorption.

The plasma concentrations of PA after its intravenous administration at dose ranges of 14.8–59.2 mg/kg also decreased in a polyexponential fashion (Figure 2B). PA showed slower CL (primarily CL_{NR}) and greater dose-normalized AUC values at the highest dose than at the lowest dose. This indicates that the elimination of PA is saturated at the highest dose. Intravenous PA over the lower dose range of 2.5–10 mg/kg showed linear PKs supported by constant CL (49.3–53.2 mL/min/kg) and dose-proportional AUC values [21]. The CL values of PA (21.4–29.3 mL/min/kg) obtained in this study (dose range of 14.8–59.2 mg/kg), which are slower than those from a previous report, again suggest the saturation of elimination at a higher dose range in this study. The CL_R of PA as a free (unbound to plasma proteins) fraction ($CL_{R,fu}$) was estimated based on the CL_R (Table 1) and free fraction of PA in plasma. Thus, the $CL_{R,fu}$ values estimated were 0.324–0.821 mL/min/kg, slower than the reported glomerular filtration rate in rats (5.24 mL/min/kg) [39]. The above data indicate that PA was primarily reabsorbed from the renal tubules in rats. Because the contribution of CL_R of PA to CL was negligible (0.941–2.55%), nonrenal elimination was concluded to be the major elimination route of PA. The V_{ss} values of PA (1100–1290 mL/kg) are greater than the reported total body water in rats (668 mL/kg) [39]. Unlike following intravenous administration, PA showed linear PKs following the oral administration of pure PA and DA-9805 at a dose range of 14.8–59.2 mg/kg as PA. The linear oral PKs of PA have been reported with a pure PA dose range of 35 to 140 mg/kg in rats [22].

The plasma concentrations of IMP after its intravenous administration at a dose range of 2.9–11.5 mg/kg also decreased in a polyexponential fashion (Figure 2C). Slowed CL (primarily CL_{NR}) and increased dose-normalized AUC values of IMP in the highest dose group suggested the saturation of its elimination at the highest dose. The almost negligible recovery from urine (Ae_{0-24h}) and CL_R of IMP (Table 1) indicates that the major elimination route of IMP is a nonrenal process. IMP showed the greatest V_{ss} values among the three components of DA-9805, which suggests that it has the highest affinity to tissue(s). Following oral administration of pure IMP, the significantly greater dose-normalized AUC and C_{max} values of IMP at the highest level (5.8 mg/kg) than those in the lower-dose groups (1.4 and 2.9 mg/kg) could be a result of the saturation of first-pass metabolism of IMP at the highest dose.

When the PKs of each component following oral administration of DA-9805 were compared to the administration of each equivalent dose of pure component, several significant and interesting differences were found. First, following the oral administration of DA-9805, significantly higher plasma concentrations, and hence, greater AUC and F values of SSa and PA, were observed than those following oral administration of each equivalent dose of pure SSa and PA. This suggests the significant influence of DA-9805 component(s) on the PKs of SSa and PA. Among the components of DA-9805, IMP shows inhibitory effects on CYP1A2 and 2B6 in both human and rat liver microsomes [42]. It also has weaker inhibitory effects on other major human (2C19, 2C9, 2D6, and 3A4) and rat (2D2 and 3A1/2)

CYP isozymes. O-demethylation of PA is the major in vivo metabolic pathway in rats [22], and the major isoform responsible for O-demethylation of PA in human liver microsomes is CYP1A2 [43]. Therefore, it is likely that IMP in DA-9805 inhibits the hepatic metabolism of PA via CYP1A2 and results in greater AUC values of PA following DA-9805 administration than after pure PA administration. SSa is also mainly metabolized in a Phase I manner [44]. Although the enzymes responsible for this Phase I metabolism of SSa have not been reported, the inhibition of SSa metabolism by IMP or other component(s) in DA-9805 could result in increased AUCs following DA-9805 administration.

Second, significantly more SSa was recovered from the GI tract at 24 h (including feces collected for 24 h) after the oral dose ($GI_{24 h}$ values in Table 2) when DA-9805 was administered compared to pure SSa administration. This may not be due to decreased absorption of SSa when DA-9805 was administered compared to when pure SSa was administered because even greater AUC and F values of SSa were observed in rats with DA-9805 administration. Possibly, other saikosaponins and sugar-containing glycosides in DA-9805 could competitively prevent the decomposition of SSa in the GI lumen such as the hydrolysis of sugar moieties by intestinal flora.

Finally, the absorption of PA and IMP seemed to be delayed following oral administration of DA-9805 supported by their delayed T_{max} values compared to the administration of each pure component. Multiple components in DA-9805 might influence the absorption rate of each component. One of the possible reasons for the slowed absorption of PA and IMP could be slowed GI motility following DA-9805 administration because both Radix Paeoniae [45,46] and Radix Bupleuri [47] have antispasmodic effects on the GI tract. Because of the delayed absorption of IMP following DA-9805 administration, the C_{max} value of IMP is lowered and might not reach the level to cause saturation of its first-pass metabolism. This explains linear PKs of IMP up to the highest oral dose, when DA-9805 was administered. By contrast, following the highest oral dose (5.8 mg/kg) of pure IMP, possible saturation of its first-pass metabolism may result in greater dose-normalized AUCs than the lower dose groups.

Enhanced exposure of SSa and PA and delayed absorption of PA and IMP when administered as DA-9805 resulted in favorable PK profiles (i.e., elevated and sustained plasma concentrations of the three active components). The different PKs of the active components when administered as DA-9805 suggest possibly superior efficacy of DA-9805 over each pure component or their simple mixture.

The binding values of SSa and IMP to plasma protein were considerable (97.3% and 96.5%, respectively), whereas PA has relatively low binding values. However, the binding values of SSa, PA, and IMP were all considerable (>90.5%) in mixed brain, striatum, and hippocampus homogenates. Note that all three components of DA-9805 showed greater binding values (smaller free fraction) in brain homogenates than in plasma, possibly enabling their higher concentrations in the brain than in plasma. This result is consistent with the tissue-to-plasma ratios of the three components being greater than unity in most brain tissues at 2 h following multiple oral administrations of DA-9805. PA and IMP pass through the blood–brain barrier [14,32]. The concentrations of IMP in the striatum and hippocampus are higher than those in other regions [32]; our results are consistent with those findings. Notably, a brain-to-plasma ratio greater than unity of SSa suggests the possibility that SSa passes through the blood–brain barrier, despite its high polarity and large molecular weight, in line with previous studies reporting pharmacological activities of SSa in CNS [10,11]. By contrast, extremely low concentrations of the three components in the CSF suggest that the distribution of the three components in the CSF is negligible.

5. Conclusions

Following the intravenous administration of each pure component of DA-9805 (SSa, PA, and IMP), all three components showed dose-dependent PKs because of the saturation of elimination at a higher dose. By contrast, the dose-proportional AUC values of SSa, PA, and IMP were observed following oral administration of each pure component (except IMP at the highest dose) or DA-9805. Compared to the oral administration of each pure compound, oral administration as DA-9805 showed an increase in the AUC of SSa and PA, possibly due to inhibition of their metabolism by IMP or other component(s) in DA-9805. A delay in the absorption of PA and IMP was also observed when they were administered as DA-9805. The binding values of SSa and IMP to plasma protein or brain homogenates were considerable, whereas PA had relatively low binding values in plasma. All three components showed greater binding values in brain homogenates than in plasma, possibly explaining the observed brain-to-plasma ratios being greater than unity following multiple oral administrations of DA-9805 in contrast to their negligible levels in the CSF. This study furthers our understanding of the comprehensive PKs of SSa, PA, and IMP in rats and comparative oral PKs between each pure component and DA-9805.

Author Contributions: Conceptualization, J.S.J., J.R., Y.W.C. and H.E.K.; funding acquisition, H.E.K.; methodology, H.E.K.; formal analysis, M.H.K. and H.E.K.; investigation, M.H.K. and H.E.K.; resources, J.S.J., J.R. and Y.W.C.; Writing-Original draft preparation, M.H.K.; Writing-Review and editing, H.E.K.

Funding: This research was supported by the Technology Innovation Program funded by the Ministry of Trade, Industry, and Energy, Republic of Korea (No. 10051960), Dong-A ST Co. Ltd, Basic Science Research Program through the National Research Foundation of Korea (NRF) funded by the Ministry of Education (2018R1A6A1A03025108), and the Research Fund 2018 of the Catholic University of Korea.

Conflicts of Interest: The authors declare no conflict of interest. J.S.J., J.R., and Y.W.C. are full-time employees of Dong-A ST Co. Ltd. The funders had no role in the design of the study; in the collection, analyses, or interpretation of data; in the writing of the manuscript, and in the decision to publish the results.

Abbreviations

Ae_{0-24h}	the percentage of the dose excreted in the urine during 24 h
AUC	area under the plasma concentration–time curve
CL	time-averaged total body clearance
CL_{NR}	time-averaged nonrenal clearance
CL_R	time-averaged renal clearance
C_{max}	maximum plasma concentration
F	the extent of absolute oral bioavailability
f_u	unbound fraction
GI_{24h}	the percentage of the dose recovered from the gastrointestinal tract at 24 h (including their contents and feces during 24 h)
IMP	imperatorin
IS	internal standard
LC-MS/MS	liquid chromatographic–tandem mass spectrometry
LLOQ	lower limit of quantification
MRT	mean residence time
PA	paeonol
PKs	pharmacokinetics
SD	standard deviation
SSa	saikosaponin a
T_{max}	time to reach C_{max}
V_{ss}	apparent volume of distribution at steady state

References

1. Amro, M.S.; Teoh, S.L.; Norzana, A.G.; Srijit, D. The potential role of herbal products in the treatment of Parkinson's disease. *Clin. Ter.* **2018**, *169*, e23–e33. [PubMed]
2. Francardo, V.; Schmitz, Y.; Sulzer, D.; Cenci, M.A. Neuroprotection and neurorestoration as experimental therapeutics for Parkinson's disease. *Exp. Neurol.* **2017**, *298*, 137–147. [CrossRef] [PubMed]
3. Park, W.H.; Kang, S.; Piao, Y.; Pak, C.J.; Oh, M.S.; Kim, J.; Kang, M.S.; Pak, Y.K. Ethanol extract of *Bupleurum falcatum* and saikosaponins inhibit neuroinflammation via inhibition of NF-κB. *J. Ethnopharmacol.* **2015**, *174*, 37–44. [CrossRef] [PubMed]

4. Lee, J.Y.; Kim, H.S.; Oh, T.H.; Yune, T.Y. Ethanol extract of *Bupleurum falcatum* improves functional recovery by inhibiting matrix metalloproteinases-2 and -9 activation and inflammation after spinal cord injury. *Exp. Neurobiol.* **2010**, *19*, 146–154. [CrossRef] [PubMed]

5. Lee, B.; Shim, I.; Lee, H.; Hahm, D.H. Effect of *Bupleurum falcatum* on the stress-induced impairment of spatial working memory in rats. *Biol. Pharm. Bull.* **2009**, *32*, 1392–1398. [CrossRef] [PubMed]

6. Kim, H.G.; Park, G.; Piao, Y.; Kang, M.S.; Pak, Y.K.; Hong, S.P.; Oh, M.S. Effects of the root bark of *Paeonia suffruticosa* on mitochondria-mediated neuroprotection in an MPTP-induced model of Parkinson's disease. *Food Chem. Toxicol.* **2014**, *65*, 293–300. [CrossRef] [PubMed]

7. Moon, Y.J.; Lee, J.Y.; Oh, M.S.; Pak, Y.K.; Park, K.S.; Oh, T.H.; Yune, T.Y. Inhibition of inflammation and oxidative stress by *Angelica dahuricae* radix extract decreases apoptotic cell death and improves functional recovery after spinal cord injury. *J. Neurosci. Res.* **2012**, *90*, 243–256. [CrossRef] [PubMed]

8. Tang, Y.H.; Zhang, Y.Y.; Zhu, H.Y.; Huang, C.G. A high-performance liquid chromatographic method for saikosaponin a quantification in rat plasma. *Biomed. Chromatogr.* **2007**, *21*, 458–462. [CrossRef] [PubMed]

9. Chen, M.F.; Huang, C.C.; Liu, P.S.; Chen, C.H.; Shiu, L.Y. Saikosaponin a and saikosaponin d inhibit proliferation and migratory activity of rat HSC-T6 cells. *J. Med. Food* **2013**, *16*, 793–800. [CrossRef] [PubMed]

10. Ye, M.; Bi, Y.F.; Ding, L.; Zhu, W.W.; Gao, W. Saikosaponin a functions as anti-epileptic effect in pentylenetetrazol induced rats through inhibiting mTOR signaling pathway. *Biomed. Pharmacother.* **2016**, *81*, 281–287. [CrossRef] [PubMed]

11. Mao, X.; Miao, G.; Tao, X.; Hao, S.; Zhang, H.; Li, H.; Hou, Z.; Tian, R.; Lu, T.; Ma, J.; et al. Saikosaponin a protects TBI rats after controlled cortical impact and the underlying mechanism. *Am. J. Transl. Res.* **2016**, *8*, 133–141. [PubMed]

12. Liu, Y.; Li, Z.; Liu, X.; Pan, R. Review on the toxic effects of Radix Bupleuri. *Curr. Opin. Complement. Alternat. Med.* **2014**, *1*, 3–7.

13. Xu, L.; Song, R.; Tian, J.X.; Tian, Y.; Liu, G.Q.; Zhang, Z.J. Analysis of saikosaponins in rat plasma by anionic adducts-based liquid chromatography tandem mass spectrometry method. *Biomed. Chromatogr.* **2012**, *26*, 808–815. [CrossRef] [PubMed]

14. Li, H.; Wang, S.; Yang, Q.; Xie, Y.; Cao, W.; Zhang, B.; Wang, J.; Wang, J.; Wang, M. LC tissue distribution study of paeonol in rats after oral administration. *Chromatographia* **2011**, *73*, 495–500. [CrossRef]

15. Li, Y.J.; Bao, J.X.; Xu, J.W.; Murad, F.; Bian, K. Vascular dilation by paeonol—A mechanism study. *Vasc. Pharmacol.* **2010**, *53*, 169–176. [CrossRef] [PubMed]

16. Lee, B.; Shin, Y.W.; Bae, E.A.; Han, S.J.; Kim, J.S.; Kang, S.S.; Kim, D.H. Antiallergic effect of the root of *Paeonia lactiflora* and its constituents paeoniflorin and paeonol. *Arch. Pharm. Res.* **2008**, *31*, 445–450. [CrossRef] [PubMed]

17. Tsai, H.Y.; Lin, H.Y.; Fong, Y.C.; Wu, J.B.; Chen, Y.F.; Tsuzuki, M.; Tang, C.H. Paeonol inhibits RANKL-induced osteoclastogenesis by inhibiting ERK, p38 and NF-kappaB pathway. *Eur. J. Pharmacol.* **2008**, *588*, 124–133. [CrossRef] [PubMed]

18. Hsieh, C.L.; Cheng, C.Y.; Tsai, T.H.; Lin, I.H.; Liu, C.H.; Chiang, S.Y.; Lin, J.G.; Lao, C.J.; Tang, N.Y. Paeonol reduced cerebral infarction involving the superoxide anion and microglia activation in ischemia-reperfusion injured rats. *J. Ethnopharmacol.* **2006**, *106*, 208–215. [CrossRef] [PubMed]

19. Wu, J.B.; Song, N.N.; Wei, X.B.; Guan, H.S.; Zhang, X.M. Protective effects of paeonol on cultured rat hippocampal neurons against oxygen-glucose deprivation-induced injury. *J. Neurol. Sci.* **2008**, *264*, 50–55. [CrossRef] [PubMed]

20. Zhong, S.Z.; Ge, Q.H.; Qu, R.; Li, Q.; Ma, S.P. Paeonol attenuates neurotoxicity and ameliorates cognitive impairment induced by D-galactose in ICR mice. *J. Neurol. Sci.* **2009**, *277*, 58–64. [CrossRef] [PubMed]

21. Tsai, T.H.; Chou, C.J.; Chen, C.F. Pharmacokinetics of paeonol after intravenous administration in rats. *J. Pharm. Sci.* **1994**, *83*, 1307–1309. [CrossRef] [PubMed]

22. Xie, Y.; Zhou, H.; Wong, Y.F.; Xu, H.X.; Jiang, Z.H.; Liu, L. Study on the pharmacokinetics and metabolism of paeonol in rats treated with pure paeonol and an herbal preparation containing paeonol by using HPLC-DAD-MS method. *J. Pharm. Biomed. Anal.* **2008**, *46*, 748–756. [CrossRef] [PubMed]

23. Xie, Y.; Jiang, Z.H.; Zhou, H.; Ma, W.Z.; Wong, Y.F.; Liu, Z.Q.; Liu, L. The pharmacokinetic study of sinomenine, paeoniflorin and paeonol in rats after oral administration of a herbal product Qingfu Guanjiesu capsule by HPLC. *Biomed. Chromatogr.* **2014**, *28*, 1294–1302. [CrossRef] [PubMed]

24. Xiao, Y.; Zhang, Y.H.; Sheng, Y.X.; Zhang, J.L. LC-MS determination and pharmacokinetic studies of paeonol in rat plasma after administration of different compatibility of Su-Xiao-Xin-Tong prescriptions. *Biomed. Chromatogr.* **2008**, *22*, 527–534. [CrossRef] [PubMed]

25. Abad, M.J.; de las Heras, B.; Silvan, A.M.; Pascual, R.; Bermejo, P.; Rodriquez, B.; Villar, A.M. Effects of furocoumarins from *Cachrys trifida* on some macrophage functions. *J. Pharm. Pharmacol.* **2001**, *53*, 1163–1168. [CrossRef] [PubMed]

26. Ban, H.S.; Lim, S.S.; Suzuki, K.; Jung, S.H.; Lee, S.; Lee, Y.S.; Shin, K.H.; Ohuchi, K. Inhibitory effects of furanocoumarins isolated from the roots of *Angelica dahurica* on prostaglandin E2 production. *Planta Med.* **2003**, *69*, 408–412. [PubMed]

27. Wang, N.; Wu, L.; Cao, Y.; Wang, Y.; Zhang, Y. The protective activity of imperatorin in cultured neural cells exposed to hypoxia re-oxygenation injury via anti-apoptosis. *Fitoterapia* **2013**, *90*, 38–43. [CrossRef] [PubMed]

28. Budzynska, B.; Boguszewska-Czubara, A.; Kruk-Slomka, M.; Skalicka-Wozniak, K.; Michalak, A.; Musik, I.; Biala, G.; Glowniak, K. Effects of imperatorin on nicotine-induced anxiety- and memory-related responses and oxidative stress in mice. *Physiol. Behav.* **2013**, *122*, 46–55. [CrossRef] [PubMed]

29. Luszczki, J.J.; Glowniak, K.; Czuczwar, S.J. Time-course and dose-response relationships of imperatorin in the mouse maximal electroshock seizure threshold model. *Neurosci. Res.* **2007**, *59*, 18–22. [CrossRef] [PubMed]

30. Zhao, G.; Peng, C.; Du, W.; Wang, S. Simultaneous determination of imperatorin and its metabolites in vitro and in vivo by a GC-MS method: Application to a bioavailability and protein binding ability study in rat plasma. *Biomed. Chromatogr.* **2014**, *28*, 947–956. [CrossRef] [PubMed]

31. Zhang, J.; Zhang, M.; Fu, S.; Li, T.; Wang, S.; Zhao, M.; Ding, W.; Wang, C.; Wang, Q. Simultaneous determination of imperatorin and its metabolite xanthotoxol in rat plasma by using HPLC-ESI-MS coupled with hollow fiber liquid phase microextraction. *J. Chromatogr. B Anal. Technol. Biomed. Life Sci.* **2014**, *945–946*, 185–192. [CrossRef] [PubMed]

32. Zhang, X.; Xie, Y.; Cao, W.; Yang, Q.; Miao, S.; Wang, S. Brain distribution study of imperatorin in rats after oral administration assessed by HPLC. *Chromatographia* **2011**, *74*, 259–265. [CrossRef]

33. Lili, W.; Yehong, S.; Qi, Y.; Yan, H.; Jinhui, Z.; Yan, L.; Cheng, G. In vitro permeability analysis, pharmacokinetic and brain distribution study in mice of imperatorin, isoimperatorin and cnidilin in Radix *Angelicae dahuricae*. *Fitoterapia* **2013**, *85*, 144–153. [CrossRef] [PubMed]

34. Li, Y.; Wang, Y.; Tai, W.; Yang, L.; Chen, Y.; Chen, C.; Liu, C. Challenges and solutions of pharmacokinetics for efficacy and safety of traditional Chinese medicine. *Curr. Drug Metab.* **2015**, *16*, 765–776. [CrossRef] [PubMed]

35. Kim, J.M.; Yoon, J.N.; Jung, J.W.; Choi, H.D.; Shin, Y.J.; Han, C.K.; Lee, H.S.; Kang, H.E. Pharmacokinetics of hederacoside C, an active ingredient in AG NPP709, in rats. *Xenobiotica* **2013**, *43*, 985–992. [CrossRef] [PubMed]

36. Kwon, M.H.; Jeong, J.S.; Ryu, J.; Cho, Y.W.; Kang, H.E. Simultaneous determination of saikosaponin a, paeonol, and imperatorin, components of DA-9805, in rat plasma by LC-MS/MS and application to a pharmacokinetic study. *J. Chromatogr. B Anal. Technol. Biomed. Life Sci.* **2017**, *1068–1069*, 289–296. [CrossRef] [PubMed]

37. Chiou, W.L. Critical Evaluation of the potential error in pharmacokinetic studies of using the linear trapezoidal rule method for the calculation of the area under the plasma level–time curve. *J. Pharmacokinet. Biopharm.* **1978**, *6*, 539–546. [CrossRef] [PubMed]

38. Gibaldi, M.; Perrier, D. *Pharmacokinetics*, 2nd ed.; Marcel-Dekker: New York, NY, USA, 1982; ISBN 9780824710422.

39. Davies, B.; Morris, T. Physiological parameters in laboratory animals and humans. *Pharm. Res.* **1993**, *10*, 1093–1095. [CrossRef] [PubMed]

40. Shimizu, K.; Amagaya, S.; Ogihara, Y. Structural transformation of saikosaponins by gastric juice and intestinal flora. *J. Pharmacobiodyn.* **1985**, *8*, 718–725. [CrossRef] [PubMed]

41. Kida, H.; Akao, T.; Meselhy, M.R.; Hattori, M. Metabolism and pharmacokinetics of orally administered saikosaponin b1 in conventional, germ-free and *Eubacterium* Sp. A-44-infected gnotobiote rats. *Biol. Pharm. Bull.* **1998**, *21*, 588–593. [CrossRef] [PubMed]

42. Cao, Y.; Zhong, Y.H.; Yuan, M.; Li, H.; Zhao, C.J. Inhibitory Effect of imperatorin and isoimperatorin on activity of cytochrome p450 enzyme in human and rat liver microsomes. *Zhongguo Zhong Yao Za Zhi* **2013**, *38*, 1237–1241. [PubMed]
43. Liu, H.X.; Hu, Y.; Liu, Y.; He, Y.Q.; Li, W.; Yang, L. CYP1A2 is the major isoform responsible for paeonol *O*-demethylation in human liver microsomes. *Xenobiotica* **2009**, *39*, 672–679. [CrossRef] [PubMed]
44. Liu, G.; Tian, Y.; Li, G.; Xu, L.; Song, R.; Zhang, Z. Metabolism of saikosaponin a in rats: Diverse oxidations on the aglycone moiety in liver and intestine in addition to hydrolysis of glycosidic bonds. *Drug Metab. Dispos.* **2013**, *41*, 622–633. [CrossRef] [PubMed]
45. Chen, L.C.; Chou, M.H.; Lin, M.F.; Yang, L.L. Effects of Paeoniae Radix, a traditional Chinese medicine, on the pharmacokinetics of phenytoin. *J. Clin. Pharm. Ther.* **2001**, *26*, 271–278. [CrossRef] [PubMed]
46. Kobayashi, M.; Ueda, C.; Aoki, S.; Tajima, K.; Tanaka, N.; Yamahara, J. Anticholinergic action of paeony root and its active constituents. *Yakugaku Zasshi* **1990**, *110*, 964–968. [CrossRef] [PubMed]
47. Jung, B.S.; Shin, M.K. *Korean Domestic Pharmaceutical Pharmacopoeia (Herbal Medicine)*; Yeongnimsa: Seoul, Korea, 2003; pp. 412–414. ISBN 9788985897044.

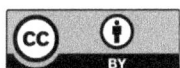

pharmaceutics

MDPI

Article

Pharmacokinetic Drug-Drug Interaction and Responsible Mechanism between Memantine and Cimetidine

Young A. Choi [1], Im-Sook Song [2] and Min-Koo Choi [1,*]

[1]   College of Pharmacy, Dankook University, Cheon-an 31116, Korea; ayha06@gmail.com
[2]   College of Pharmacy and Research Institute of Pharmaceutical Sciences, Kyungpook National University, Daegu 41566, Korea; isssong@knu.ac.kr
*   Correspondence: minkoochoi@dankook.ac.kr; Tel.: +82-43-550-1432

Received: 27 June 2018; Accepted: 3 August 2018; Published: 6 August 2018

Abstract: A sensitive and simple chromatography-tandem mass spectrometry (LC-MS/MS) method was developed to evaluate memantine in rat plasma. Memantine and propranolol (internal standard) in rat plasma was extracted using a methanol precipitation method. The standard curve value was 0.2–1000 ng/mL and selectivity, linearity, inter-day and intra-day accuracy and precision were within acceptance criteria. Using this validated method, drug-drug interactions between memantine and cimetidine was measured following co-administration of memantine and cimetidine intravenously and orally. Plasma exposure of memantine was increased by 1.6- and 3.0-fold by co-medication with cimetidine intravenously and orally, respectively. It suggested that the drug interaction occurred during the gut absorption process, which was consistent with the results showing that the intestinal permeability of memantine in the presence of cimetidine was 3.2-fold greater than that of memantine alone. Inhibition of cimetidine on hepatic elimination of memantine rather than renal excretion was also attributed to the drug-drug interaction between memantine and cimetidine, which explained the decreased clearance of memantine by co-medication with cimetidine. In conclusion, the newly developed simple and sensitive LC-MS/MS analytical method was applied to investigate the pharmacokinetic drug-drug interactions of memantine. Plasma exposure of memantine by co-administration with cimetidine was increased because of its enhanced intestinal permeability and the decreased metabolic activity of memantine.

Keywords: mematine; drug interaction; liquid chromatography-tandem mass spectrometry; pharmacokinetics

---

1. Introduction

Alzheimer's disease is among the most common dementia and is progressed by memory loss, confusion, impaired judgement and disorientation [1]. Currently drugs that can completely cure Alzheimer's disease are not available [2]. Accessible medications focus on symptomatic treatment and only reduce disease progression [2]. Memantine (Namenda®) is N-methyl-D-aspartate antagonist in the brain [3] which has been approved by US Food and Drug Administration (FDA) to treat moderate to severe dementia. Memantine also inhibits the neurodegenerative effects of glutamate [4] and protects neuron cells [5]. Based on this mode of action, memantine showed promising clinical and preclinical effects on several psychiatric disorders such as bipolar disorder, depression, schizophrenia and anxiety disorders as mono or add-on therapy [6]. Therefore, memantine has been prescribed alone or in combination with other cognitive drugs such as donepezil (Aricept®), rivastigmine (Exelon®) and galantamine (Razadyne®) as well as anti-psychotic drugs [6,7]. It has been reported that no drug-drug interaction between memantine and donepezil, rivastigmine and galantamine was observed [8–10]. However, it may interact with other *N*-methyl-D-aspartate receptor ligands such as dextromethorphan, ketamine and phencyclidine and anti-psychotic drugs such as amantadine and dopamine antagonists [6]. Drug-drug interaction may change the pharmacokinetic features and therapeutic response of memantine. In addition, Dizziness and vomiting are common adverse events of memantine, which may be associated with the high plasma concentrations of memantine [5].

Because of its pharmacokinetic-pharmacodynamic relationship, the therapeutic drug monitoring of Alzheimer's disease drugs as well as anti-psychotic drugs is increasingly necessary for studying individual variations, metabolic and kinetic alterations in some patients, responsible mechanisms for decreasing effectiveness and to make a decision to adherence or changing existed therapy [11]. Moreover, to investigate the mechanisms responsible for the possible interaction between memantine and other drugs which may cause the high plasma concentration of memantine, it is necessary to establish an accurate, sensitive and simple bioanalysis method for the detection of memantine in diverse matrices.

Therefore, the aim of this study was to develop and validate a sensitive and simple liquid chromatography tandem mass spectrometry (LC-MS/MS) method for measuring memantine focusing on lowering the required plasma volume and simplifying the overall process. The method was fully validated according to the FDA Guideline for Bioanalytical Method for its linearity, selectivity, accuracy, precision, recovery, stability and matrix effects [12].

To examine application of this analytical method, we investigated pharmacokinetic drug–drug interactions between memantine and cimetidine. To understand the underlying mechanisms of the drug-drug interaction between memantine and cimetidine, we administered memantine with or without cimetidine intravenously as well as orally. Cimetidine was selected because it inhibits cytochrome P 450 (Cyp)-mediated metabolism and the organic cation transporter (Oct)-mediated transport process [13,14]. In addition to Cyp and Oct inhibition, cimetidine, an H2 receptor antagonist, is used to treat peptic ulcers and is the most prescribed over-the-counter drug that is easily accessed by patients [15,16]. Cimetidine is well-absorbed from the gut through the paracellular transport and mainly excreted via the renal route in rats (70% of oral dose was eliminated via the renal route for 72 h) with limited metabolism and low plasma protein binding (approximately 20%) [17,18], suggesting that a high plasma concentration of cimetidine is maintained. Thus, the plausibility of concomitant administration of memantine and cimetidine and drug-drug interaction between memantine and cimetidine seems to be high.

2. Materials and Methods

2.1. Materials

Memantine, cimetidine and propranolol was purchased from Sigma-Aldrich (St. Louis, MO, USA). Methanol and water was of HPLC grade (Burdick & Jackson Korea, Seoul, Korea). All other reagents and solvents were of reagent or analytical grade.

2.2. Animals

Male Sprague-Dawley rats (7–8 weeks, 220–250 g) were purchased from Samtako (Osan, Kyunggi-do, Korea). They were acclimatized to the circumstances for 5 days with water and food ad libitum. Rats were provided a cereal-based maintenance diet, altromin 1320 pellet formula (Altromin, Lage, Germany). Energy density of this diet is about 3227 kcal/kg consisting of 11% of fat, 24% of protein and 65% of carbohydrates. All rats were housed in light (light: 07:00–19:00, dark: 19:00–07:00), temperature ($22 \pm 2\,^\circ$C) and humidity (55 ± 5%)-controlled room.

All animal procedures were approved by the Animal Care and Use Committee of Kyungpook National University (2015-0098) and conducted in accordance with the National Institutes of Health guidance for the care and the use of laboratory animals.

2.3. LC-MS/MS Analysis of Memantine

Memantine in each sample was determined by an Agilent 6430 Triple Quadrupole LC-MS/MS system (Agilent, Wilmington, DE, USA). The isocratic mobile phase consisting a mixture of water and methanol (15:85, v/v) containing 0.1% formic acid was used at a flow rate of 0.20 mL/min to elute memantine and propranolol peak from the rat plasma matrix. The separation was performed on a Polar RP column (150 × 4.6 mm, 5 µm particle size; Pheonomenex, Torrance, CA, USA).

Mass transition was monitored using multiple reaction monitoring (MRM) mode at m/z 180.1 → 163.1 for memantine and m/z 260.0 → 116.0 for propranolol (internal standard, IS) in positive ion mode with a collision energy of 10–15 eV. The analytical data were quantified using mass Hunter (version B.06.00, Agilent, Wilmington, DE, USA).

2.4. Method Validation

2.4.1. Selectivity

The representative MRM chromatograms of the standard lower limit of quantification (LLoQ) concentrations of memantine or propranolol (IS) and plasma samples obtained from a rat 10 h after the oral administration of memantine (5 mg/kg) were compared with those of blank plasma [19].

2.4.2. Linearity of Standard Curves

The calibration curve (0.2, 0.5, 2, 10, 50, 200, 1000 ng/mL) was prepared using an internal standard method. Aliquots of standard curve samples (50 µL) were added to 250 µL of methanol containing 20 ng/mL of propranolol (IS). After vortex-mixing and centrifugation for 10 min at 13,200 rpm, an aliquot (2 µL) of the supernatant was injected into the LC-MS/MS system. Linearity of the calibration standard was calculated from the peak response ratio of memantine to IS with the weight adjusted method ($1/x^2$).

2.4.3. Precisions and Accuracy

The precision and accuracy of inter- and intra-day assays were assessed from five measurements of the quality control (QC) samples (0.6, 20, 500 ng/mL) of memantine. Precision was evaluated from the relative standard deviation (RSD) of five measurements. The accuracy of inter-day and intra-day assays was calculated by dividing the measured QC concentration by the spiked QC concentration. Analytical sample preparations were identical during the validation process.

2.4.4. Matrix Effect and Recovery

Matrix effects were monitored by dividing the peak areas of QC samples in water by those in blank plasma [20]. Recovery was calculated by comparing the peak response of QC in the post-extraction spiked samples with those of the pre-extraction spiked samples [20].

2.4.5. Stability

The stability of memantine and IS in the rat plasma was tested from the low and high QC samples exposed to different conditions [19]. Short-term stability was calculated by comparing QC samples that were stored for 12 h at 25 °C with the untreated QC samples. The freeze-thaw stability was analyzed by comparing QC samples that underwent three freeze–thaw cycles (−80 °C to 25 °C as one cycle) with the untreated QC samples. Post-preparative stability was evaluated by analyzing the extracted QC samples maintained in the autosampler at 6 °C for 24 h compared with the untreated QC samples [19].

2.5. Pharmacokinetic (PK) Interaction Study

Before oral administration or rat jejunum resection, the rats were fasted for 12 h but water ad libitum. On the day of study, the femoral arteries and femoral veins of rats were cannulated with PE50 tubing (Jungdo, Seoul, Korea) under anesthesia with isoflurane (30 mmol/kg).

Cimetidine solution (10 mg/kg/mL in water, four rats) or vehicle solution (1 mL/kg of water, four rats) was injected intravenously to rats at 10 Am and, 5 min later, memantine solution (3 mg/kg/mL in water) was injected intravenously to the same rat. Blood samples (250 μL) were collected from the femoral artery at 0, 0, 0.25, 0.5, 0.75, 1, 1.5, 2, 3, 6, 9, 24 h after intravenous bolus injection of memantine and/or cimetidine. Blood samples were centrifuged for 10 min at 13,200 rpm and aliquots of plasma samples (50 μL) were stored at −80 °C until the analysis. Urine samples were collected for 24 h and pooled urine samples were weighed. 50 μL aliquot of urine samples was stored at −80 °C until the analysis.

Similarly, cimetidine solution (50 mg/kg, dissolved in 2 mL water, four rats) or vehicle solution (2 mL/kg of water, four rats) was administered orally to rats at 10 Am and 30 min later, memantine solution (5 mg/kg, dissolved in 2 mL water) was administered orally to the same rat. Blood samples (250 μL) were collected from the femoral artery at 0, 0.083, 0.25, 0.5, 1, 2, 3, 6, 9, 24 h after oral administration of memantine and/or cimetidine. Blood samples were centrifuged for 10 min at 13,200 rpm and aliquots of plasma samples (50 μL) were stored at −80 °C until the analysis.

Memantine concentrations in plasma and urine samples were analyzed using a LC-MS/MS system.

2.6. Intestinal Permeability Test

Apparent permeability (P_{app}) of memantine in the presence or absence of cimetidine was determined with slight modification of a method of Kwon et al. [21]. Briefly, the rat jejunum segments mounted on the inserts of the Ussing chambers were acclimatized with Hank's balanced salt solution (HBSS) for 15 min. Carbogen gas (5% CO_2/ 95% O_2) was bubbled into the Ussing chambers at a rate of 150 drops/min during the experiment for the jejunum segment viability. The experiments started with changing the HBSS with preheated HBSS containing memantine (0.5 mg/mL) with or without cimetidine (5 mg/mL) to the apical (A) side of jejunum. Aliquots (400 μL) of HBSS in the basal side (B) were withdrawn at 0, 30, 60, 90 and 120 min and compensated with an equal volume of fresh, preheated HBSS. Aliquots of 50 μL of samples were analyzed using a LC-MS/MS system applied to the same sample preparation method.

For system feasibility, P_{app} of caffeine, propranolol, ofloxacin and atenolol were monitored as marker compounds for high, moderate and low permeable drugs. P_{app} value of caffeine and propranolol, positive controls of high permeability, was 36.8×10^{-6} and 23.7×10^{-6} cm/s, respectively, which is consistent with the findings of other studies [22]. P_{app} value of ofloxacin and atenolol, a positive control of moderate and poor permeability, respectively, was 4.5×10^{-6} and 0.04×10^{-6} cm/s, respectively, which corroborates with the findings of other studies [23].

2.7. Microsomal Stability

The metabolic stability of memantine (1 μM) in the presence or absence or cimetidine (0, 2 and 20 μM) in the rat liver microsomes was measured as previously described [24]. Briefly, memantine solution (1 μM) in 100 mM potassium phosphate buffer (pH 7.4) containing 0.5 mg of liver microsomes (from Sprague-Dawley rats; Corning, Tewksbury, MA, USA) and an NADPH-generating system incubated at 37 °C for 0, 15, 30, 45 and 60 min in a shaking water bath. The reaction was quenched by adding ice-cold methanol containing 20 ng/mL of propranolol (250 μL). After undergoing the sample preparation procedure, memantine concentration was measured.

We also measured the metabolic stability of 1 µM metformin and 1 µM propranolol by the same procedure to ensure system feasibility [24]. The percent of remaining metformin and propranolol after 60 min incubation in the rat liver microsomes was 63.4% and 12.2%, respectively.

2.8. Data Analysis and Statistics

PK parameters were calculated using the WinNonlin 2.0 (Pharsight Co., Certara, NJ, USA) and the data are expressed as the means ± standard deviation (SD).

A value of $p < 0.05$ was determined to be statistically significant, using a Mann Whitney test between the two means for unpaired data.

3. Results

3.1. Validation of Analytical Method

3.1.1. Selectivity

Representative MS/MS chromatograms memantine and IS (Figure 1) showed that the memantine and IS peaks were well-separated with no interfering peaks at the respective retention times. The selectivity of the analytes was confirmed in six different rat blank plasma and rat plasma samples obtained after memantine administration. The retention times of memantine and IS were 3.62 and 3.14 min, respectively and the total run time was 4.0 min.

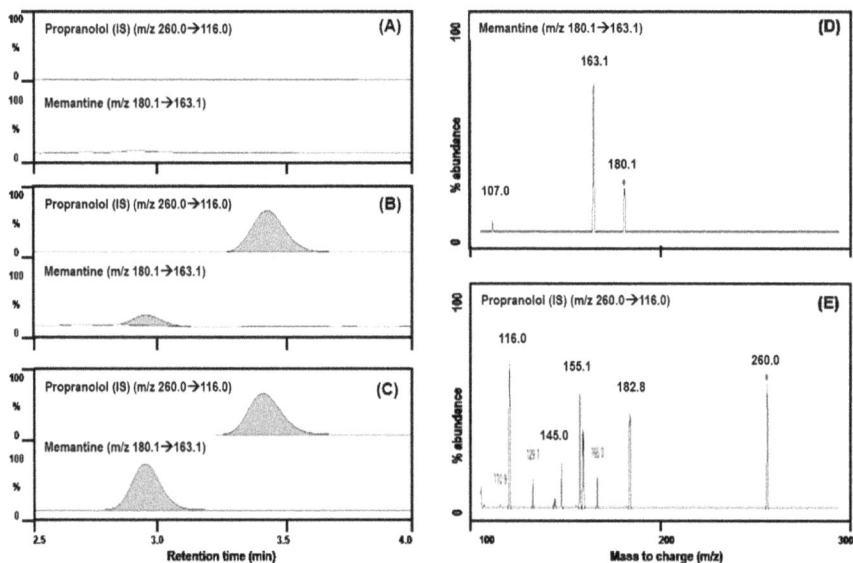

Figure 1. Representative MS/MS chromatograms of memantine and IS in rat (**A**) double blank plasma, (**B**) blank plasma spiked with memantine at lower limit of quantification (LLoQ; 0.2 ng/mL) and propranolol and (**C**) plasma samples following single oral administration of memantine is shown in the left panel. Product ion spectra of memantine (**D**) and propranolol (**E**) are shown in the right panel.

3.1.2. Precision and Accuracy

The precision and accuracy of intra-day and inter-day assays are shown in Table 1. For inter-day validation, the precision was in the range of 8.10 to 11.4%. The accuracy ranged from 101.2 to 108.6%. In intra-day validation, the precision and accuracy ranged from 1.68 to 14.1% and 109.9 to 113.8%, respectively (Table 1).

Table 1. Intra-day and inter-day precision and accuracy of memantine.

Memantine	Spiked (ng/mL)	Inter-day			Intra-day		
		Measured (ng/mL)	Accuracy (%)	Precision (%)	Measured (ng/mL)	Accuracy (%)	Precision (%)
Low QC	0.6	0.62 ± 0.05	101.2	8.10	0.68 ± 0.10	113.8	14.1
Medium QC	20	20.6 ± 2.13	108.6	10.3	21.98 ± 0.37	109.9	1.68
High QC	500	497.6 ± 56.9	104.2	11.4	555.6 ± 23.5	111.2	4.23

Data represent the means ± SD of five measurements.

3.1.3. Matrix Effect and Recovery

The mean recoveries of memantine in the low, medium and high QC samples ranged from 87.5 to 91.2% with an RSD of less than 3.70%. The matrix effects ranged from 91.1 to 108.2% with an RSD of less than 12.6%. These results indicate that no significant interference occurred during the ionization and methanol precipitation process. The matrix effect of the IS at 20 ng/mL was 102.9% and the recovery of IS was 87.7% (Table 2).

Table 2. Matrix effect and recovery of memantine.

Compounds		Spiked (ng/mL)	Recovery (%)	Matrix Effect (%)
Propranolol	IS	20	87.7 ± 1.96 (2.2)	102.9 ± 1.20 (1.2)
Memantine	Low QC	0.6	90.7 ± 3.11 (3.4)	108.2 ± 13.7 (12.6)
	Medium QC	20	91.2 ± 3.38 (3.7)	92.7 ± 5.43 (5.9)
	High QC	500	87.5 ± 3.18 (3.6)	91.1 ± 7.55 (8.3)

Data represent the means ± SD of five measurements.

3.1.4. Stability

The stabilities of memantine and propranolol are summarized in Table 3. Low and high QC samples were stable after being exposed to three freeze-thaw cycles and stable for at least 12 h at 25 °C. Post-preparative samples were stable after storage at 24 h in the autosampler after sample preparation.

Table 3. Stability of memantine.

Spiked (ng/mL)	Measured (ng/mL)	Accuracy (%)	Precision (%)
Bench-top stability for 12 h in plasma			
Low QC (0.6)	0.67 ± 0.10	112.2	14.9
High QC (500)	532.7 ± 27.6	106.6	5.2
Three freeze-thaw cycles			
Low QC (0.6)	0.51 ± 0.05	85.1	10.7
High QC (500)	539.3 ± 16.4	107.9	3.1
Post treatment stability for 24 h			
Low QC (0.6)	0.59 ± 0.04	98.4	7.6
High QC (500)	540.1 ± 13.7	108	2.5

Data represent the means ± SD of five measurements.

3.2. PK Interaction of Memantine and Cimetidine in Rats

The PK profiles of memantine following intravenous injection (3 mg/kg) in the presence or absence of cimetidine (10 mg/kg) are shown in Figure 2A and PK profiles of memantine following oral administration (5 mg/kg) in the presence or absence of cimetidine (50 mg/kg) are shown in Figure 2B. Their related PK parameters are presented in Table 4. The pharmacokinetic parameters of memantine were comparable to those reported previously [3,7,25].

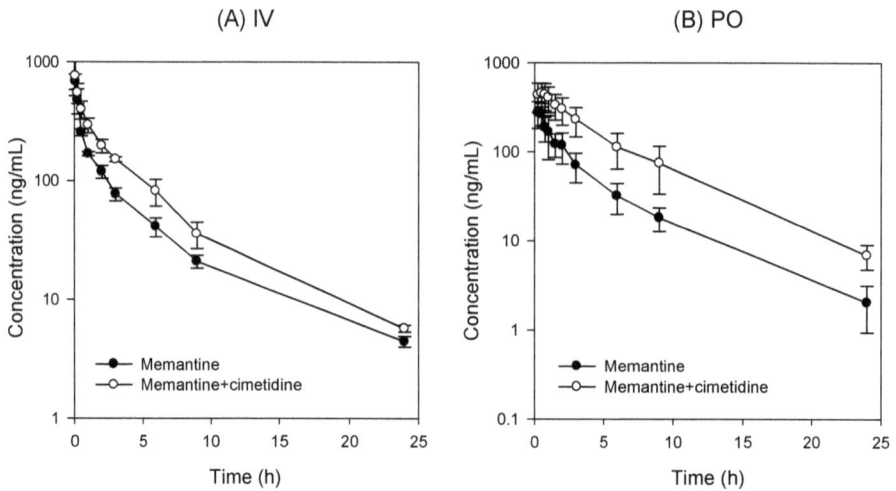

Figure 2. Plasma concentration-time profile of memantine after single intravenous (IV; **A**) and oral (PO; **B**) administration of memantine (3 and 5 mg/kg, respectively) in the presence (○) or absence (●) of cimetidine (10 and 50 mg/kg, respectively) in rats. Data points are the means ± SD of four rats.

Table 4. PK parameters of memantine after single intravenous (IV) and oral (PO) administration of memantine in the presence or absence of cimetidine in rats.

PK Parameters		IV		PO	
		Memantine (3 mg/kg)	Memantine (3 mg/kg) + Cimetidine (10 mg/kg)	Memantine (5 mg/kg)	Memantine (5 mg/kg) + Cimetidine (50 mg/kg)
C_{max}	µg/mL	686.84 ± 100.75	759.04 ± 240.18	293.45 ± 90.90	486.78 ± 140.75 *
T_{max}	h			0.35 ± 0.14	0.50 ± 0.18
AUC_{24h}	µg·h/mL	1089.58 ± 116.55	1724.52 ± 241.36 *	811.38 ± 238.01	2392.69 ± 950.06 *
AUC_{∞}	µg·h/mL	1121.98 ± 116.74	1765.56 ± 237.78 *	825.60 ± 241.92	2439.28 ± 951.72 *
$t_{1/2}$	h	5.06 ± 0.38	4.98 ± 0.59	4.51 ± 0.92	4.70 ± 0.75
$V_{d,ss}$	L/kg	19.70 ± 3.32	12.50 ± 3.16		
CL	mL/min/kg	44.87 ± 4.40	28.67 ± 3.92 *		
CL/F	mL/min/kg			107.63 ± 28.83	39.06 ± 16.00 *
CL_{renal}	mL/min/kg	12.88 ± 3.89	10.64 ± 5.73		

Data were expressed as mean ± SD from four rats per group. *: $p < 0.05$ compared with the memantine group. C_{max}: maximum plasma concentration; T_{max}: time to reach C_{max}. AUC_{24h} or AUC_{∞}: Area under plasma concentration-time curve from zero to 24 h or infinity. $t_{1/2}$: elimination half-life; $V_{d,ss}$: volume of distribution at steady-state CL or CL/F: systemic clearance; CL_{renal}: renal clearance.

There was no significant difference in the C_{max}, $t_{1/2}$ and $V_{d,ss}$ values of memantine between two groups (memantine alone vs. memantine + cimetidine). However, the AUC value of memantine + cimetidine was increased by 1.6-fold compared to that of memantine alone and, consequently, the CL of memantine decreased by co-injection with cimetidine.

Interestingly, the drug–drug interaction between memantine and cimetidine administered orally was greater than that of intravenous injection. For example, the AUC value of memantine + cimetidine was increased by 3.0-fold compared to that of memantine alone without changing the T_{max} and $t_{1/2}$ values. These results suggest that a major drug–drug interaction between memantine and cimetidine occurred during the absorption process. Moreover, systemic clearance (CL and CL/F) of memantine was decreased by co-administration of memantine and cimetidine by both the oral and intravenous routes, suggesting that memantine elimination is affected by the presence of cimetidine.

To investigate the underlying mechanism of the drug interaction in the absorption process, we investigated the effect of cimetidine on the intestinal permeability of memantine.

For the elimination process, we investigated the changes in metabolic stability in the rat liver microsomes because renal elimination (CL_{renal}) was not significantly altered by the presence of cimetidine (Table 4) and, therefore, non-renal clearance of memantine (calculated by subtracting CL_{renal} from CL) was decreased by the presence of cimetidine.

3.3. Effect of Cimetidine on the Intestinal Permeability of Memantine

To mimic the intestinal situation that occurred when memantine and cimetidine were concomitantly administered to rats via oral route, the concentrations of memantine and cimetidine were determined based on the oral dose of these drugs used in pharmacokinetic analysis and fluid volume of the stomach. For example, memantine and cimetidine were administered at doses of 5 and 50 mg/kg (dissolved in 2 mL/kg water), respectively, to rats with stomach fluid volumes of 3.4–4.6 mL [26], which resulted in 8–10-fold dilution.

The apparent permeability of memantine (0.5 mg/mL) in the presence of cimetidine (5 mg/mL) was significantly increased compared to that of memantine alone (Figure 3).

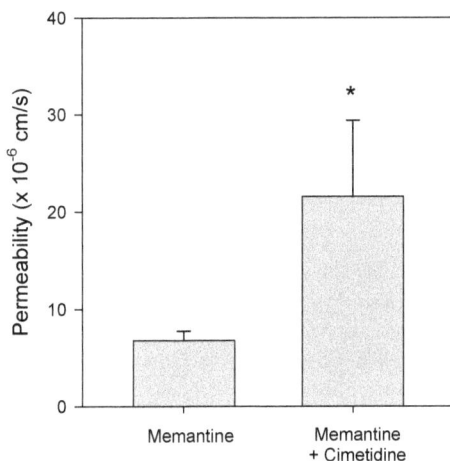

Figure 3. The apparent permeability (P_{app}) of memantine (0.5 mg/mL) in the absence or presence of cimetidine (5 mg/mL) was measured in rat jejunum using the Ussing system. Bar represents the mean $\pm$ SD of three independent experiments. * $p < 0.05$ compared with the memantine group.

3.4. Effect of Cimetidine on the Metabolic Stability of Memantine

Approximately 45% of memantine was degraded after 1 h incubation of memantine in the rat liver microsomes (Figure 4), which is consistent with the results of a previous study showing that memantine exhibits rat-specific Cyp-dependent moderate to high intrinsic clearance [3]. Adding 2 and 20 µM cimetidine and 1 µM memantine to the rat liver microsomes showed that the metabolic rate of memantine decreased with increasing concentrations of cimetidine (Figure 4).

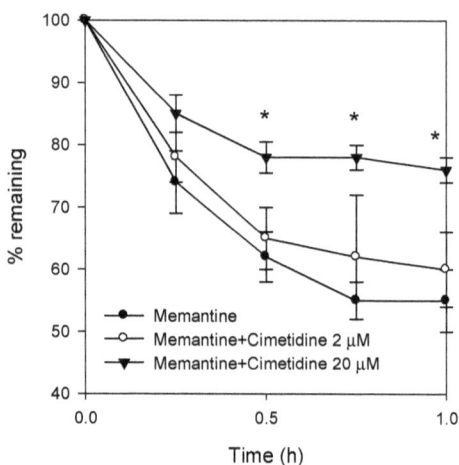

Figure 4. The effect of cimetidine on the metabolic stability of memantine with rat liver microsomes. Memantine (1 μM) in the absence or presence of cimetidine (0, 2 and 20 μM) was incubated with 0.5 mg rat liver microsomes for 60 min at 37 °C. Data represents the mean ± SD of three independent experiments. * $p < 0.05$ compared with the memantine group.

4. Discussion

The newly developed analytical method for memantine using an LC-MS/MS system showed comparable sensitivity (i.e., LLoQ 0.2 ng/mL) as previously published methods (i.e., LLoQ 0.1–1 ng/mL) despite the use of a small volume (50 μL) of plasma samples compared with previous methods [7,27–31]. Additionally, previously established methods used solid-phase extraction or liquid-liquid extraction which requires costly reagents and large volume of plasma samples (100–1000 μL) [27–31]. Noetzli et al. applied the protein-precipitation method and sample preparations were processed by evaporation and reconstitution [29]. However, we used a protein-precipitation method involving methanol containing an internal standard rather than previously described solid-phase extraction or liquid–liquid extraction methods and then directly injected an aliquot of the supernatant after the centrifugation of protein-precipitated plasma samples. Finally, we developed and fully validated a rapid, simple and sensitive analytical method for memantine in biological samples with total run time of 4.0 min. This method can easily be applied in the bioanalysis and pharmacokinetic study of memantine in small experimental animals. Moreover, following appropriate validation, the present method can be extended to determine the routine drug monitoring of memantine in human plasma and thus applied to clinical pharmacokinetic studies.

Memantine showed non-linear pharmacokinetic properties in a single oral dose range of 1–10 mg/kg. Beconi et al. reported that the active process mediated by rat-specific Cyp and active tubular secretion modulated the non-linear pharmacokinetics of memantine [3]. Cimetidine (as a perpetrator) increased the plasma concentration of the victim drug by inhibiting Cyp-mediated metabolism [14] and organic cation-mediated renal tubular secretion [13,14].

Based on these pharmacokinetic properties, the pharmacokinetics drug-drug interaction between memantine and cimetidine could be summarized as follows: (1) the AUC increase of memantine by co-administration with cimetidine was much greater following oral administration of memantine and cimetidine than that following intravenous injection. This suggests that the drug interaction was dominantly induced during the gut absorption process, which was supported by the increased permeability of memantine following addition of cimetidine (Figure 3). Although the intestinal absorption process of memantine has not been fully postulated, memantine absorption increased from 36.3% to 84.9% when oral dose increased from 1 mg/kg to 10 mg/kg, suggesting the presence of active process [3]. The involvement of pH-dependent transport mechanism via Octn1 has been reported in the distribution of memantine [32,33] and cimetidine could efficiently increase the influx of memantine through the inhibition of Octn1 by the inhibition of inwardly directed proton gradient and increase of gut pH [32,33]. (2) The AUC increase of memantine by co-administration of memantine and cimetidine intravenously may be attributed to the decreased clearance of memantine because of the decreased metabolic activity of memantine in the presence of cimetidine (Figure 4). This was also consistent with the previous reports that the intrinsic clearance calculated as moderate to high for rats, in which rat Cyp2c11 is responsible for the memantine metabolism [3] and cimetidine could inhibit hepatic Cyp2C6 and Cyp2C11 enzymes [34]. (3) Inhibition of organic cation-mediated renal tubular secretion of memantine by co-administration with cimetidine was not observed in this study, possibly because the renal clearance of memantine was not significantly decreased by the presence of cimetidine (Table 4). In conclusion, taken together, the pharmacokinetic interaction between memantine and cimetidine in rats was occurred not only at hepatic metabolism but also at intestinal membrane.

The clinical drug-drug between memantine and cimetidine was not investigated yet. However, approximately 48% of memantine was excreted as its unchanged form via renal route in human, in which multidrug and toxin extrusion protein (MATE) 1 was known to be involved [6,35]. The remaining 50% of memantine is metabolized into N-glucuronide conjugate, 6-hydroxy memantine and 1-nitroso deaminated memantine [6]. Since cimetidine acts as inhibitors of MATE1 and CYP enzymes [14,34], possibility of clinical drug-drug interaction between memantine and cimetidine should be carefully considered at high dose administration of cimetidine with memantine.

Author Contributions: Conceptualization, Y.A.C. and M.-K.C.; Methodology, Y.A.C. and I.-S.S.; Investigation, Y.A.C., I.-S.S. and M.-K.C.; Writing-Original Draft Preparation, Y.A.C. and I.-S.S.; Supervision, M.-K.C.; Writing-Review & Editing, M.-K.C.

Funding: This research received no external funding.

Conflicts of Interest: The authors declare no conflicts of interest.

References

1. Jahn, H. Memory loss in Alzheimer's disease. *Dialogues Clin. Neurosci.* **2013**, *15*, 445–454. [PubMed]
2. Greig, N.H.; Lahiri, D.K. Advances in understanding alzheimer's disease, and the contributions of current alzheimer research: Ten years on and beyond. *Curr. Alzheimer Res.* **2014**, *11*, 107–109. [CrossRef] [PubMed]
3. Beconi, M.G.; Howland, D.; Park, L.; Lyons, K.; Giuliano, J.; Dominguez, C.; Munoz-Sanjuan, I.; Pacifici, R. Pharmacokinetics of memantine in rats and mice. *PLoS Curr.* **2011**, *3*. [CrossRef] [PubMed]
4. Molinuevo, J.L.; Llado, A.; Rami, L. Memantine: Targeting glutamate excitotoxicity in alzheimer's disease and other dementias. *Am. J. Alzheimer's Dis. Other Dement.* **2005**, *20*, 77–85. [CrossRef] [PubMed]
5. McShane, R.; Areosa Sastre, A.; Minakaran, N. Memantine for dementia. *Cochrane Database Syst. Rev.* **2006**. [CrossRef] [PubMed]
6. Sani, G.; Serra, G.; Kotzalidis, G.D.; Romano, S.; Tamorri, S.M.; Manfredi, G.; Caloro, M.; Telesforo, C.L.; Caltagirone, S.S.; Panaccione, I.; et al. The role of memantine in the treatment of psychiatric disorders other than the dementias: A review of current preclinical and clinical evidence. *CNS Drugs* **2012**, *26*, 663–690. [CrossRef] [PubMed]
7. Bhateria, M.; Ramakrishna, R.; Pakala, D.B.; Bhatta, R.S. Development of an lc-ms/ms method for simultaneous determination of memantine and donepezil in rat plasma and its application to pharmacokinetic study. *J. Chromatogr. B Anal. Technol. Biomed. Life Sci.* **2015**, *1001*, 131–139. [CrossRef] [PubMed]
8. Periclou, A.P.; Ventura, D.; Sherman, T.; Rao, N.; Abramowitz, W.T. Lack of pharmacokinetic or pharmacodynamic interaction between memantine and donepezil. *Ann. Pharmacother.* **2004**, *38*, 1389–1394. [CrossRef] [PubMed]
9. Figiel, G.S.; Koumaras, B.; Meng, X.; Strigas, J.; Gunay, I. Long-term safety and tolerability of rivastigmine in patients with alzheimer's disease switched from donepezil: An open-label extension study. *Prim. Care Companion J. Clin. Psychiatry* **2008**, *10*, 363–367. [CrossRef] [PubMed]

10. Yao, C.; Raoufinia, A.; Gold, M.; Nye, J.S.; Ramael, S.; Padmanabhan, M.; Walschap, Y.; Verhaeghe, T.; Zhao, Q. Steady-state pharmacokinetics of galantamine are not affected by addition of memantine in healthy subjects. *J. Clin. Pharmacol.* **2005**, *45*, 519–528. [CrossRef] [PubMed]

11. Lostia, A.M.; Mazzarini, L.; Pacchiarotti, I.; Lionetto, L.; De Rossi, P.; Sanna, L.; Sani, G.; Kotzalidis, G.D.; Girardi, P.; Simmaco, M.; et al. Serum levels of risperidone and its metabolite, 9-hydroxyrisperidone: Correlation between drug concentration and clinical response. *Ther. Drug Monit.* **2009**, *31*, 475–481. [CrossRef] [PubMed]

12. Zimmer, D. New us fda draft guidance on bioanalytical method validation versus current fda and ema guidelines: Chromatographic methods and isr. *Bioanalysis* **2014**, *6*, 13–19. [CrossRef] [PubMed]

13. Ito, S.; Kusuhara, H.; Yokochi, M.; Toyoshima, J.; Inoue, K.; Yuasa, H.; Sugiyama, Y. Competitive inhibition of the luminal efflux by multidrug and toxin extrusions, but not basolateral uptake by organic cation transporter 2, is the likely mechanism underlying the pharmacokinetic drug-drug interactions caused by cimetidine in the kidney. *J. Pharmacol. Exp. Ther.* **2012**, *340*, 393–403. [CrossRef] [PubMed]

14. Matsushima, S.; Maeda, K.; Inoue, K.; Ohta, K.Y.; Yuasa, H.; Kondo, T.; Nakayama, H.; Horita, S.; Kusuhara, H.; Sugiyama, Y. The inhibition of human multidrug and toxin extrusion 1 is involved in the drug-drug interaction caused by cimetidine. *Drug Metab. Dispos. Boil. Fate Chem.* **2009**, *37*, 555–559. [CrossRef] [PubMed]

15. Hoffman, A.; Perlstein, I.; Habib, G.; Pinto, E.; Gilhar, D. The effect of cimetidine on the pharmacodynamics of theophylline-induced seizures and ethanol hypnotic activity. *Pharmacol. Toxicol.* **1999**, *85*, 130–132. [CrossRef] [PubMed]

16. Rafi, J.A.; Frazier, L.M.; Driscoll-Bannister, S.M.; O'Hara, K.A.; Garnett, W.R.; Pugh, C.B. Effect of over-the-counter cimetidine on phenytoin concentrations in patients with seizures. *Ann. Pharmacother.* **1999**, *33*, 769–774. [CrossRef] [PubMed]

17. Kurata, T.; Muraki, Y.; Mizutani, H.; Iwamoto, T.; Okuda, M. Elevated systemic elimination of cimetidine in rats with acute biliary obstruction: The role of renal organic cation transporter OCT2. *Drug Metab. Pharmacokinet.* **2010**, *25*, 328–334. [CrossRef] [PubMed]

18. Piyapolrungroj, N.; Zhou, Y.S.; Li, C.; Liu, G.; Zimmermann, E.; Fleisher, D. Cimetidine absorption and elimination in rat small intestine. *Drug Metab. Dispos. Boil. Fate Chem.* **2000**, *28*, 65–72.

19. Guo, P.; Dong, L.; Yan, W.; Wei, J.; Wang, C.; Zhang, Z. Simultaneous determination of linarin, naringenin and formononetin in rat plasma by lc-ms/ms and its application to a pharmacokinetic study after oral administration of bushen guchi pill. *Biomed. Chromatogr.* **2015**, *29*, 246–253. [CrossRef] [PubMed]

20. Huang, P.; Zhang, L.; Chai, C.; Qian, X.C.; Li, W.; Li, J.S.; Di, L.Q.; Cai, B.C. Effects of food and gender on the pharmacokinetics of ginkgolides a, b, c and bilobalide in rats after oral dosing with ginkgo terpene lactones extract. *J. Pharm. Biomed. Anal.* **2014**, *100*, 138–144. [CrossRef] [PubMed]

21. Kwon, M.; Ji, H.K.; Goo, S.H.; Nam, S.J.; Kang, Y.J.; Lee, E.; Liu, K.H.; Choi, M.K.; Song, I.S. Involvement of intestinal efflux and metabolic instability in the pharmacokinetics of platycodin d in rats. *Drug Metab. Pharmacokinet.* **2017**, *32*, 248–254. [CrossRef] [PubMed]

22. Levin, V.A. Relationship of octanol/water partition coefficient and molecular weight to rat brain capillary permeability. *J. Med. Chem.* **1980**, *23*, 682–684. [CrossRef] [PubMed]

23. Stewart, B.H.; Chan, O.H.; Lu, R.H.; Reyner, E.L.; Schmid, H.L.; Hamilton, H.W.; Steinbaugh, B.A.; Taylor, M.D. Comparison of intestinal permeabilities determined in multiple in vitro and in situ models: Relationship to absorption in humans. *Pharm. Res.* **1995**, *12*, 693–699. [CrossRef] [PubMed]

24. Choi, M.K.; Lee, J.; Nam, S.J.; Kang, Y.J.; Han, Y.; Choi, K.; Choi, Y.A.; Kwon, M.; Lee, D.; Song, I.S. Pharmacokinetics of jaspine b and enhancement of intestinal absorption of jaspine b in the presence of bile acid in rats. *Mar. Drugs* **2017**, *15*, 279. [CrossRef] [PubMed]

25. Lee, S.H.; Kim, S.H.; Noh, Y.H.; Choi, B.M.; Noh, G.J.; Park, W.D.; Kim, E.J.; Cho, I.H.; Bae, C.S. Pharmacokinetics of memantine after a single and multiple dose of oral and patch administration in rats. *Basic Clin. Pharmacol. Toxicol.* **2016**, *118*, 122–127. [CrossRef] [PubMed]

26. McConnell, E.L.; Basit, A.W.; Murdan, S. Measurements of rat and mouse gastrointestinal ph, fluid and lymphoid tissue, and implications for in-vivo experiments. *J. Pharm. Pharmacol.* **2008**, *60*, 63–70. [CrossRef] [PubMed]

27. Qiu, H.W.; Xia, L.; Gong, L.M.; Ruan, L.M.; Zhao, Y.G. Rapid determination of memantine in human plasma by using nanoring carboxyl-functionalized paramagnetic molecularly imprinted polymer d-mu-spe and uflc-ms/ms. *Drug Test. Anal.* **2015**, *7*, 535–543. [CrossRef] [PubMed]

28. Suresh, P.S.; Mullangi, R.; Sukumaran, S.K. Highly sensitive lc-ms/ms method for determination of galantamine in rat plasma: Application to pharmacokinetic studies in rats. *Biomed. Chromatogr.* **2014**, *28*, 1633–1640. [CrossRef] [PubMed]

29. Noetzli, M.; Ansermot, N.; Dobrinas, M.; Eap, C.B. Simultaneous determination of antidementia drugs in human plasma: Procedure transfer from hplc-ms to uplc-ms/ms. *J. Pharm. Biomed. Anal.* **2012**, *64–65*, 16–25. [CrossRef] [PubMed]

30. Konda, R.K.; Challa, B.R.; Chandu, B.R.; Chandrasekhar, K.B. Bioanalytical method development and validation of memantine in human plasma by high performance liquid chromatography with tandem mass spectrometry: Application to bioequivalence study. *J. Anal. Methods Chem.* **2012**, *2012*. [CrossRef] [PubMed]

31. Almeida, A.A.; Campos, D.R.; Bernasconi, G.; Calafatti, S.; Barros, F.A.; Eberlin, M.N.; Meurer, E.C.; Paris, E.G.; Pedrazzoli, J. Determination of memantine in human plasma by liquid chromatography-electrospray tandem mass spectrometry: Application to a bioequivalence study. *J. Chromatogr. B Anal. Technol. Biomed. Life Sci.* **2007**, *848*, 311–316. [CrossRef] [PubMed]

32. Mehta, D.C.; Short, J.L.; Nicolazzo, J.A. Memantine transport across the mouse blood-brain barrier is mediated by a cationic influx h+ antiporter. *Mol. Pharm.* **2013**, *10*, 4491–4498. [CrossRef] [PubMed]

33. Yabuuchi, H.; Tamai, I.; Nezu, J.; Sakamoto, K.; Oku, A.; Shimane, M.; Sai, Y.; Tsuji, A. Novel membrane transporter octn1 mediates multispecific, bidirectional, and ph-dependent transport of organic cations. *J. Pharmacol. Exp. Ther.* **1999**, *289*, 768–773. [PubMed]

34. Levine, M.; Law, E.Y.; Bandiera, S.M.; Chang, T.K.; Bellward, G.D. In vivo cimetidine inhibits hepatic CYP2C6 and CYP2C11 but not cyp1a1 in adult male rats. *J. Pharmacol. Exp. Ther.* **1998**, *284*, 493–499. [PubMed]

35. Muller, F.; Weitz, D.; Derdau, V.; Sandvoss, M.; Mertsch, K.; Konig, J.; Fromm, M.F. Contribution of mate1 to renal secretion of the nmda receptor antagonist memantine. *Mol. Pharm.* **2017**, *14*, 2991–2998. [CrossRef] [PubMed]

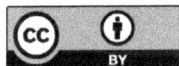

pharmaceutics

MDPI

Article

Exploring the Metabolism of Loxoprofen in Liver Microsomes: The Role of Cytochrome P450 and UDP-Glucuronosyltransferase in Its Biotransformation

Riya Shrestha [1], Pil Joung Cho [1], Sanjita Paudel [1], Aarajana Shrestha [2], Mi Jeong Kang [2], Tae Cheon Jeong [2], Eung-Seok Lee [2] and Sangkyu Lee [1,*]

[1]   BK21 Plus KNU Multi-Omics based Creative Drug Research Team, College of Pharmacy, Research Institute of Pharmaceutical Sciences, Kyungpook National University, Daegu 41566, Korea; riya.shrestha07@gmail.com (R.S.); whvlfwjd@naver.com (P.J.C.); sanjitapdl99@gmail.com (S.P.)

[2]   College of Pharmacy, Yeungnam University, Gyeongsan 38541, Korea; aarajanashrestha1@gmail.com (A.S.); jkang@ynu.ac.kr (M.J.K.); taecheon@ynu.ac.kr (T.C.J.); eslee@ynu.ac.kr (E.-S.L.)

*   Correspondence: sangkyu@knu.ac.kr; Tel.: +82-53-950-8571; Fax: +82-53-950-8557

Received: 29 June 2018; Accepted: 30 July 2018; Published: 2 August 2018

Abstract: Loxoprofen, a propionic acid derivative, non-steroidal anti-inflammatory drug (NSAID) is a prodrug that is reduced to its active metabolite, trans-alcohol form (Trans-OH) by carbonyl reductase enzyme in the liver. Previous studies demonstrated the hydroxylation and glucuronidation of loxoprofen. However, the specific enzymes catalyzing its metabolism have yet to be identified. In the present study, we investigated metabolic enzymes, such as cytochrome P450 (CYP) and UDP-glucuronosyltransferase (UGT), which are involved in the metabolism of loxoprofen. Eight microsomal metabolites of loxoprofen were identified, including two alcohol metabolites (M1 and M2), two mono-hydroxylated metabolites (M3 and M4), and four glucuronide conjugates (M5, M6, M7, and M8). Based on the results for the formation of metabolites when incubated in dexamethasone-induced microsomes, incubation with ketoconazole, and human recombinant cDNA-expressed cytochrome P450s, we identified CYP3A4 and CYP3A5 as the major CYP isoforms involved in the hydroxylation of loxoprofen (M3 and M4). Moreover, we identified that UGT2B7 is the major UGT isoform catalyzing the glucuronidation of loxoprofen and its alcoholic metabolites. Further experimental studies should be carried out to determine the potency and toxicity of these identified metabolites of loxoprofen, in order to fully understand of mechanism of loxoprofen toxicity.

Keywords: loxoprofen; CYP; UGT; human liver microsomes; LC-HR/MS

1. Introduction

Loxoprofen, 2-(4-((2-Oxocyclopentyl)methyl)phenyl) propionic acid, is a non-selective non-steroidal anti-inflammatory drug (NSAID) developed in Japan by Daiichi Sankyo Co. Ltd. in 1986 [1]. Loxoprofen is mainly used to treat pain and inflammation related to musculoskeletal and joint disorders, such as rheumatoid arthritis, osteoarthritis [2,3], and post-operative pain [1]. Loxoprofen is a prodrug metabolized in the liver by carbonyl reductase enzyme to its active trans-alcohol metabolite (Trans-OH), 2-(4-((trans-2-hydroxycyclopentyl)-methyl)-phenyl) propionic acid (Figure 1a) [1,4]. The active metabolite exhibits anti-inflammatory activity by inhibiting the cyclooxygenase enzymes, thus impairing the formation of the chemical prostaglandin, which is responsible for pain and inflammation [5,6]. Although it has been reported to be safer than its counterparts and is one of the most prescribed anti-inflammatory drugs in Japan, loxoprofen has shown diverse adverse drug reactions (ADRs) and has recorded the highest rate of adverse effects in Korea in the first half of 2017 [7–10]. Some of the ADRs of loxoprofen are gastro-intestinal disorder, nausea, hypersensitivity, blood disorders (leukopenia and hemolytic anemia), renal disorders, drug induced liver injury, shock, and anaphylaxis [1]. In addition, the potential drug-drug interaction of loxoprofen with aspirin, enoxacin, and valacyclovir has been reported [10–12]. Thus, the ADRs of loxoprofen might be attributed to its drug-drug interactions with other marketed drugs.

(a)

(b)

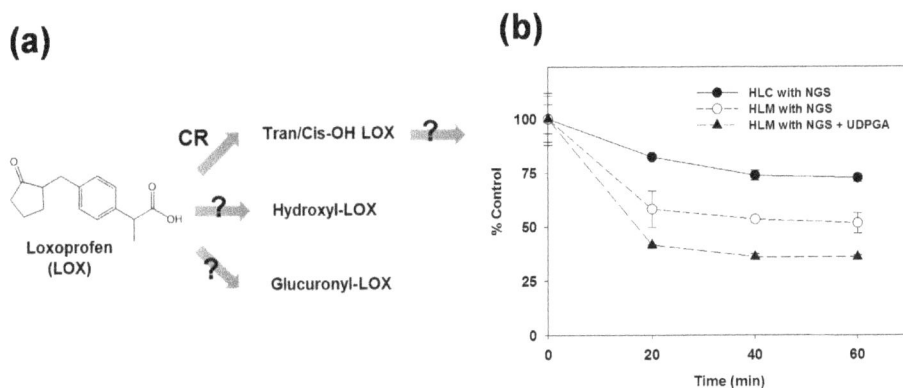

Figure 1. Chemical structure of loxoprofen and its metabolites (**a**). Metabolic stability of 5 μM of loxoprofen in 0.25 mg/mL of human liver cytosols (HLC) in the presence of β-reduced nicotinamide adenine dinucleotide phosphate (β-NADPH) regeneration system (NGS) and 0.25 mg/mL of human liver microsomes (HLMs) in the presence of NGS and uridine 5′-diphosphoglucuronic acid trisodium (UDPGA) incubated at 37 °C for 60 min (**b**). The data are represented as mean ± standard error (S.E) of the triplicate samples.

The reaction phenotyping of a drug is an essential part of the drug discovery and development process, which helps in preventing the ADRs derived from drug–drug interactions. While the pharmacokinetic profiling of loxoprofen and its active metabolites has been widely studied [5,13–19], only few studies have investigated its metabolic characteristics [15,20,21]. A previous study identified four hydroxylated and four glucuronide conjugates of loxoprofen after oral administration to monkey [21]. The in vivo metabolites of loxoprofen had been profiled in the plasma, urine, and skin of rats [15]. However, to the best of our knowledge, no detailed studies on the in vitro metabolism of loxoprofen in the human liver microsomes (HLMs) have been documented (Figure 1a).

In the present study, we investigated the loxoprofen metabolism in human, mouse, dog, rat, and monkey liver microsomes so as to investigate any possible in vitro metabolite formation of loxoprofen by microsomal enzymes. We also identified the possible cytochrome P450 (CYP) and UDP-glucuronosyltransferase (UGT) isoforms involved in the biotransformation of loxoprofen in HLMs. We identified four microsomal enzymes that produce metabolites of loxoprofen, including the active trans-alcohol metabolite. We found that CYP3A4 and CYP3A5 are the major CYP isoforms involved in the hydroxylation of loxoprofen. Similarly, we identified two glucuronide metabolites of loxoprofen that are mainly produced by UGT2B7 and UGT1A6.

2. Materials and Methods

2.1. Materials

Loxoprofen was purchased from Tokyo Chemicals Industry (Tokyo, Japan). Trans-OH and Cis-OH loxoprofen (purities 96.5% and 97.9%, respectively) were chemically synthesized from loxoprofen [22]. The β-reduced nicotinamide adenine dinucleotide phosphate (β-NADPH) regeneration system (NGS) was purchased from Promega Corp. (Madison, WI, USA). Pooled HLMs (mixed gender) were purchased from Sekisui Xeno Tech, LLC (Kansas City, MO, USA). Mixed Gender Corning UltraPool 150-donor liver cytosols; mouse, rat, dog, and monkey liver microsomes (RLM, MLM, DLM, and MoLM, respectively); and purified human recombinant cDNA encoding CYPs and UGTs were purchased from Corning Gentest (Woburn, MA, USA). Alamethicin and Uridine 5′-diphosphoglucuronic acid trisodium (UDPGA) were obtained from Sigma-Aldrich (St. Louis, MO, USA). Mass spectrometry (MS) grade water and acetonitrile (ACN) were acquired from Fischer Scientific (Pittsburgh, PA, USA).

2.2. Metabolic Stabilities in Human Liver Microsomes and the Cytosols

To properly understand the metabolism of loxoprofen, its metabolic stability was compared between human liver cytosols (HLCs) and HLMs in the presence of NGS and UDPGA. The phase I metabolic stability was performed by incubating loxoprofen (5 μM) with 1 mg/mL of HLC or HLMs in 0.1 M phosphate buffer (pH 7.4) at 37 °C, with the addition of NGS to give a total reaction volume of 100 μL. The reaction was terminated at 0, 20, 40, and 60 min time points by the addition of ice cold 100% ACN, containing tolbutamide as an internal standard. The sample was vortexed and kept on ice for complete protein denaturation. Following centrifugation for 10 min at 13,000 × *g* at 4 °C, the supernatant was transferred to high performance liquid chromatography (HPLC) vials and analyzed using a TSQ vantage mass spectrometer (Thermo Fisher Scientific, Waltham, MA, USA).

Similarly, for the Phase II metabolic stability of loxoprofen, 1 mg/mL of HLM was treated with 25 μg/mL of alamethicin and kept on ice for 20 min. Then, 5 μM (final concentration) of loxoprofen was added to the reaction mixture and pre-incubated for 5 min at 37 °C in the presence of NGS. The reaction was finally initiated by the addition of cofactor UDPGA (5 mM), and incubated at 37 °C. The samples were then subjected to the same post-reaction procedure as that for Phase I metabolic stability.

2.3. Biotransformation of Loxoprofen in Microsomes and the Cytosols

To perform the metabolite profiling, loxoprofen (20 μM) was incubated with 1 mg/mL of HLC or HLM, MLM, RLM, DLM, and MoLM, with the addition of 0.1 M of phosphate buffer (pH 7.4), in the presence or absence of NGS at 37 °C for 60 min. The final reaction volume was 200 μL and the reaction was terminated by adding 400 μL of 100% ACN. The samples were centrifuged at 13,000× *g* at 4 °C for 10 min, and the supernatants (550 μL) were taken and dried under vacuum using a Labonco speed-vac concentrator (Kansas City, MO, USA) at 35 °C. The dried sample was stored at −80 °C until use. The dried samples were reconstituted with 20% ACN (MS grade) and vortexed for at least 10 min. The samples were then centrifuged and 10 μL of the supernatant was analyzed using high-resolution mass spectrometry coupled with liquid chromatography (LC-HR/MS), and the metabolites were identified by studying the chromatographs and spectrums of the *m/z* of all of the possible Phase I metabolites.

For the UGT-mediated metabolism of loxoprofen, 1 mg/mL of a liver preparation was treated with 25 μg/mL (final concentration) of alamethicin for 20 min. Then, 20 μM of loxoprofen and 0.1 M phosphate buffer (pH 7.4) were added and pre-incubated for 5 min after addition of NGS. The reaction was started by incubating the reaction mixture at 37 °C in presence or absence of 5 mM UDPGA in a reaction volume of 200 μL. After 60 min, the reaction was quenched with 400 μL of 100% MS grade ACN, vortexed, and centrifuged at 13,000 × *g* at 4 °C for 10 min. The supernatant (550 μL) was removed and dried in a speed-vac at 35 °C. The dried samples were reconstituted with 20% ACN (MS grade) and underwent similar procedures as mentioned for the Phase I metabolism.

2.4. Metabolism of Loxoprofen in Chemically-Induced Microsomes and CYP Enzyme Inhibitors

To better understand the CYP-mediated metabolism of loxoprofen, we prepared microsomes enriched with specific CYPs after a selective chemical induction [23]. Four selective inducers were administered to male Sprague-Dawley rats, 3-methylcholanthrene (3-MC) for CYP1A, phenobarbital for CYP2B, dexamethasone for CYP3A, and acetone for CYP2E (Appendix A). Loxoprofen (20 μM) was incubated with 1 mg/mL of enriched microsomes, with the addition of 0.1 M phosphate buffer (pH 7.4) in the presence of NGS at 37 °C for 60 min. The effect of SKF-525A (non-selective CYP inhibitor) and ketoconazole (CYP3A4/5 selective inhibitor) on the metabolism of loxoprofen was investigated in the pooled HLMs. The incubations were performed with an inhibitor (25 and 50 μM for SKF-525A, 1 and 10 μM for ketoconazole, respectively), HLMs (1 mg/mL), and loxoprofen (20 μM) in 0.1 M phosphate buffer (pH 7.4), in the presence of NGS at 37 °C for 60 min.

2.5. Recombinant cDNA-Expressed CYPs and UGTs Metabolism of Loxoprofen

To identify the metabolic enzymes for loxoprofen, loxoprofen was incubated with purified CYP and UGT isoforms. For the CYP metabolism study, 5 μM of loxoprofen was incubated with 5 pmol of 10 CYP isoforms (CYP1A1, 1A2, 2B6, 2C8, 2C9, 2C19, 3A4, 3A5, 2D6, and 2E1) at 37 °C for 60 min. The reaction volume was 200 μL. The reaction was stopped by the addition of 400 μL of 100% ACN and centrifugation at 13,000 × *g* for 10 min. The supernatant (550 μL) was dried, reconstituted with 20% ACN, and analyzed in LC-MS.

To detect the glucuronide metabolites of loxoprofen, 5 μM of loxoprofen, Trans-OH, or Cis-OH loxoprofen was incubated with 0.1 mg/mL of five purified UGT isoforms (UGT1A1, 1A3, 1A4, 1A6, 1A9, and 2B7) in presence of 5 mM of UDPGA with a reaction volume of 200 μL at 37 °C for 60 min. The reaction was stopped by 100% ACN and then processed according to the procedure mentioned in the previous paragraph.

2.6. Instrument

The LC-MS/MS system consisted of the Thermo Scientific™ Dionex™ Ultimate™ 3000 UHPLC system (Dionex Softron GmbH, Germering, Germany), equipped with an HPG-3200SD Standard binary pump, WPS 3000 TRS analytical autosampler, and a TCC-3000 SD Column compartment. The LC system was coupled with a high-resolution mass spectrometer, the Thermo Scientific™ Q Exactive™ Focus quadrupole-Orbitrap MS (Thermo Fisher Scientific, Bremen, Germany). A heated electrospray ionization source II (HESI-II) probe was used as the ion generator, with nitrogen used as the auxiliary, sheath, and sweep gas. The mass spectrometer was calibrated in both positive and negative mode using a Pierce™ LTQ Velos ESI Positive Ion Calibration Solution and Pierce™ ESI Negative Ion Calibration Solution (Pierce Biotechnology, Rockford, IL, USA) respectively to ensure the mass accuracy of the mass spectrometer. The mass spectrometer was operated in negative ion mode, with sheath gas, and auxiliary gas set to 35 and 12 aux units, respectively. The other parameters were set as follows: the spray voltage to 2.5 KV, capillary temperature to 320 °C, S-lens RF level to 50, and aux gas heater temperature to 200 °C. For the metabolic profiling, a reverse-phase liquid chromatography column (Kinetex® C18 column (150 mm × 2.1 mm, 2.6-μm, Phenomenex, Torrance, CA, USA) was employed at 40 °C. The mobile phase consisted of 100% MS grade water with 0.1% formic acid as solvent A, and 100% MS ACN with 0.1% formic acid as solvent B. The gradient elution was used at a flow rate of 250 μL/min for adequate compound separation, starting with 10% of solvent B for 0.5 min, gradually increasing to 50% in 21.0 min, again increased to 95% over a minute, and kept constant for 3 min before equilibrating the column with 10% solvent B for 5 min.

3. Results

3.1. Microsomal Metabolism of Loxoprofen

To determine the importance of the microsomal metabolism of loxoprofen, the metabolic stability test was performed in HLC or HLMs in the presence of NGS or UDPGA (Figure 1b). The comparison of the Phase I metabolic stability of the 5 μM loxoprofen between HLC and HLMs showed a marked decrease in the stability of loxoprofen in HLMs compared to that in HLC. Moreover, the metabolic stability of loxoprofen decreased further when it was incubated with UDPGA to stimulate glucuronide conjugation (Phase 2 metabolism). Although the major bioactivation of loxoprofen is mediated by cytosolic carbonyl reductase enzymes, our metabolic stability study suggested that loxoprofen undergoes extensive metabolism in HLMs.

The metabolic stability is linked to the type of metabolites produced in the cytosols and microsomes. In fact, more diverse metabolites were produced in the microsomes compared to those in the cytosols. In Figure 2, the representative extraction chromatograms obtained following the incubation of loxoprofen in HLC and HLMs are shown. Six different metabolites of loxoprofen were identified, including two alcohol metabolites (M1 and M2), two mono-hydroxylated metabolites (M3 and M4), and two conjugates with glucuronide (M5 and M6). In particular, the metabolism of loxoprofen in HLC in presence of NGS produced only the two alcohol metabolites (reduction of ketone to alcohol); M1, the active Trans-OH metabolite, $C_{15}H_{19}O_3$ (m/z 247.1335) at a retention time of 14.6 min, and M2, the cis-alcohol (Cis-OH) metabolite, $C_{15}H_{19}O_3$ (m/z 247.1334) at a retention time of 15.0 min (Figure 2a). The bioactivation of loxoprofen to its active (trans-alcohol) metabolite, M1, was about five times higher than that of its cis isoform.

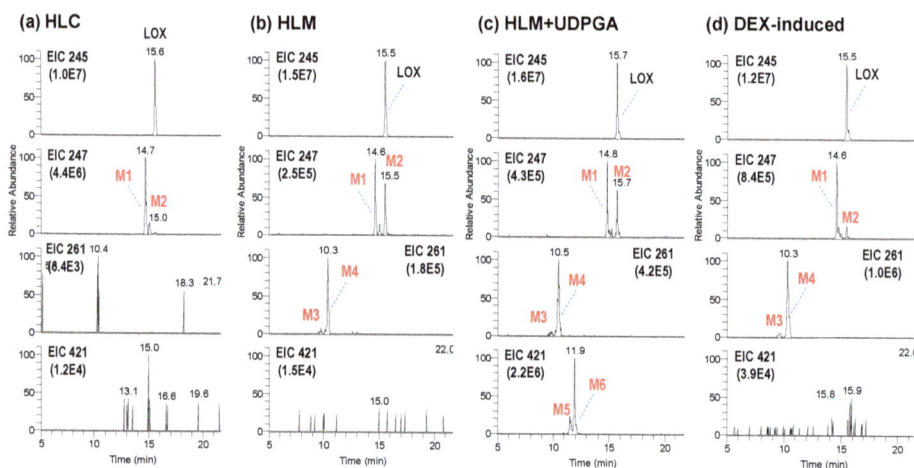

Figure 2. The extracted ion chromatograph (EIC); DEX, dexamethasone EIC of loxoprofen and its metabolites in human liver cytosols (HLC) (**a**) and human liver microsomes (HLM) (**b**) in presence of β-NADPH regeneration system (NGS), HLMs in presence of NGS and UDPGA (**c**), and dexamethasone (DEX)-induced rat liver microsomes (**d**) in the presence of NGS.

Two peaks of hydroxylated metabolites, M3 and M4 (m/z 261.1129 and 261.1128, $C_{15}H_{17}O_4$) were observed at 9.8 and 10.3 mins, respectively, after the incubation of HLM in the presence of NGS. The yields of alcohol metabolites and hydroxylated metabolites were similar in the control HLMs (Figure 2b). In the presence of UDPGA, two glucuronide metabolites, M5 and M6 (m/z 421.1498 and 421.1500, $C_{21}H_{25}O_9$) at retention times of 11.4 and 11.7 min, respectively, were generated (Figure 2d). M5 and M6 were hypothesized to be the acyl glucuronides of loxoprofen.

The in vitro metabolic profile of loxoprofen in MLM, DLM, RLM, and MoLM were found to be similar to that obtained in the HLMs (Figure 3a). A higher Phase I metabolism was observed in MLMs compared to the microsomes from the other species, while a higher glucuronidation was observed in the DLMs compared to the microsomes from the other species (Figure 3b).

3.2. Structure Elucidation of Microsomal Metabolites In Vitro

Full MS and CID MS/MS scans were performed in negative ion mode for the characterization of metabolites structures using high resolution mass spectrometry coupled with ultra-high performance liquid chromatography (LC-HRMS). The structure of the metabolites was confirmed from the MS/MS fragmentation pattern with exact mass measurement of the precursor and product ions having mass accuracy <5 ppm.

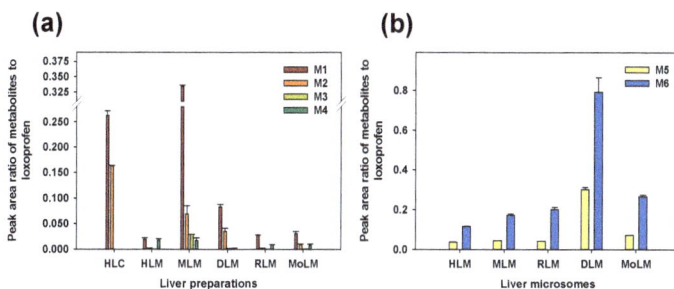

Figure 3. Formation of Phase 1 metabolites (**a**) and Phase 2 conjugates (M5 and M6) (**b**) in the liver microsomes of five mammalian species. The data are represented as mean ± S.E of area ratio of metabolites to loxoprofen of triplicate samples. HLC—human liver cytosols; HLM—human liver microsomes; MLM—mouse liver microsomes; DLM—dog liver microsomes; RLM—rat liver microsomes; MoLM—monkey liver microsomes.

M1 and M2 were identified as Trans-OH and Cis-OH metabolites, respectively. The stereochemistry of two alcoholic metabolites were confirmed by comparing the MS^2 fragmentation pattern and chromatographic retention time of chemically synthesized standard compounds (data not shown). The major product ions at m/z 217.1228 ($C_{14}H_{17}O_2$) and 191.1070 ($C_{12}H_{15}O_2$) showed that fragmentation occurred at the cyclopentanol ring of the loxoprofen alcohol metabolites. MS/MS fragmentation of M3 and M4 produced a major ion ($C_5H_7O_2$) of m/z 99.0440 ($C_5H_7O_2$), which suggested that the hydroxylation occurred at the cyclopentanone ring of loxoprofen. M5 and M6 were hypothesized to be the acyl glucuronides of loxoprofen, which were supported by major product ions at m/z 245.1179 ($C_{15}H_{17}O_3$), 193.0346 ($C_6H_9O_7$), and 83.0490 (C_5H_7O) (Figure A1).

3.3. Reaction Phenotyping for Phase 1 and Phase 2

To investigate the possible CYP isozymes involved in the loxoprofen metabolism, the products formed during the incubation of loxoprofen with the control, 3-methylcholanthrene, phenobarbital (PB), dexamethasone (DEX), and acetone-induced RLMs were determined and displayed in Figure 4a. The production of M4 was increased in the DEX-induced RLMs by 15-fold compared to that in the uninduced control microsomes. Metabolite M3 was produced in PB and DEX-induced microsomes at higher levels compared to that in the uninduced microsomes. We also observed an increase in M3 and M4 formation in the DEX-induced RLMs compared to with that in the control HLMs (Figure 4a). The formation of M3 and M4 was significantly inhibited by SKF-525A, a non-specific CYP inhibitor, indicating that the Phase 1 metabolism of loxoprofen depended on CYP (Figure 4b) [24]. M1 (Trans-OH form) and M2 (Cis-OH form) are products of a reductase; therefore, the formation of M1 and M2 were not inhibited by SKF-525A treatment.

Additionally, the metabolism of loxoprofen dependent on the CYP3A subfamily was confirmed by incubation with a selective CYP3A inhibitor in HLMs (Figure 4c). Ketoconazole, a selective inhibitor of CYP3A4, strongly inhibited the formation of M3 and M4 in a concentration-dependent manner, whereas the formation of M1 and M2 was not affected by ketoconazole. The selective formation of M3 and M4 were finally confirmed by incubation with ten different CYP isoforms (CYP1A1, 1A2, 2B6, 2C8, 2C9, 2C19, 3A4, 3A5, 2D6, and 2E1) (Figure 4d). M3 and M4 were predominantly generated by CYP3A4 and 3A5 in HLMs.

Following the incubation of loxoprofen with six UGT enzyme isoforms (UGT1A1, 1A3, 1A4, 1A6, 1A9, and 2B7), we found that the UGT2B7 isoform predominantly mediated the glucuronidation of loxoprofen to its glucuronide metabolites, M5 and M6. M5 was detected only in the UGT2B7 isoform, whereas UGT1A4, 1A6, 1A3, and 1A9 contributed to the formation of M6 to a minor extent.

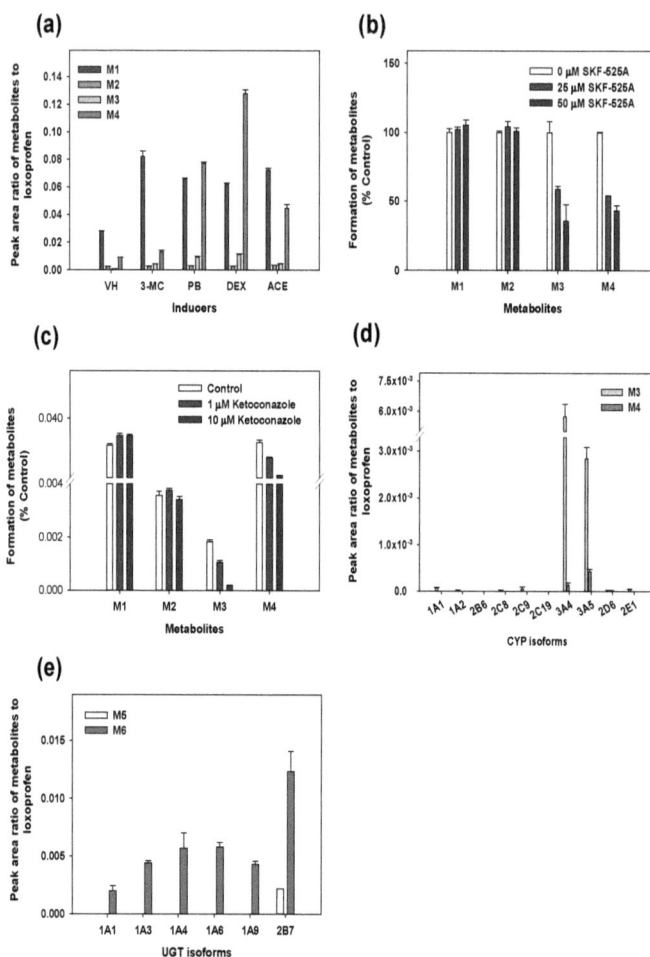

Figure 4. Formation of metabolites expressed as peak area ratio of metabolites to loxoprofen in chemically-induced rat liver microsomes (**a**). Effect of the non-selective cytochrome P450 (CYP) inhibitor, SKF 525-A (25 and 50 μM) (**b**), and the CYP3A4 selective inhibitor, ketoconazole (1 and 10 μM) (**c**), on the metabolism of loxoprofen in human liver microsomes after incubation with 20 μM loxoprofen in presence of a β-NAPDH regeneration system (NGS) for 60 min at 37 °C. The formation of Phase 1 metabolites and Phase 2 conjugates after the incubation of 5 μM loxoprofen with human recombinant cDNA-expressed CYP isoforms in the presence of NGS (**d**), and UDP-glucuronosyltransferases (UGTs) isoforms in the presence of NGS and uridine 5′-diphosphoglucuronic acid (**e**) at 37 °C for 60 min. The data are represented as mean ± standard error (S.E.) of the triplicate samples. VH—vehicle control (untreated rat liver microsomes); 3-MC—3-methylcholanthrene; PB—phenobarbital; DEX—dexamethasone; ACE—acetone.

The previous in vivo study on the metabolism of loxoprofen reported the formation of two glucuronide conjugates of the alcohol metabolites of loxoprofen (Lox-OH-glucuronide) in monkey, mouse and dog urine (15, 16). Although we were unable to detect these metabolites after the incubation of loxoprofen with purified UGT enzyme isoforms, we incubated chemically synthesized Trans-OH or Cis-OH standard with six UGT isoforms (UGT1A1, 1A3, 1A4, 1A6, 1A9, and 2B7) in the presence of NGS and UDPGA, which yielded two Lox-OH-glucuronides, M7 and M8, of m/z 423.1652 primarily by UGT2B7 isoform at retention time of 11.2 and 11.7 mins (Figure 5). The CID MS/MS fragmentation of M7 and M8 resulted in product ions at m/z 247.1327 ($C_{15}H_{19}O_3$, after loss of a glucuronide ion) and 193.0345 ($C_6H_9O_7$) (Figure A1). From this fragmentation pattern, we proposed that M7 and M8 are the acyl glucuronide conjugates of the alcohol metabolites of loxoprofen. The final postulated metabolic pathway was shown in Figure 6.

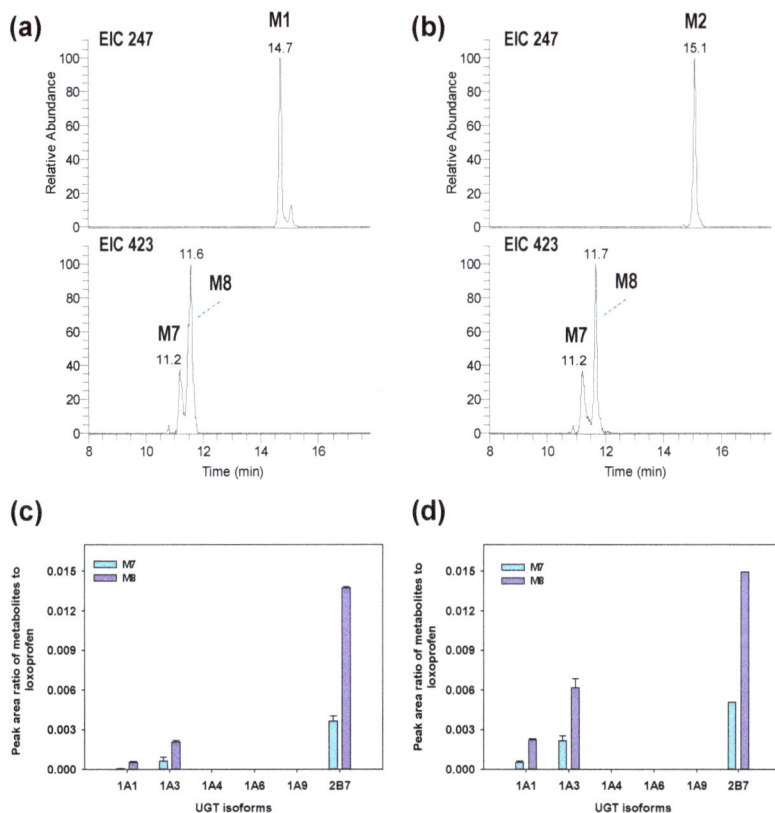

Figure 5. EIC of chemically synthesized Trans-OH (**a**) and Cis-OH standard (**b**) and their glucuronyl conjugates in human recombinant cDNA-expressed UGT2B7 on a Kinetex® C-18 column. The formation of glucuronide metabolites, M7 and M8, expressed as a peak area ratio of metabolites to loxoprofen, after incubating 5 μM of chemically synthesized standards of Trans-OH (**c**) and Cis-OH (**d**) in presence of uridine 5′-diphosphoglucuronic acid in six different UDP-glucuronosyltransferase (UGT) isoforms (UGT1A1, 1A3, 1A4, 1A6, 1A9, and 2B7) at 37 °C for 60 min. The data is represented as mean ± S.E of the duplicate samples.

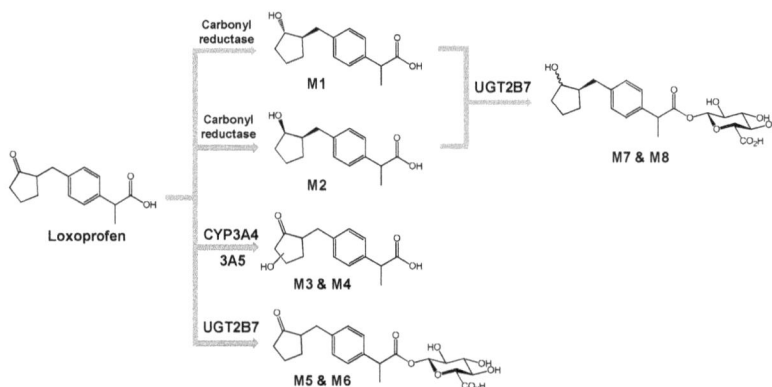

Figure 6. Metabolic pathway of loxoprofen in human liver microsomes.

4. Discussion

Loxoprofen is a popular drug of choice for musculoskeletal pain relief in many East-Asian countries. However, until now, the microsomal metabolic profile of loxoprofen was unknown. The active metabolite of loxoprofen, the Trans-OH form, exhibits anti-inflammatory properties by inhibiting cyclooxygenase enzymes. However, not only is the non-selective inhibition of cyclooxygenase enzymes of loxoprofen associated with adverse effects, but also, other ADRs of loxoprofen have been reported [9,10]. To prevent the toxicity caused by the drug–drug interaction, the metabolic profiling of loxoprofen should be clarified. In the present study, we investigated the metabolic pathway of loxoprofen in the liver microsomes from five mammalian species and identified the enzymes involved in the metabolism of loxoprofen in HLMs.

In the liver microsomes of the five mammalian species, we identified two hydroxylated metabolites (M3 and M4) and two glucuronide metabolites (M5 and M6). A comparison of the metabolic activity among five mammalian species revealed a higher Phase I metabolism in the mouse liver microsomes compared with that in the other species, probably reflecting its higher CYP content (pmol/mg protein) [25]. The dog liver microsomes produced higher levels of the glucuronide metabolites compared to those produced by the other species. Previous studies showed that the UGT1A1 and UGT2B7 substrates were highly metabolized by several-fold to their glucuronide metabolites in the dog liver compared with that in the human liver [26,27].

Incubation with chemically induced microsomes, a CYP3A4/5 selective inhibitor, and human recombinant cDNA-expressed CYPs (Figure 3a,d,e), showed that CYP3A4 and CYP3A5 are the primary CYP isoforms responsible for the microsomal hydroxylation of loxoprofen. CYP3A is the major CYP subfamily involved in the metabolism of more than 60% of drugs metabolized by CYP enzymes [28]. Many toxicities associated with modulation of CYP3A activity have been reported [29,30]. The metabolism of tacrolimus by the CYP3A subfamily in human liver microsomes was inhibited by loxoprofen to a lesser extent [31]. From previous studies, it is found that the polymorphism of the CYP3A subfamily either has no effect or shows a decrease in the expression or activity of the CYP3A subfamily. However, there have been a number of drugs that are known to induce CYP3A4 isoforms in humans, such as rifampicin, phenytoin, St. John's wort, and carbamazepine [32]. Previous study showed that the induction of the CYP3A4 isoform by rifampicin increased the acetaminophen induced toxicity [33]. The induction of the CYP3A4 isoform might alter the metabolic pathway of loxoprofen, leading to the reduced anti-inflammatory activity of loxoprofen, and thus a proper dose adjustment should be made to maintain the optimal therapeutic level of the drug. Therefore, it is important to further investigate the interaction between the loxoprofen and CYP3A activity modulators, which could result in drug–drug interactions.

The structure of loxoprofen contains a carboxylic acid moiety in its aliphatic chain. Drugs with a carboxylic acid moiety have long been associated with idiosyncratic drug toxicity; mainly drug induced liver injury caused by the formation of reactive metabolites like acyl glucuronide, acyl-co-A thioester, and acyl glutathione thioester derivatives [34–36]. Generally, glucuronidation is the detoxification and elimination pathway for xenobiotics [37]; however, the electrophilic acyl glucuronide can specifically and covalently bind to proteins like albumin. Neoantigens are formed to govern the immune-mediated reactions caused by the covalent binding of proteins to reactive acyl glucuronides, resulting in the toxicities associated with carboxylic acid containing drugs, which are mainly hypersensitivity reactions [38]. In the present study, we found that the metabolic conversion of loxoprofen to the acyl glucuronide metabolites occurred at a rate similar to that of its active metabolites (M1 and M2). The generated acyl glucuronide might be linked to loxoprofen-induced toxicities, and UGT2B7 was identified as the primary UGT isoform involved in the glucuronidation of loxoprofen and its alcoholic metabolites (M1 and M2) in HLMs. UGT2B7 is a major isoform involved in the metabolism of many NSAID drugs [39,40]. Although the UGT2B7 variants UGT2B7*1 and UGT2B7*2 have been found to be about 10-fold higher in Japanese than in Caucasians, this UGT2B7 polymorphism showed no significant alteration in the enzyme activity. The concomitant administration of drugs inducing UGT2B7 isoform, like phenobarbital and rifampicin, with loxoprofen, could lead to deleterious adverse effects from the increase in acyl glucuronide formation [41,42]. Owing to the formation of four acyl glucuronides, it is of utmost importance to investigate the toxicity of the acyl glucuronides of loxoprofen.

5. Conclusions

Using LC-HR/MS, four in vitro Phase I metabolites of loxoprofen (two alcohol metabolites and two hydroxylated metabolites) were identified in human, mouse, dog, rat, and monkey liver microsomes. CYP3A4 and 3A5 enzymes were found to be the major enzyme involved in the hydroxylation of loxoprofen, and UGT2B7 was found to be the main enzyme involved in its acyl-conjugation. We postulated that further studies should be carried to assess the potency and toxicity of these identified metabolites of loxoprofen, in order to gain a proper understanding of the mechanism of loxoprofen toxicity.

Author Contributions: Conceptualization, R.S. and S.L.; methodology, R.S., P.J.C., and S.P.; formal analysis, R.S.; resources, A.S., M.J.K., T.C.J., and E.-S.L.; data curation, R.S. and S.L.; writing (original draft preparation), R.S.; writing (review and editing), S.L.; funding acquisition, S.L.

Funding: This work was supported by the Korea Institute of Planning and Evaluation for Technology in Food, Agriculture, Forestry, and Fisheries (IPET), through the Export Promotion Technology Development Program, funded by the Ministry of Agriculture, Food, and Rural Affairs (MAFRA) (grant number 316017-3).

Acknowledgments: In this section you can acknowledge any support given that is not covered by the author contribution or funding sections. This may include administrative and technical support, or donations in kind (e.g., materials used for experiments).

Conflicts of Interest: The authors report no conflict of interest. The authors alone are responsible for the content and writing of this article.

Appendix A.

Appendix A.1. Supplemental Methods

Animal Treatment and Preparation of Liver Microsomes

Specific pathogen-free male Sprague-Dawley rats (250–280 g) were obtained from Charles River, Korea (Seoul, Korea). The animals were received at 5–6 weeks of age and were acclimated for at least one week. Upon arrival, the animals were randomized and housed as five animals per cage. The animal quarters were strictly maintained at 23 ± 3 °C and $50 \pm 10\%$ relative humidity. A 12 h light and dark cycle was used with an intensity of 150–300 Lux. All of the animal procedures were based on the guidelines recommended by the Society of Toxicology (USA) in 1989. For the preparation of enriched microsomes, specific pathogen-free male Sprague-Dawley rats (270–300 g) were pretreated with either 3-methylcholanthrene (3MC, 40 mg/kg, i.p., three days) in corn oil, PB (80 mg/kg, i.p., three days) in saline, dexamethasone (DEX, 50 mg/kg, i.p., three days) in corn oil, or acetone (ACE, 5 mL/kg, p.o., once). Twenty-four hours after the last dose, or two days after the last dose in the case of ACE, the enriched liver microsomes were isolated.

Instrument for Metabolic Stability

For the metabolic stability, a TSQ vantage triple quadrupole mass spectrometer equipped with a HESI-II Spray source was used, coupled to a Shimadzu Prominence UFLC system (Kyoto, Japan), incorporating a DGU-20A5 degasser, an LC-20AD Pump, an SIL-20A autosampler, and a CTO-20A column oven. The analytes were separated using a Kinetex® C18 column (150 mm × 2.1 mm, 2.6-μm, Phenomenex, Torrance, CA, USA). The mobile phase consisted of 100% ACN with 0.1% formic acid (mobile phase A) and 0.1% aqueous formic acid (mobile phase B) at a flow rate of 0.25 mL/min at 40 °C. The gradient conditions were as follows: 20% of B for 0.5 min, 20–99% of B at 0.5–2 min, 99% of B at 2–7 min, 99–20% of B at 7–7.5 min, and 20% of B at 7.5–12 min. For the qualification and quantitation of loxoprofen and its metabolites, instruments were set for $[M-H]^-$ ion. The MS operating conditions were as follows: electrospray ionization in negative mode, spray voltage, 3000 V; capillary temperature, 350 °C; vaporizer temperature, 300 °C; sheath gas pressure, 35 Arb; auxiliary gas pressure, 10 Arb; ion sweep gas pressure, 2.0 Arb. The data were analyzed using the Xcalibur software (Thermo Fisher Scientific Inc., Waltham, MA, USA).

Appendix A.2. Supplemental Data

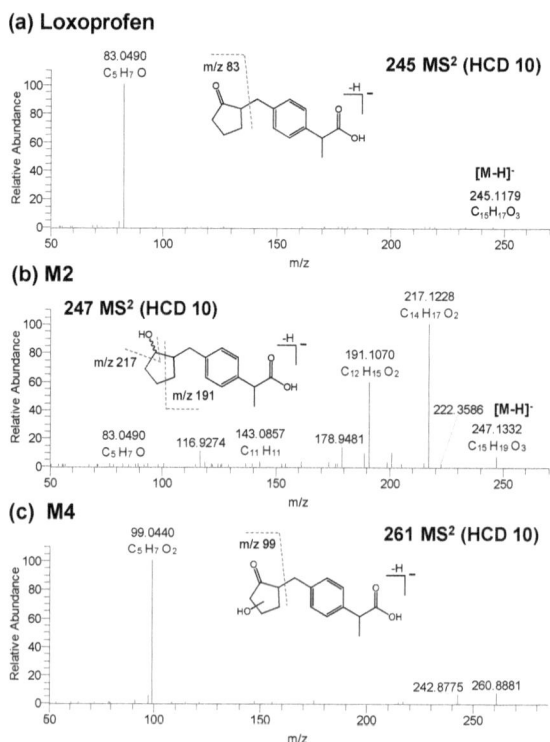

Figure A1. *Cont.*

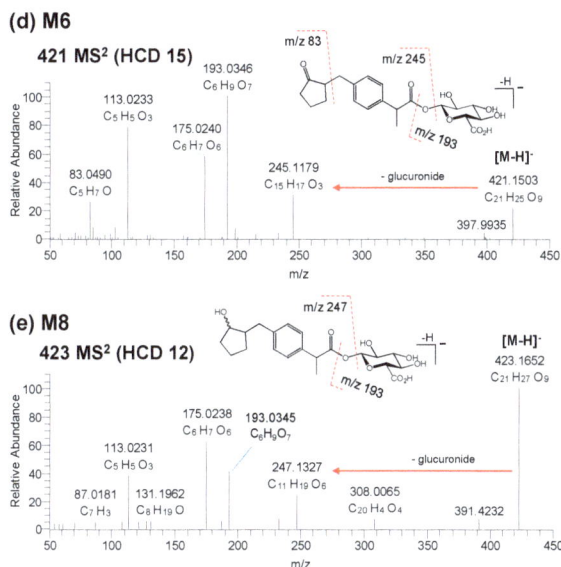

Figure A1. Collision-induced dissociation (CID) spectra of de-protonated loxoprofen (**a**), M2 (**b**), M4 (**c**), M6 (**d**), and M8 (**e**).

References

1. Greig, S.L.; Garnock-Jones, K.P. Loxoprofen: A review in pain and inflammation. *Clin. Drug. Investig.* **2016**, *36*, 771–781. [CrossRef] [PubMed]
2. Asami, T.; Yamanouchi, N.; Asami, A.; Tanaka, H.; Nogami, N. The effectiveness of patches containing loxoprofen sodium hydrate (lx-p) in the conservative therapy of muscular back pain—Clinical results using the japanese orthopaedic association back pain evaluation questionnaire (joabpeq). *Jpn. J. Compr. Rehabil. Sci.* **2013**, *4*, 22–29.
3. Waikakul, S.; Soparat, K. Effectiveness and safety of loxoprofen compared with naproxen in nonsurgical low back pain. *Clin. Drug. Investig.* **1995**, *10*, 59–63. [CrossRef]
4. Nagashima, H.; Tanaka, Y.; Watanabe, H.; Hayashi, R.; Kawada, K. Optical inversion of (2R)-to (2S)-isomers of 2-[4-(2-administration oxocyclopentylmethyl)-phenyl] propionic acid (loxoprofen), a new anti-inflammatory agent, and its monohydroxy metabolites in the rat. *Chem. Pharm. Bull.* **1984**, *32*, 251–257. [CrossRef] [PubMed]
5. Koo, T.S.; Kim, D.H.; Ahn, S.H.; Kim, K.P.; Kim, I.W.; Seo, S.Y.; Suh, Y.G.; Kim, D.D.; Shim, C.K.; Chung, S.J. Comparison of pharmacokinetics of loxoprofen and its active metabolites after an intravenous, intramuscular, and oral of loxoprofen in rats: Evidence for extrahepatic metabolism. *J. Pharm. Sci.* **2005**, *94*, 2187–2197. [CrossRef] [PubMed]
6. Sakamoto, C.; Kawai, T.; Nakamura, S.; Sugioka, T.; Tabira, J. Comparison of gastroduodenal ulcer incidence in healthy japanese subjects taking celecoxib or loxoprofen evaluated by endoscopy: A placebo-controlled, double-blind 2-week study. *Aliment. Pharmacol. Ther.* **2013**, *37*, 346–354. [CrossRef] [PubMed]
7. Sekiguchi, H.; Inoue, G.; Nakazawa, T.; Imura, T.; Saito, W.; Uchida, K.; Miyagi, M.; Takahira, N.; Takaso, M. Loxoprofen sodium and celecoxib for postoperative pain in patients after spinal surgery: A randomized comparative study. *J. Orthop. Sci.* **2015**, *20*, 617–623. [CrossRef] [PubMed]
8. Kaniwa, N.; Ueta, M.; Nakamura, R.; Okamoto-Uchida, Y.; Sugiyama, E.; Maekawa, K.; Takahashi, Y.; Furuya, H.; Yagami, A.; Matsukura, S. Drugs causing severe ocular surface involvements in japanese patients with stevensejohnson syndrome/toxic epidermal necrolysis. *Allergol. Int.* **2015**, *64*, 379–381. [CrossRef] [PubMed]

9.   Ueharaguchi, Y. Loxoprofen/piperacillin acute generalised exanthematous pustulosis. *Reactions* **2011**, *1355*, 11.

10.   Yue, Z.; Shi, J.; Jiang, P.; Sun, H. Acute kidney injury during concomitant use of valacyclovir and loxoprofen: Detecting drug–drug interactions in a spontaneous reporting system. *Pharmacoepidemiol. Drug Saf.* **2014**, *23*, 1154–1159. [CrossRef] [PubMed]

11.   Taniguchi, Y.; Deguchi, Y.; Noda, K. Interaction between enoxacin, a new antimicrobial, and nimesulide, a new non-steroidal anti-inflammatory agent in mice. *Inflamm. Res.* **1996**, *45*, 376–379. [CrossRef] [PubMed]

12.   Shibata, K.; Akagi, Y.; Nozawa, N.; Shimomura, H.; Aoyama, T. Influence of nonsteroidal anti-inflammatory drugs on aspirin's antiplatelet effects and suggestion of the most suitable time for administration of both agents without resulting in interaction. *J. Pharm. Health Care Sci.* **2017**, *3*, 9. [CrossRef] [PubMed]

13.   Yamakawa, N.; Suemasu, S.; Watanabe, H.; Tahara, K.; Tanaka, K.-I.; Okamoto, Y.; Ohtsuka, M.; Maruyama, T.; Mizushima, T. Comparison of pharmacokinetics between loxoprofen and its derivative with lower ulcerogenic activity, fluoro-loxoprofen. *Drug Metab. Pharmacokinet.* **2013**, *28*, 118–124. [CrossRef] [PubMed]

14.   Lee, H.W.; Ji, H.Y.; Sohn, D.H.; Kim, S.M.; Lee, Y.B.; Lee, H.S. Liquid chromatography-tandem mass spectrometry method of loxoprofen in human plasma. *Biomed. Chromatogr.* **2009**, *23*, 714–718. [CrossRef] [PubMed]

15.   Sawamura, R.; Kazui, M.; Kurihara, A.; Izumi, T. Absorption, distribution, metabolism and excretion of loxoprofen after dermal application of loxoprofen gel to rats. *Xenobiotica* **2014**, *44*, 1026–1038. [CrossRef] [PubMed]

16.   Sawamura, R.; Sakurai, H.; Wada, N.; Nishiya, Y.; Honda, T.; Kazui, M.; Kurihara, A.; Shinagawa, A.; Izumi, T. Bioactivation of loxoprofen to a pharmacologically active metabolite and its disposition kinetics in human skin. *Biopharm. Drug Dispos.* **2015**, *36*, 352–363. [CrossRef] [PubMed]

17.   Jhee, O.H.; Lee, M.H.; Shaw, L.M.; Lee, S.E.; Park, J.H.; Kang, J.S. Pharmacokinetics and bioequivalence study of two brands of loxoprofen tablets in healthy volunteers. *Arzneimittelforschung* **2007**, *57*, 542–546. [CrossRef] [PubMed]

18.   Cho, H.-Y.; Park, C.-H.; Lee, Y.-B. Direct and simultaneous analysis of loxoprofen and its diastereometric alcohol metabolites in human serum by on-line column switching liquid chromatography and its application to a pharmacokinetic study. *J. Chromatogr. B Analyt. Technol. Biomed. Life Sci.* **2006**, *835*, 27–34. [CrossRef] [PubMed]

19.   Kanazawa, H.; Tsubayashi, A.; Nagata, Y.; Matsushima, Y.; Mori, C.; Kizu, J.; Higaki, M. Stereospecific analysis of loxoprofen in plasma by chiral column liquid chromatography with a circular dichroism-based detector. *J. Chromatogr. A* **2002**, *948*, 303–308. [CrossRef]

20.   Kim, I.-W.; Chung, S.-J.; Shim, C.-K. Altered metabolism of orally administered loxoprofen in human subjects after an oral administration of loxoprofen for three consecutive days followed by a seven-day washout. *J. Pharm. Sci.* **2002**, *91*, 973–979. [CrossRef] [PubMed]

21.   Tanaka, Y.; Nishikawa, Y.; Hayashi, R. Species differences in metabolism of sodium 2-[4-(2-oxocyclopentylmethyl)-phenyl] propionate dihydrate (loxoprofen sodium), a new anti-inflammatory agent. *Chem. Pharm. Bull.* **1983**, *31*, 3656–3664. [CrossRef] [PubMed]

22.   Naruto, S.; Terada, A. Synthesis of the 8 possible optically-active isomers of 2-[4-(2-hydroxycyclopentylmethyl) phenyl] propionic acid. *Chem. Pharm. Bull.* **1983**, *31*, 4319–4323. [CrossRef]

23.   Kim, D.O.; Lee, S.K.; Jeon, T.W.; Jin, C.H.; Hyun, S.H.; Kim, E.J.; Moon, G.I.; Kim, J.A.; Lee, E.S.; Lee, B.M.; et al. Role of metabolism in parathion-induced hepatotoxicity and immunotoxicity. *J. Toxicol. Environ. Health A* **2005**, *68*, 2187–2205. [CrossRef] [PubMed]

24.   Emoto, C.; Murase, S.; Sawada, Y.; Jones, B.C.; Iwasaki, K. In vitro inhibitory effect of 1-aminobenzotriazole on drug oxidations catalyzed by human cytochrome P450 enzymes: A comparison with SKF-525A and ketoconazole. *Drug Metab. Pharmacokinet.* **2003**, *18*, 287–295. [CrossRef] [PubMed]

25.   Pasanen, M. Species differences in CYP enzymes. *Monografías de la Real Academia Nacional de Farmacia* **2014**, *XIV*, 63–90.

26.   Sharer, J.E.; Shipley, L.A.; Vandenbranden, M.R.; Binkley, S.N.; Wrighton, S.A. Comparisons of phase i and phase ii in vitro hepatic enzyme activities of human, dog, rhesus monkey, and cynomolgus monkey. *Drug Metab. Dispos* **1995**, *23*, 1231–1241. [PubMed]

27. Soars, M.G.; Riley, R.J.; Findlay, K.A.; Coffey, M.J.; Burchell, B. Evidence for significant differences in microsomal drug glucuronidation by canine and human liver and kidney. *Drug Metab. Dispos* **2001**, *29*, 121–126. [PubMed]
28. Gibson, G.; Plant, N.; Swales, K.; Ayrton, A.; El-Sankary, W. Receptor-dependent transcriptional activation of cytochrome P4503A genes: Induction mechanisms, species differences and interindividual variation in man. *Xenobiotica* **2002**, *32*, 165–206. [CrossRef] [PubMed]
29. Honig, P.K.; Wortham, D.C.; Zamani, K.; Conner, D.P.; Mullin, J.C.; Cantilena, L.R. Terfenadine-ketoconazole interaction. *JAMA* **1993**, *269*, 1513–1518. [CrossRef] [PubMed]
30. Huang, S.M.; Strong, J.M.; Zhang, L.; Reynolds, K.S.; Nallani, S.; Temple, R.; Abraham, S.; Habet, S.A.; Baweja, R.K.; Burckart, G.J. New era in drug interaction evaluation: Us food and drug administration update on CYP enzymes, transporters, and the guidance process. *J. Clin. Pharmacol.* **2008**, *48*, 662–670. [CrossRef] [PubMed]
31. Iwasaki, K.; Matsuda, H.; Nagase, K.; Shiraga, T.; Tokuma, Y.; Uchida, K. Effects of twenty-three drugs on the metabolism of FK506 by human liver microsomes. *Res. Commun. Chem. Pathol. Pharmacol* **1993**, *82*, 209. [PubMed]
32. Klaassen, C. *Casarett & Doull's Toxicology: The Basic Science of Poisons*, 8th ed.; McGraw-Hill Education: New York, NY, USA, 2013.
33. Cheng, J.; Ma, X.; Krausz, K.W.; Idle, J.R.; Gonzalez, F.J. Rifampicin-activated human PXR and CYP3A4 induction enhance acetaminophen-induced toxicity. *Drug Metab. Dispos.* **2009**, *37*, 1611–1621. [CrossRef] [PubMed]
34. Darnell, M.; Weidolf, L. Metabolism of xenobiotic carboxylic acids: Focus on coenzyme a conjugation, reactivity, and interference with lipid metabolism. *Chem. Res. Toxicol.* **2013**, *26*, 1139–1155. [CrossRef] [PubMed]
35. Lassila, T.; Hokkanen, J.; Aatsinki, S.M.; Mattila, S.; Turpeinen, M.; Tolonen, A. Toxicity of carboxylic acid-containing drugs: The role of acyl migration and coa conjugation investigated. *Chem. Res. Toxicol.* **2015**, *28*, 2292–2303. [CrossRef] [PubMed]
36. Skonberg, C.; Olsen, J.; Madsen, K.G.; Hansen, S.H.; Grillo, M.P. Metabolic activation of carboxylic acids. *Expert Opin. Drug Metab. Toxicol.* **2008**, *4*, 425–438. [CrossRef] [PubMed]
37. Kroemer, H.K.; Klotz, U. Glucuronidation of drugs. *Clin. Pharmacokinet.* **1992**, *23*, 292–310. [CrossRef] [PubMed]
38. Regan, S.L.; Maggs, J.L.; Hammond, T.G.; Lambert, C.; Williams, D.P.; Park, B.K. Acyl glucuronides: The good, the bad and the ugly. *Biopharm. Drug Dispos.* **2010**, *31*, 367–395. [CrossRef] [PubMed]
39. Kuehl, G.E.; Lampe, J.W.; Potter, J.D.; Bigler, J. Glucuronidation of nonsteroidal anti-inflammatory drugs: Identifying the enzymes responsible in human liver microsomes. *Drug Metab. Dispos.* **2005**, *33*, 1027–1035. [CrossRef] [PubMed]
40. Jinno, N.; Tagashira, M.; Tsurui, K.; Yamada, S. Contribution of cytochrome P450 and UDT-glucuronosyltransferase to the metabolism of drugs containing carboxylic acid groups: Risk assessment of acylglucuronides using human hepatocytes. *Xenobiotica* **2014**, *44*, 677–686. [CrossRef] [PubMed]
41. Kiang, T.K.; Ensom, M.H.; Chang, T.K. UDP-glucuronosyltransferases and clinical drug-drug interactions. *Pharmacol. Ther.* **2005**, *106*, 97–132. [CrossRef] [PubMed]
42. Soars, M.G.; Petullo, D.M.; Eckstein, J.A.; Kasper, S.C.; Wrighton, S.A. An assessment of UDP-glucuronosyltransferase induction using primary human hepatocytes. *Drug Metab. Dispos.* **2004**, *32*, 140–148. [CrossRef] [PubMed]

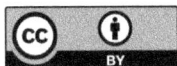

pharmaceutics

MDPI

Article

A Simple and Sensitive Liquid Chromatography with Tandem Mass Spectrometric Method for the Simultaneous Determination of Anthraquinone Glycosides and Their Aglycones in Rat Plasma: Application to a Pharmacokinetic Study of *Rumex acetosa* Extract

Hossain Mohammad Arif Ullah [†], Junhyeong Kim [†], Naveed Ur Rehman, Hye-Jin Kim, Mi-Jeong Ahn * and Hye Jin Chung *

College of Pharmacy and Research Institute of Pharmaceutical Sciences, Gyeongsang National University, Jinju 52828, Korea; arifpha@ymail.com (H.M.A.U.); jhk6914@naver.com (J.K.); naveed.rehman50@gmail.com (N.U.R.); black200203@gmail.com (H.-J.K.)
* Correspondence: amj5812@gnu.ac.kr (M.-J.A.); hchung@gnu.ac.kr (H.J.C.);
   Tel.: +82-55-772-2425 (M.-J.A.); +82-55-772-2430 (H.J.C.)
† These authors contributed equally to this work.

Received: 24 June 2018; Accepted: 18 July 2018; Published: 20 July 2018

check for updates

Abstract: *Rumex acetosa* (*R. acetosa*) has been used in folk remedies for gastrointestinal disorders and cutaneous diseases. *Rumex* species, in particular, contain abundant anthraquinones. Anthraquinone glycosides and aglycones show different bioactive effects.   However, information on the pharmacokinetics of anthraquinone glycosides is limited, and methods to quantify anthraquinone glycosides in plasma are rarely available. A simple and sensitive liquid chromatography-tandem mass spectrometric bioanalytical method for the simultaneous determination of both anthraquinone glycosides and their aglycones, including emodin, emodin-8-*O*-β-D-glucoside, chrysophanol, chrysophanol-8-*O*-β-D-glucoside, physcion, and physcion-8-*O*-β-D-glucoside , in a low volume of rat plasma (20 µL) was established. A simple and rapid sample preparation was employed using methanol as a precipitating agent with appropriate sensitivity. Chromatographic separation was performed on HPLC by using a biphenyl column with a gradient elution using 2 mM ammonium formate (pH 6) in water and 2 mM ammonium formate (pH 6) in methanol within a run time of 13 min. The anthraquinones were detected on triple-quadrupole mass spectrometer in negative ionization mode using multiple-reaction monitoring. The method was validated in terms of selectivity, linearity, accuracy, precision, recovery, and stability. The values of the lower limit of quantitation of anthraquinones were 1–20 ng/mL. The intra-batch and inter-batch accuracies were 96.7–111.9% and the precision was within the acceptable limits. The method was applied to a pharmacokinetic study after oral administration of *R. acetosa* 70% ethanol extract to rats at a dose of 2 g/kg.

Keywords: anthraquinone; glycoside; aglycone; LC-MS/MS; plasma; protein precipitation

---

1. Introduction

   Rumex acetosa L. (*R. acetosa*), belonging to the Polygonaceae family, is a perennial herb that is listed in the Korean Food Code (Korea Food and Drug Administration) as a food material and has been used in folk remedies for gastrointestinal disorders and cutaneous diseases [1]. Extracts of *R. acetosa* have been reported to have various biological activities, including anti-ulcerogenic, anti-inflammatory, anti-proliferative, and anti-viral effects [2–4]. They contain a number of bioactive compounds, including anthraquinones, flavonoids, and polysaccharides [5]. In particular, *Rumex* species contain abundant anthraquinones, including emodin, chrysophanol, and physcion in all parts of the plant, in free and glycoside forms [6]. A difference in anthraquinone physiological activity between these forms has been described [7]. Previous studies reported a number of quantitative methods of anthraquinones in plasma [8–10]. However, we found that most of these studies focused on determining aglycones (free anthraquinones). Methods to quantify anthraquinone glycosides in plasma are rarely available.

As interest in natural drugs has increased in the pharmaceutical industry, research is underway to develop potential applications of *R. acetosa*, which has already proven its efficacy. Therefore, a simple and sensitive analytical method to examine bioactive anthraquinones in biological samples is needed to evaluate the potential of new treatments.

The aim of this study is to establish a simple, rapid, and sensitive liquid chromatography-tandem mass spectrometry (LC-MS/MS) method to simultaneously quantify emodin (E), emodin-8-*O*-β-D-glucoside (EG), chrysophanol (C), chrysophanol-8-*O*-β-D-glucoside (CG), physcion (P), and physcion-8-*O*-β-D-glucoside (PG) in rat plasma within one chromatographic run. The method was applied to determine pharmacokinetic parameters after oral administration of *R. acetosa* 70% ethanol extract in rat. The results of this study might be helpful in the development of a new type of medicine using *R. acetosa*.

2. Materials and Methods

2.1. Materials

The plant of *R. acetosa* L. (Polygonaceae) was collected from the Sancheong province of Korea in April 2014 and identified by Mi-Jeong Ahn of the College of Pharmacy, Gyeongsang National University (Jinju, Korea). The voucher specimen (APG-1403) was deposited in the Herbarium of the College of Pharmacy, Gyeongsang National University. The standards of the six anthraquinones (E, EG, C, CG, P, and PG) were isolated from the whole part of *R. acetosa* and their structures (Figure 1) were elucidated using spectroscopy such as MS and nuclear magnetic resonance spectroscopy (data not shown) [11]. The purity of anthraquinone compounds isolated from *R. acetosa* was confirmed to be more than 95% by NMR and HPLC-UV. Diclofenac used as an internal standard (IS) was purchased from Sigma Aldrich (St. Louis, MO, USA). HPLC-grade acetonitrile, methanol, and water were products of Fisher Scientific Korea Ltd. (Seoul, Korea). All reagents were analytical grade.

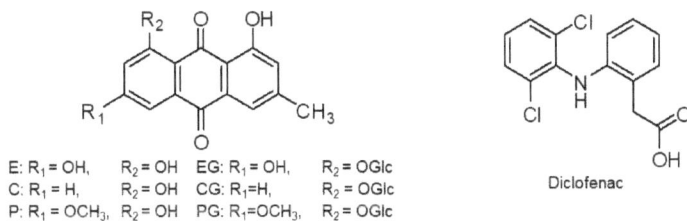

E: R$_1$ = OH,   R$_2$ = OH   EG: R$_1$ = OH,   R$_2$ = OGlc
C: R$_1$ = H,   R$_2$ = OH   CG: R$_1$=H,   R$_2$ = OGlc
P: R$_1$ = OCH$_3$, R$_2$ = OH   PG: R$_1$=OCH$_3$, R$_2$ = OGlc

Diclofenac

Figure 1. The chemical structures of six anthraquinones and diclofenac (internal standard). E, emodin; EG, emodin-8-*O*-β-D-glucoside; C, chrysophanol; CG, chrysophanol-8-*O*-β-D-glucoside; P, physcion; PG, physcion-8-*O*-β-D-glucoside.

2.2. Chromatographic Condition

The analysis was performed on an Agilent 1260 series (Agilent Technologies, Waldbronn, Germany) HPLC system. Chromatographic separation of the samples was carried out on a Kinetex Biphenyl column (100 × 3.0 mm, 2.6 μm, 110 Å, Phenomenex, Torrance, CA, USA). The mobile phase consisted of 2 mM ammonium formate (pH 6) in water (A) and 2 mM ammonium formate (pH 6) in methanol (B). The gradient program was used at a flow rate of 0.3 mL/min while maintaining the column temperature at 40 °C. The mobile phase initial composition of 25% B was maintained for 2 min. It was then increased linearly from 25% to 95% B for 0.5 min and held for 7 min. The gradient was then changed back to the initial condition for 0.5 min and kept at the initial condition for 3 min. The total analysis time was 13 min for each sample. The injection volume was 15 μL.

2.3. Mass Spectrometric Condition

The mass spectrometric detection was performed on an Agilent 6460 triple-quadruple mass spectrometer (Agilent Technologies, Singapore) with an electrospray ionization source. It was operated in the negative ion detection mode because of its higher sensitivity than that in the positive ionization mode on multiple reaction monitoring (MRM). The data were acquired and processed using Mass Hunter Workstation B.06.00 software (Agilent Technologies, Singapore). The mass spectrometric parameters of each compound are summarized in Table 1 [12]. The MS spectra of the six anthraquinones are shown in Figure 2. The source parameters were also optimized as follows: a drying gas flow and temperature at 6 L/min and 350 °C were used, respectively; the sheath gas flow and temperature were maintained at 12 L/min and 350 °C, respectively; the nebulizing gas (N_2) pressure was set at 25 psi; and the capillary and nozzle voltages were set at 3500 V and 500 V, respectively.

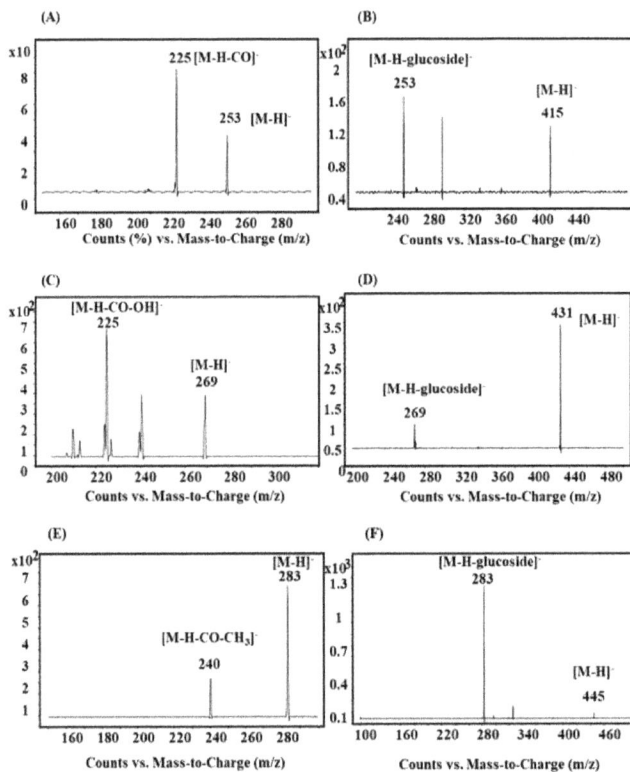

Figure 2. MS/MS scan spectra of six anthraquinones. (**A**) chrysophanol; (**B**) chrysophanol-8-*O*-β-D-glucoside; (**C**) emodin; (**D**) emodin-8-*O*-β-D-glucoside; (**E**) physcion; (**F**) physcion-8-*O*-β-D-glucoside.

Table 1. Summary of the MS/MS parameters.

Compounds	MRM Transition (*m/z*) [a] Precursor Ion → Product Ion	Fragmentor (V)	Collision Energy (V)
E	269 → 225	145	20
EG	431 → 269	150	24
C	253 → 225	175	22
CG	415 → 253	89	13
P	283 → 240	157	16
PG	445 → 283	95	5
IS (Diclofenac)	294 → 250	65	1

[a] MRM transitions refer to the reference [12]. MRM, multiple reaction monitoring; E, emodin; EG, emodin-8-*O*-β-D-glucoside; C, chrysophanol; CG, chrysophanol-8-*O*-β-D-glucoside; P, physcion; PG, physcion-8-*O*-β-D-glucoside; IS, internal standard.

2.4. Preparation of R. acetosa Extract

The dried plant material (100 g) was ground and extracted with 70% ethanol. The extract was filtered using filter papers (Whatman No. 40) and concentrated through a rotary evaporator. The concentrate was lyophilized and stored at −80 °C. The exact amount was weighed and used as the samples for the animal studies. The contents of E, EG, C, CG, P, and PG in *R. acetosa* extract were 0.94 ± 0.15%, 1.29 ± 0.06%, 0.68 ± 0.09%, 0.77 ± 0.12%, 0.17 ± 0.02%, and 0.41 ± 0.05% (*w/w*), respectively. The values were expressed as mean ± standard deviation.

2.5. Preparation of the Calibration Standard and Quality Control (QC) Samples

The primary stock solutions of E, EG, C, CG, P, PG, and IS were prepared in dimethyl sulfoxide at a concentration of 1 mg/mL and stored at −80 °C. The mixture stock solutions to obtain the standard solutions were serially diluted in methanol. The IS stock solution of 5 ng/mL was prepared in methanol. The calibration standards were prepared by spiking 10 μL of above standard solutions into 90 μL of blank rat plasma to yield concentration ranges of 1–300 ng/mL for E, 20–300 ng/mL for P and C, 1–150 ng/mL for EG, 10–150 ng/mL for CG and PG. Twenty microliters of aliquots were prepared and stored at −80 °C until analysis.

The QC samples were prepared in the same way as the calibration samples for E, EG, C, CG, P, and PG in rat plasma at low, middle, and high concentrations. All the solutions were kept at −80 °C.

2.6. Sample Preparation

To 20 μL aliquot of the rat plasma samples, 60 μL of 5 ng/mL IS in methanol was added. The mixture was vortexed for 30 s and kept at 4 °C for 30 min. The mixture was centrifuged at 10,000× *g* for 10 min. The supernatant was transferred to an HPLC vial, and 15 μL of the processed sample was injected onto the LC-MS/MS system.

2.7. Method Validation

The method validation was performed according to the United States Food and Drug Administration's guidance on bioanalytical method validation [13].

2.7.1. Selectivity

The selectivity study was performed by comparing the chromatograms of the six different rat plasma samples to investigate the interference near the retention time of the analytes and the IS.

2.7.2. Calibration Curves and Sensitivity

The linearity of each calibration curve was determined by plotting the peak area ratio of the analyte to IS versus the plasma concentrations. The least-square method was used to achieve a linear regression equation. Sensitivity was defined by calculating the lower limit of detection and the lower limit of quantification (LLOQ) based on a signal-to-noise ratio of greater than 3 and 10, respectively. Besides signal-to-noise ratio, LLOQ values with acceptable precision and accuracy values were chosen. The criteria of precision and accuracy at LLOQ are within 20% relative standard deviation (RSD) for precision and between 80–120% for accuracy.

2.7.3. Precision and Accuracy

Precision and accuracy were investigated by analyzing six replicates of four QC levels on the same batch (intra-batch) and five different batches (inter-batch) of four QC levels (LLOQ, low QC, middle QC, and high QC). The intra- and inter-batch precision was expressed by RSD (%), and accuracy was evaluated by expressing it as a percentage of the theoretical value (the mean calculated concentration/nominal concentration) × 100%. The acceptance criteria are within 15% RSD except 20% at LLOQ for precision and ±15% of nominal concentrations except ±20% at LLOQ for accuracy.

2.7.4. Extraction Recovery and Matrix Effect

The extraction recovery was evaluated by comparing the peak area of the extracted sample with that of the post-extracted sample at three replicates of three QC levels. The matrix effect of the analytes was investigated by comparing the peak area of the post-extracted sample with the peak area obtained by the corresponding standard solutions in pH 7.4 buffer at three QC levels. Matrix effects were determined using the equation below.

$$\left(\frac{\text{peak area of the analytes for the sample spiked with the target compounds after extraction}}{\text{peak area of the analytes for the standard solutions}} \right) \times 100\%$$

2.7.5. Stability

The stability of the analytes in rat plasma was evaluated by analyzing triplicates of three QC levels at room temperature for 4 h (short-term stability), −80 °C for one month (long-term stability), three freeze-thaw cycles from −80 °C to room temperature (freeze and thaw stability), and 4 °C for 24 h (processed sample stability). The stability of analytes in stock solution was also evaluated. The peak areas obtained from freshly prepared stock solutions were compared with stock solutions stored for 4 h at room temperature.

2.8. Pharmacokinetic Study

Male Sprague-Dawley rats (8-week-old, weighing 250 ± 10 g) were obtained from Koatech (Pyeongtaek, Korea). They were housed and acclimated in the Animal Laboratory, Gyeongsang National University, under controlled temperature and humidity and regular 12 h light cycle, freely accessible to food and water for 7 days before the experiment. The rats were cannulated into the carotid artery and allowed to recover for one day. Before the pharmacokinetic study, all rats were fasted for 12 h with free access to water. *R. acetosa* extract suspended in a solution (ethanol:polysorbate 80:water = 1:2:7, *v/v/v*) was orally administered to the three rats at a dose of 2 g/kg. The calculated doses of compounds based on the contents in the extract were 18.8, 25.8, 13.6, 15.4, 3.4, and 8.2 mg/kg for E, EG, C, CG, P, and PG, respectively. Blood samples (100 μL) were collected via the cannulated carotid vessel at 0, 15, 30, 45 min, 1, 2, 3, 4, 6, 8, 12, and 24 h after oral administration. To collect plasma, the blood samples were immediately centrifuged at 10,000× g for 5 min. All plasma samples were stored at −80 °C until analysis. All experimental procedures of the animal study were approved (GNU-130618-R0038) by the Animal Care and Use Committee of Gyeongsang National University, Korea.

3. Results

3.1. Method Validation

3.1.1. Specificity and Selectivity

The representative MRM chromatograms of blank rat plasma and that spiked with six anthraquinones and IS are shown in Figure 3. No interference from endogenous substances near the retention time of the analytes or the IS was observed.

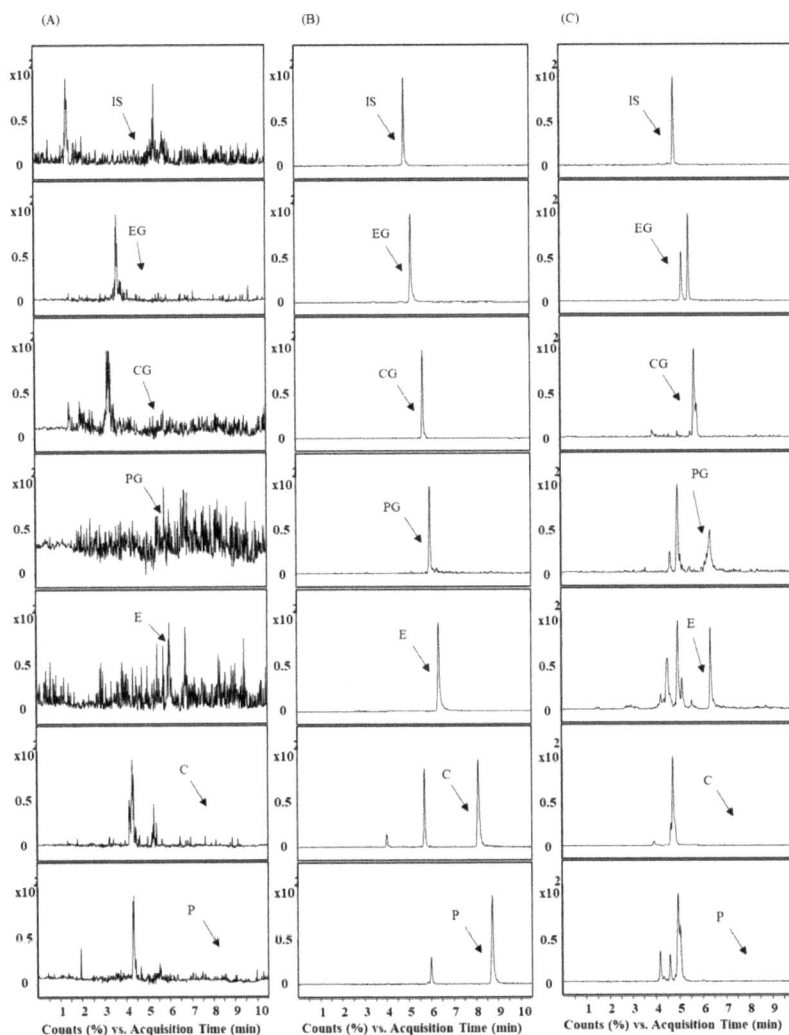

Figure 3. Representative MRM chromatograms of IS, EG, CG, PG, E, C, and P in rat plasma. (**A**) blank plasma; (**B**) blank plasma spiked with six anthraquinones (250 ng/mL for aglycones and 125 ng/mL for glycosides) and IS; (**C**) plasma sample obtained from rats 45 min after oral administration of *R. acetosa* extract (2 g/kg).

3.1.2. Linearity and Sensitivity

The calibration curves showed good linearity over their corresponding ranges for the analytes ($R^2 > 0.9934$).

3.1.3. Precision and Accuracy

The intra- and inter-batch precision and accuracies are presented in Table 2. The RSD values for the intra- and inter-batch were below 13.5%, except for EG at LLOQ (18.9%). The accuracies were between 85% and 115%. All results showed acceptable accuracy and precision.

Table 2. Accuracy and precision of anthraquinones in rat plasma ($n = 6$). RSD: relative standard deviation.

Analyte	Nominal Concentration (ng/mL)	Intra-Batch			Inter-Batch		
		Mean Calculated Concentration (ng/mL)	Accuracy (%)	RSD (%)	Mean Calculated Concentration (ng/mL)	Accuracy (%)	RSD (%)
P	20	20.5	102.5	8.83	21.3	106.4	11.2
	60	58.0	96.7	4.69	63.4	105.6	7.72
	150	156	104.2	3.98	158	105.3	5.90
	300	308	102.6	2.80	312	104.1	5.54
E	1	1.10	110.1	13.5	1.05	104.6	11.1
	3	3.31	110.3	6.87	3.12	103.9	6.87
	150	155	103.4	2.32	154	102.8	2.66
	300	309	103.0	3.45	299	99.8	2.28
C	20	21.8	109.2	9.23	19.8	98.9	2.98
	60	64.1	106.9	7.79	59.3	98.9	5.75
	150	153	101.9	4.91	155	103.1	6.85
	300	303	101.1	3.94	321	107.0	4.20
PG	10	10.2	102.1	10.7	10.2	102.3	12.1
	30	32.1	107.1	6.83	31.7	105.7	5.72
	75	80.3	107.1	5.38	80.5	107.3	4.95
	150	160	106.5	4.13	159	106.2	4.89
EG	1	1.10	110.1	18.9	1.05	105.2	9.10
	3	3.35	111.8	5.49	3.27	108.9	12.9
	75	77.3	103.0	1.59	78.5	104.6	3.85
	150	156	104.1	1.24	153.9	102.6	4.34
CG	10	11.2	111.9	8.34	11.0	109.9	8.00
	30	31.5	105.0	4.13	31.6	105.4	5.79
	75	76.3	101.7	2.72	76.5	102.0	3.16
	150	154	102.9	3.87	157	104.5	2.12

3.1.4. Extraction Recovery and Matrix Effect

The extraction recoveries and matrix effects of the anthraquinone compounds are shown in Table 3. The matrix effects were consistent among different concentrations for each compound. The recoveries ranged from 96.0% to 112.7% for the analytes at the QC levels. The matrix effects were constant for each analyte with different concentrations.

3.1.5. Stability

The stability of stock solution was determined. As compared with fresh stock solutions, the mean concentration of analytes ($n = 3$) in stock solutions stored at room temperature for 4 h were 99.2, 94.8, 95.9, 102.4, 100.4, and 101.7% for P, E, C, PG, EG, and CG, respectively. There was no detectable degradation of compounds in dimethyl sulfoxide and methanol stored at room temperature for 3 months based on HPLC-UV chromatogram. The stability results of the analytes in rat plasma under different conditions are shown in Table 4.

Table 3. Extraction recovery and matrix effect of anthraquinones in rat plasma (*n* = 3).

Analyte	Nominal Concentration (ng/mL)	Extraction Recovery (%)		Matrix Effect (%)	
		Mean	RSD	Mean	RSD
P	60	106.5	4.85	185.6	2.29
	150	106.4	1.23	185.1	3.13
	300	98.6	1.49	183.9	3.92
E	3	101.3	2.74	70.1	6.65
	150	105.6	0.82	87.0	1.46
	300	100.4	1.90	92.3	2.77
C	60	112.7	8.71	143.0	1.04
	150	102.1	1.07	144.3	1.62
	300	96.6	1.04	144.6	4.11
PG	30	106.4	13.0	42.5	8.41
	75	107.4	5.60	44.3	6.07
	150	96.6	3.14	51.4	2.33
EG	3	97.6	3.48	286.5	4.29
	75	100.5	0.77	277.6	3.60
	150	97.6	1.25	277.8	2.84
CG	30	96.0	1.36	113.8	6.64
	75	96.6	6.01	121.9	3.24
	150	96.5	6.89	126.7	2.02

Table 4. Stability of anthraquinones in rat plasma (*n* = 3).

Analyte	Conc. (ng/mL)	Short Term Stability (%)		Long Term Stability (%)		Freeze and Thaw Stability (%)		Processed Sample Stability (%)	
		Accuracy	RSD	Accuracy	RSD	Accuracy	RSD	Accuracy	RSD
P	60	104.9	2.05	107.3	5.31	103.6	8.18	102.2	9.10
	150	98.9	5.64	100.1	2.34	103.9	4.48	101.6	2.87
	300	103.8	2.39	98.0	2.00	104.2	3.21	102.7	5.76
E	3	103.2	3.46	106.8	4.25	107.5	2.38	108.2	5.26
	150	100.7	2.55	107.8	1.87	104.5	4.32	108.0	5.96
	300	101.8	2.44	107.7	0.93	102.0	3.47	104.6	3.60
C	60	103.5	6.23	104.3	8.67	89.7	0.76	101.5	9.60
	150	98.6	1.07	97.9	7.67	91.8	3.94	103.7	5.43
	300	101.2	2.97	102.6	2.98	92.4	8.25	102.3	6.47
PG	30	98.9	9.48	97.7	5.64	101.5	9.06	98.8	6.33
	75	91.8	6.60	98.5	5.36	94.3	6.57	92.7	4.64
	150	96.7	1.62	97.1	2.85	93.6	2.16	96.8	1.19
EG	3	99.8	5.11	102.9	4.02	100.4	6.39	91.5	3.11
	75	108.5	2.79	107.9	1.54	112.3	3.60	107.9	2.88
	150	98.9	1.81	102.8	2.14	100.9	1.69	100.3	4.14
CG	30	97.6	9.29	97.5	4.04	98.3	4.81	91.1	2.45
	75	96.9	0.56	100.6	1.38	101.0	2.23	100.2	7.38
	150	101.8	5.27	101.5	2.52	97.0	5.66	96.7	5.93

3.2. Pharmacokinetics Study

The validated LC-MS/MS method was applied to the pharmacokinetic study after oral administration of *R. acetosa* extract at a dose of 2 g/kg to the rats. The concentrations of EG and P were not high enough to determine the pharmacokinetic parameters. The concentrations of C and PG were below the LLOQ from 6 h after administration of extract, CG and E could be detected until 8 and 24 h, respectively. The mean plasma concentration–time profiles of the analytes are presented in Figure 4. The major pharmacokinetic parameters of C, E, CG, and PG calculated by non-compartmental analysis are listed in Table 5. The data were expressed as mean ± standard deviation. The concentrations of emodin fluctuated and were insufficient to calculate the half-life of elimination ($t_{1/2}$). Meanwhile, rapid absorption of aglycones was observed because of the higher lipophilic character with T_{max} of 0.25 (0.25–0.5) h and 0.25 (0.25–0.75) h, compared with that of glycosides.

Table 5. The pharmacokinetic parameters of anthraquinones after oral administration of *R. acetosa* extract to rats at a dose of 2 g/kg ($n = 3$).

Analyte	AUC_{0-last} [a] (ng h/mL)	C_{max} (ng/mL)	T_{max} [b] (h)	MRT (h)	$t_{1/2}$ (h)
C	265.6 ± 70.9	155.6 ± 86.0	0.25 (0.25–0.5)	2.4 ± 0.2	3.9 ± 0.6
E	1165 ± 336.1	123.5 ± 41.7	0.25 (0.25–0.75)	7.7 ± 3.0	NA
CG	158.0 ± 12.3	28.7 ± 4.7	2 (0.75–2)	2.4 ± 0.08	4.8 ± 0.5
PG	82.8 ± 13.8	20.5 ± 1.4	0.75 (0.5–2)	2.7 ± 0.6	6.2 ± 3.9

The values were expressed as mean ± standard deviation except T_{max}. [a] The last measured time points for C, E, CG, and PG were 6, 24, 8, and 6 h. [b] Median (range). AUC_{0-last}, total area under the plasma concentration–time curve from time zero to last measured time; C_{max}, maximum plasma concentration; T_{max}, time to reach C_{max}; MRT, mean residence time; $t_{1/2}$, half-life; NA, not available.

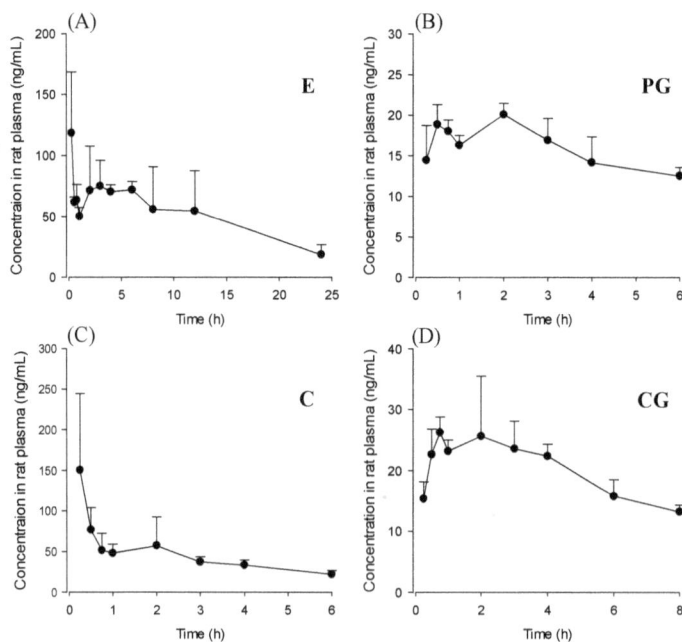

Figure 4. Mean plasma concentration–time profiles after oral ($n = 3$) administration of *R. acetosa* extract (2 g/kg) to SD male rats. Bars represent standard deviation. (**A**) emodin; (**B**) physcion-8-*O*-β-D-glucoside; (**C**) chrysophanol; (**D**) chrysophanol-8-*O*-β-D-glucoside.

4. Discussion

The objective of this study was to develop a bioanalytical method that simultaneously quantified the bioactive glycosides and aglycones of anthraquinones. The developed LC-MS/MS method could quantify six anthraquinones simultaneously in rat plasma in an accurate, reproducible, and simple way. Reported bioanalytical methods which simultaneously determine both aglycones and glycosides of anthraquinones are rarely available. In this study, simultaneous determination achieved by using biphenyl column. The column could prolong retention time of hydrophilic glycosides compare to C18 column at the same mobile phase composition.

There was no interfering peak when the compound mixture was spiked to blank rat plasma. However, there were small peaks appeared near CG and PG peaks after oral administration of plant extract. It is suggested that those peaks came from the extract or the metabolites of components in the extract. It is known that emodin is extensively glucuronized after absorption [14] and the molecular weight of emodin glucuronide is same as PG. There is some possibility that emodin glucuronide could interfere PG. However, the MS/MS fragment pattern of emodin glucuronide is different from PG. Emodin glucuronide might cause little interference. We could quantify CG and PG by adjusting the baselines because the interfering peaks were small.

A simple and rapid sample preparation was utilized on a low volume of rat plasma sample (20 μL) by using methanol as a precipitating agent with appropriate sensitivity compare to the reported methods [8,12,15]. The comparison with reported analytical methods for aglycones and glycosides of anthraquinones was shown in Table 6.

Table 6. Comparison with reported analytical methods for aglycones and glycosides of anthraquinone.

Analytical Condition		Our Method	Lin et al. [8]	Wang et al. [12]	Ma et al. [15]
Sample volume		20 μL	25 μL	25 μL	100 μL
Sample preparation		Protein precipitation	Solid phase extraction	Liquid-liquid extraction	Liquid-liquid extraction
Target compounds		E, C, P, EG, CG, PG	EG, E	E, C, P, EG, CG, PG	EG, E
	E	1	1	2	9.6
	C	20	-	50	-
LLOQ (ng/mL)	P	20	-	50	-
	EG	1	1	2	33.7
	CG	10	-	2	-
	PG	10	-	1	-

The method was acceptably validated and used to perform a pharmacokinetic study of anthraquinones after oral administration of *R. acetosa* in rats. As shown in Figure 4, C, E, CG, and PG could be detected in every rat from the first sampling time, 15 min. All of the studied anthraquinones were absorbed rapidly from rat gastrointestinal tract. Median T_{max} value of C and E was 15 min (Table 5). This result was consistent with reported values [8,10]. Emodin could be detected for the longest time among four compounds even though the concentrations fluctuated. The fluctuated concentration was also reported in other pharmacokinetic studies of emodin in rats [9,15]. This was possibly due to enterohepatic circulation [16]. In some other works [17], emodin rapidly and extensively metabolized to form its glucuronide and the parent form was almost undetectable after administration of emodin even the doses were similar (40 mg/kg) to our study (18.8 mg/kg for E and 25.8 mg/kg for EG). Free emodin could be measured until 24 h after oral administration because of the low LLOQ level of emodin using the method developed in this work.

Generally, plant glycosides have been considered to be hydrolyzed to aglycones by microflora in the gastrointestinal tract before absorption [18]. Glycosides have large molecular weights and low lipophilicity, so they might be difficult to be absorbed. However, recent studies show that emodin glycoside can be absorbed in an intact form after oral administration of plant extract [8]. The absorption of the glycosides of anthraquinones in an intact form was confirmed by studying in vivo absorption in rats in this study. Pharmacokinetics of anthraquinone aglycones and their glycosides after oral administration of *R. acetosa* was first evaluated. CG and PG were detected in rat plasma after oral administration of *R. acetosa* extract. Interestingly, the T_{max} of C and that of CG were different after oral administration of the extract. It might be due to different lipophilicity. Glycosides and aglycones have been proposed to have different degrees of absorption and metabolic patterns. Note that second peaks in the plasma concentrations of aglycones were observed. This could be due to delayed absorption of aglycones hydrolyzed from glycosides by microflora in the gastrointestinal tract and enterohepatic circulation of anthraquinones [16]. A number of published studies have reported pharmacokinetics of anthraquinones. However, we found that most of these studies focused on determining aglycones. Pharmacokinetics of anthraquinone glycosides is rarely available. Wang et al. [12] recently reported the pharmacokinetics of anthraquinone aglycones and their glycosides in hyperlipidemic hamsters after administration of rhubarb. The plasma concentration-time profile patterns of anthraquinones were similar to our study even though the composition (dose ratio of compounds) of rhubarb extract might be quite different from *R. acetosa* extract and physiological differences between rats and hamsters probably exist. T_{max} values of glycosides were slightly longer than aglycones. Similar to our results, emodin glucoside was not detected even though emodin could be detected until 36 h. It is suggested that emodin glycoside probably rapidly hydrolyzed to emodin and was poorly absorbed as an intact form in the gastrointestinal tract.

Our pharmacokinetic study has some limitations. The number of animals ($n = 3$) is not enough to achieve statistically significant pharmacokinetic parameters after administration of an herbal product. The pharmacokinetic parameters obtained in this study might b not sufficient to represent the animal population. Nevertheless, this study showed the possibility that our bioanalytical method could be used in pharmacokinetic studies of *R. acetosa* extract. Another issue to consider is that *R. acetosa* extract contained a number of other compounds besides anthraquinones. Further studies with a large sample size and studies of the effects of other compounds on the pharmacokinetics of anthraquinones are needed for better understanding of the pharmacokinetics of anthraquinones.

5. Conclusions

A simple and sensitive LC-MS/MS method for the determination of the glycosides and aglycones of anthraquinones in rat plasma was developed. The method was acceptably validated and applied to a pharmacokinetic study of anthraquinones after oral administration of *R. acetosa* extract in rats. The absorption of the glycosides of anthraquinones in an intact form was confirmed in the pharmacokinetic study. The results of this study could be relevant to a better understanding of the pharmacokinetics and pharmacodynamics of anthraquinone glycosides and aglycones.

Author Contributions: Conceptualization, M.-J.A. and H.J.C.; Formal analysis, J.K.; Funding acquisition, M.-J.A. and H.J.C.; Investigation, H.M.A.U., J.K., N.U.R., and H.-J.K; Methodology, H.J.C.; Project administration, H.J.C.; Writing—original draft, H.M.A.U.; Writing—review and editing, J.K., M.-J.A. and H.J.C.

Funding: This work was supported by the National Research Foundation of Korea (NRF) grant funded by the Korean government (MSIP; Ministry of Science, ICT & Future Planning) [Project No. 2017R1C1B5017343] and the R&D Program for Forest Science Technology (Project No. 2017036A00-1719-BA01) provided by Korea Forest Service (Korea Forestry Promotion Institute).

Conflicts of Interest: The authors declare no conflict of interest.

Abbreviations

LC-MS/MS	liquid chromatography-tandem mass spectrometry
MRM	multiple reaction monitoring
E	emodin
EG	emodin-8-O-β-D-glucoside
C	chrysophanol
CG	chrysophanol-8-O-β-D-glucoside
P	physcion
PG	physcion-8-O-β-D-glucoside

References

1. Lee, N.-J.; Choi, J.-H.; Koo, B.-S.; Ryu, S.-Y.; Han, Y.-H.; Lee, S.-I.; Lee, D.-U. Antimutagenicity and cytotoxicity of the constituents from the aerial parts of *Rumex acetosa*. *Biol. Pharm. Bull.* **2005**, *28*, 2158–2161. [CrossRef] [PubMed]
2. Kucekova, Z.; Mlcek, J.; Humpolicek, P.; Rop, O.; Valasek, P.; Saha, P. Phenolic compounds from *Allium schoenoprasum*, *Tragopogon pratensis* and *Rumex acetosa* and their antiproliferative effects. *Molecules* **2011**, *16*, 9207–9217. [CrossRef] [PubMed]
3. Gescher, K.; Hensel, A.; Hafezi, W.; Derksen, A.; Kühn, J. Oligomeric proanthocyanidins from *Rumex acetosa* L. inhibit the attachment of herpes simplex virus type-1. *Antivir. Res.* **2011**, *89*, 9–18. [CrossRef] [PubMed]
4. Bae, J.-Y.; Lee, Y.S.; Han, S.Y.; Jeong, E.J.; Lee, M.K.; Kong, J.Y.; Lee, D.H.; Cho, K.J.; Lee, H.-S.; Ahn, M.-J. A comparison between water and ethanol extracts of *Rumex acetosa* for protective effects on gastric ulcers in mice. *Biomol. Ther.* **2012**, *20*, 425–430. [CrossRef] [PubMed]
5. Bicker, J.; Petereit, F.; Hensel, A. Proanthocyanidins and a phloroglucinol derivative from *Rumex acetosa* L. *Fitoterapia* **2009**, *80*, 483–495. [CrossRef] [PubMed]
6. Fairbairn, J.W.; Reigal, E. Chemotaxonomy of anthraquinones in *Rumex*. *Phytochemistry* **1972**, *11*, 263–268. [CrossRef]
7. Uddin, Z.; Song, Y.H.; Curtis-Long, M.J.; Kim, J.Y.; Yuk, H.J.; Park, K.H. Potent bacterial neuraminidase inhibitors, anthraquinone glucosides from *Polygonum cuspidatum* and their inhibitory mechanism. *J. Ethnopharmacol.* **2016**, *193*, 283–292. [CrossRef] [PubMed]
8. Lin, L.; Ni, B.; Lin, H.; Cao, S.; Yang, C.; Zhao, Y.; Xue, D.; Ni, J. Simultaneous determination and pharmacokinetic study of P-hydroxybenzaldehyde, 2,3,5,4′-tetrahydroxystilbene-2-*O*-β-glucoside, emodin-8-*O*-β-D-glucopyranoside, and emodin in rat plasma by liquid chromatography tandem mass spectrometry after oral administration of *Polygonum multiflorum*. *Anal. Methods* **2015**, *7*, 244–252. [CrossRef]
9. Wu, W.; Yan, R.; Yao, M.; Zhan, Y.; Wang, Y. Pharmacokinetics of anthraquinones in rat plasma after oral administration of a rhubarb extract. *Biomed. Chromatogr.* **2014**, *28*, 564–572. [CrossRef] [PubMed]
10. Yan, D.; Ma, Y. Simultaneous quantification of five anthraquinones in rat plasma by high-performance liquid chromatography with fluorescence detection. *Biomed. Chromatogr.* **2007**, *21*, 502–507. [CrossRef] [PubMed]
11. Vasas, A.; Orbán-Gyapai, O.; Hohmann, J. The genus rumex: Review of traditional uses, phytochemistry and pharmacology. *J. Ethnopharmacol.* **2015**, *175*, 198–228. [CrossRef] [PubMed]
12. Wang, M.; Hu, G.; Tian, Y.; Zhang, Z.; Song, R. Influence of wine-processing on the pharmacokinetics of anthraquinone aglycones and glycosides from rhubarb in hyperlipidemic hamsters. *RSC Adv.* **2016**, *6*, 24871–24879. [CrossRef]
13. US Food and Drug Administration. *Guidance for Industry: Bioanalytical Method Validation, Draft Guidance*; US Food and Drug Administration: Silver Spring, MD, USA, 2013.
14. Dong, X.; Fu, J.; Yin, X.; Cao, S.; Li, X.; Lin, L.; Huyiligeqi; Ni, J. Emodin: A review of its pharmacology, toxicity and pharmacokinetics. *Phytother. Res.* **2016**, *30*, 1207–1218. [CrossRef] [PubMed]
15. Ma, J.; Zheng, L.; He, Y.S.; Li, H.J. Hepatotoxic assessment of *Polygoni multiflori* radix extract and toxicokinetic study of stilbene glucoside and anthraquinones in rats. *J. Ethnopharmacol.* **2015**, *162*, 61–68. [CrossRef] [PubMed]
16. Shia, C.S.; Tsai, S.Y.; Lin, J.C.; Li, M.L.; Ko, M.H.; Chao, P.-D.L.; Huang, Y.C.; Hou, Y.C. Steady-state pharmacokinetics and tissue distribution of anthraquinones of Rhei rhizoma in rats. *J. Ethnopharmacol.* **2011**, *137*, 1388–1394. [CrossRef] [PubMed]
17. Shia, C.S.; Hou, Y.C.; Tsai, S.Y.; Huieh, P.H.; Leu, Y.L.; Chao, P.D. Differences in pharmacokinetics and ex vivo antioxidant activity following intravenous and oral administrations of emodin to rats. *J. Pharm. Sci.* **2010**, *99*, 2185–2195. [CrossRef] [PubMed]
18. Moreau, J.P.; Moreau, S.; Skinner, S. Comparative physiological disposition of some anthraquinone glycosides and aglycones. *Biopharm. Drug Dispos.* **1985**, *6*, 325–334. [CrossRef] [PubMed]

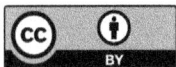

![pharmaceutics logo] *pharmaceutics*

MDPI

Article

Bioavailability of Eurycomanone in Its Pure Form and in a Standardised *Eurycoma longifolia* Water Extract

Norzahirah Ahmad [1,*], Dodheri Syed Samiulla [2], Bee Ping Teh [1], Murizal Zainol [1], Nor Azlina Zolkifli [1], Amirrudin Muhammad [1], Emylyn Matom [1], Azlina Zulkapli [3], Noor Rain Abdullah [1], Zakiah Ismail [1] and Ami Fazlin Syed Mohamed [1]

[1]   Herbal Medicine Research Centre, Institute for Medical Research, Jalan Pahang, Kuala Lumpur 50588, Malaysia; bpteh_km@yahoo.com (B.P.T.); murizal@imr.gov.my (M.Z.); norazlina@imr.gov.my (N.A.Z.); amiruddin@imr.gov.my (A.M.); emylynm@gmail.com (E.M.); noorrain@imr.gov.my (N.R.A.); drzakiah@gmail.com (Z.I.); ami@imr.gov.my (A.F.S.M.)

[2]   Aurigene Discovery Technologies Limited, Electronic City, Hosur Road, Bangalore 560100, Karmataka, India; samiulla_d@aurigene.com

[3]   Medical Resource Research Centre, Institute for Medical Research, Jalan Pahang, Kuala Lumpur 50588, Malaysia; azlina@imr.gov.my

*   Correspondence: norzahirah@imr.gov.my; Tel.: +603-2616-2633; Fax: +603-2693-4114

Received: 22 May 2018; Accepted: 20 June 2018; Published: 11 July 2018

Abstract: *Eurycoma longifolia* is one of the commonly consumed herbal preparations and its major chemical compound, eurycomanone, has been described to have antimalarial, antipyretic, aphrodisiac, and cytotoxic activities. Today, the consumption of *E. longifolia* is popular through the incorporation of its extract in food items, most frequently in drinks such as tea and coffee. In the current study, the characterisation of the physicochemical and pharmacokinetic (PK) attributes of eurycomanone were conducted via a series of in vitro and in vivo studies in rats and mice. The solubility and chemical stability of eurycomanone under the conditions of the gastrointestinal tract environment were determined. The permeability of eurycomanone was investigated by determining its distribution coefficient in aqueous and organic environments and its permeability using the parallel artificial membrane permeability assay system and Caco-2 cultured cells. Eurycomanone's stability in plasma and its protein-binding ability were measured by using an equilibrium dialysis method. Its stability in liver microsomes across species (mice, rat, dog, monkey, and human) and rat liver hepatocytes was also investigated. Along with the PK evaluations of eurycomanone in mice and rats, the PK parameters for the Malaysian Standard (MS: 2409:201) standardised water extract of *E. longifolia* were also evaluated in rats. Both rodent models showed that eurycomanone in both the compound form and extract form had a half-life of 0.30 h. The differences in the bioavailability of eurycomanone in the compound form between the rats (11.8%) and mice (54.9%) suggests that the PK parameters cannot be directly extrapolated to humans. The results also suggest that eurycomanone is not readily absorbed across biological membranes. However, once absorbed, the compound is not easily metabolised (is stable), hence retaining its bioactive properties, which may be responsible for the various reported biological activities.

Keywords: eurycomanone; *Eurycoma longifolia*; bioavailability; pharmacokinetic

1. Introduction

Eurycomanone is uniquely found in *Eurycoma longifolia* Jack (family Simaroubaceae), which is a herbaceous tree found mainly in Southeast Asia. Eurycomanone is reported to be the most abundant phytochemical quassinoid in *E. longifolia* roots [1–8]. The MS: 2409:201 of producing a freeze-dried standardised water extract of *E. longifolia* uses eurycomanone as the chemical marker.

The eurycomanone level must be consistently present at 0.80–1.50% w/v, alongside other markers such as total polysaccharides, total protein, and total glycosaponin, where their levels are expected at >20%. Traditionally, *E. longifolia* was used for ailments such as fever, wounds, and ulcers, as well as an afterbirth remedy or as a general tonic [9,10]. Biological activities of *E. longifolia* previously reported, such as male fertility enhancement [4,11] and antimalarial [12–17], cytotoxic [14,15,18], antiproliferative [19,20], and antiulcer [21] effects, are largely attributed to the quassinoids group, specifically eurycomanone.

Studies identifying eurycomanone as the compound responsible for these reported activities mainly focused on in vitro systems. Previous investigation into the physicochemical properties of several quassinoids of *E. longifolia* [16] revealed that eurycomanone and 13-α-(21)-epoxyeurycomanone possessed the necessary characteristics contributing to *E. longifolia*'s effect. Favourable physicochemical properties such as solubility, lipophilicity, chemical stability, permeability, plasma stability, and plasma protein binding act as indicators of the marker's behavior in the body. The behaviour of eurycomanone in the body is of interest as the consumption of *E. longifolia* in the forms of water extracts incorporated into health supplements and beverages are the common strategies for marketed *E. longifolia*-based products. Oral consumption of *E. longifolia* in these various forms exposes its active ingredients to varying environment, which may affect their bioavailability in the body.

Bioavailability measures the delivery of an active ingredient to its site of action in order to cause the predicted effect(s). First-pass metabolism in the liver can markedly reduce the amount of eurycomanone available to the site of action, which can be predicted in vitro by assessing its metabolic stability prior to its administration orally. Previously reported eurycomanone bioavailability in rats was studied using extracts with differing amounts of eurycomanone [7,22,23].

Experimentally based data on eurycomanone's bioavailability will be highly essential if a standardised extract is to be clinically tested. Nevertheless, to date, no bioavailability study on the standardised water extract form has been previously conducted. This study investigates the bioavailability of eurycomanone in its pure form and in a standardised water extract of *E. longifolia*.

2. Materials and Methods

2.1. Chemicals and Reagents

Standardised water extract of *E. longifolia* used conformed to the MS: 2409:201 and contained eurycomanone (1.36%), total protein (30.5%), total polysaccharide (37.8%), and glycosaponin (52%). Eurycomanone (94.8% purity) was obtained from ChromaDex Inc. (Irvine, CA, USA). Propranolol, estriol, metoprolol tartrate, diethylstil bestrol, erythromycin, atenolol, carbamazepine, propantheline bromide, enalapril, dasatinib, midazolam, terfinadine, alamethicin, uridine 5′-diphospho-glucuronosyltransferase (UDPGA), nicotinamide adenine dinucleotide phosphate (NADPH), N-methyl-2-pyrrolidone (NMP), 2-hydroxypropyl-beta-cyclodextrin (HPCD), and chemicals used in reagents and buffer preparations were purchased from Sigma Chemical Co. (St. Louis, MO, USA). Plasma and microsomes from mice and rats were prepared in-house, whilst plasma and microsomes from dog, monkey, and human were purchased from Thermo Fisher Scientific (Waltham, MA, USA). Solvents such as methanol, formic acid, acetonitrile (ACN), and DMSO used were of LC-MS and HPLC grade and were purchased from Fisher Chemicals (Waltham, MA, USA).

2.2. Animal Experiments

2.2.1. Eurycomanone Assessment

The ethical approval for the animal experiments conducted in India was granted from the Animal Ethics Committee, Aurigene Discovery Technologies, Bangalore, India. Eight male Wistar rats (12 weeks old; weighing 250–350 g) and eight Caeserean Derived-1 (CD-1) mice (weighing 20–30 g) were obtained from the Animal House, Aurigene Discovery Technologies, Bangalore, India. They were supplied with standard rodent diets and drinking water ad libitum. Each rodent species (i.e., rats and mice) were divided into two groups. One group (n = 3 for each rodent species) was administered with eurycomanone via the intravenous route (IV) and another group (n = 3 for each rodent species) via the oral route (PO) using oral gavage intubation needle. Two animals of each of the species were used as a control and they received reverse osmosis water. All rats underwent jugular vein cannulation surgery 72 h prior to the administration of the eurycomanone.

2.2.2. Standardised Water Extract of *E. longifolia* (SWE) Assessment

The animal experiment conducted in Malaysia was approved by the Animal Care and Use Committee, Ministry of Health Malaysia (ACUC Number: ACUC/KKM/02(1/2014)). Ten male Sprague Dawley rats (12 weeks old; weighing 250–400 g) were obtained from the Laboratory Animal Resource Unit, Institute for Medical Research, Kuala Lumpur, Malaysia. They were supplied with standard rodent diets and drinking water ad libitum. One group (n = 4) was administered with SWE via the IV route and another group (n = 4) via the PO route using oral gavage intubation needle. Two rats were used as the control and they were administered reverse osmosis water. All rats underwent jugular vein cannulation surgery 72 h prior to the administration of SWE. All animals were maintained in a 12-h light and dark cycle, the temperature was maintained between 22 ± 3 °C, and the relative humidity between 50–65%.

2.3. Sample Preparation

Eurycomanone (rats: 1.5 mg/mL for IV route and 3.0 mg/mL for PO route; mice: 0.5 mg/mL for IV route and 1.0 mg/mL for PO route) samples were prepared fresh on the day of dosing. For the IV administration, eurycomanone was dissolved in 3% NMP and 97% of 10% HPCD in saline. For the oral administration, eurycomanone was dissolved in 3% NMP and 97% of 30% HPCD in saline. Both samples were sonicated before use. The SWE (5 mg/mL for IV route, 10 mg/mL for PO route) was prepared fresh on the day of dosing. For the IV administration, the SWE was dissolved in reverse osmosis water and filtered (0.2 μm pore size) before administration. The SWE for the PO administration was prepared using the same method, except without filtering. The animals were not fasted and doses given were based on the body weights prior to dosing.

2.4. Specimen Collection

Blood specimens (approximately 0.30–0.40 mL via the jugular vein cannula for rats and 0.10–0.20 mL via submanibular bleeding for mice) were collected at time points 0.083 (IV group only), 0.25, 0.5, 1, 2, 4, 6, and 8 h post-dosing with eurycomanone. At the experiment end point, the animals were euthanized by excess isoflurane inhalation followed by cervical dislocation. In the experiment using SWE, the rats were placed in metabolic cages (Techniplast, West Chester, PA, USA) and blood (approximately 0.30–0.40 mL collected via the jugular vein cannula), urine, and faeces specimens were collected at the same time points with the above plus one additional time point of 24 h. Kidney and liver specimens were collected at necropsy, where the rats were euthanized by CO_2 inhalation followed by cervical dislocation. All blood specimens were centrifuged (10,000 rpm, 10 min) to obtain plasma and were stored at −80 °C until processed. Urine and faeces specimens were collected into plastic containers on wet ice while the organ specimens were snap-frozen in liquid nitrogen and maintained at −80 °C until processed.

2.5. Specimen Preparation for LC-MS/MS Analysis

Plasma specimens (100 μL), collected from the eurycomanone experiment were added with the internal standard solution (10 μL). Plasma proteins were precipitated with ACN (300 μL), vortex-mixed for 5 min, and centrifuged at 4000 rpm for 7 min. The supernatant was collected and evaporated using a nitrogen evaporator for 20 min at 50 °C. Thereafter, they were reconstituted with the mobile phase (500 µL) and transferred into LC-MS vials for analysis.

Plasma specimens (200 µL) from the SWE experiment were added with the internal standard solution (50 µL). Plasma proteins were precipitated with ACN (400 µL), vortex-mixed for 5 min, and centrifuged at 4000 rpm for 7 min. The supernatant was collected and evaporated to dryness using nitrogen evaporator at 60 °C. Thereafter, they were reconstituted with 80 µL of 30% methanol: 70% (0.1% formic acid) and transferred into LC-MS vials for analysis.

Urine specimens (200 µL) were added with ACN (400 µL), vortex-mixed for 5 min, and centrifuged at 4000 rpm for 7 min. The supernatant was collected and evaporated to dryness using a nitrogen evaporator at 60 °C. Thereafter, they were reconstituted with 80 µL of 10% methanol: 90% (0.1% formic acid) and transferred into LC-MS vials for analysis.

Faeces specimens were weighed, ultrapure water (at 8 times the weighed samples) was added, and samples were homogenised. The homogenised faeces samples (200 µL) were added with ACN (400 µL), vortex-mixed for 5 min, and centrifuged at 4000 rpm for 7 min. The supernatant was collected and evaporated to dryness using a nitrogen evaporator at 60 °C. Thereafter, they were reconstituted with 80 µL of 5% methanol: 95% (0.1% formic acid) and transferred into LC-MS vials for analysis.

Tissue specimens (kidneys and livers) were blotted with filter paper, weighed, and minced. Ultrapure water (at 3 times the weighed tissue samples) were added and samples were homogenised. The homogenised tissue specimens (200 µL) were added with ACN (400 µL), vortex-mixed for 5 min, and centrifuged at 4000 rpm for 7 min. The supernatant was collected and evaporated to dryness using a nitrogen evaporator at 60 °C. Thereafter, they were reconstituted with 80 µL of 5% methanol: 95% (0.1% formic acid) and transferred into LC-MS vials for analysis.

2.6. LC-MS/MS Analysis

Eurycomanone detection in the pure eurycomanone experiments was done via the LC-MS/MS system consisting of an Agilent 1260 Infinity HPLC system and an AB SCIEX API 4000™ Triple-Quadrupole mass spectrometer equipped with TurboIonSpray® probe and atmospheric pressure chemical ionization (APCI) (AB Sciex LLC, Framingham, MA, USA). Electrospray ionization (ESI) was performed in positive ion mode. The analytical column was Agilent Zorbax Eclipse-C18 (4.6 mm I.D. × 150 mm, 3.5 µm). The mobile phase consisted of 0.1% formic acid (solvent A) and 90% ACN with 0.1% formic acid (solvent B). The flow rate was set at 1.2 mL/min and the injection volume was 50 µL with the run time of 3.5 min. The mass transitions, monitored using multiple-reaction monitoring (MRM) detections, were $409 \rightarrow 221.1/143.1$ for eurycomanone. Eurycomanone detection in the SWE experiments were done via an LC-MS system consisting of Agilent 1100 series HPLC and mass spectrometer detector system with APCI-ESI ionization mode (Agilent Technologies, Santa Clara, CA, USA).

For plasma specimens, the analytical column used was Agilent Zorbax Eclipse XDB-Phenyl (2.1 mm I.D. × 50 mm, 5 µm). The mobile phase consisted of 35% methanol: 65% (0.1% formic acid). The flow rate was set at 0.2 mL/min and the injection volume was 2 µL with the run time of 5 min. For urine samples, the analytical column was Agilent Zorbax Eclipse XDB-Phenyl (2.1 mm I.D. × 50 mm, 3.5 µm). The mobile phase consisted of 10% methanol: 90% (0.1% formic acid). The flow rate was set at 0.2 mL/min and the injection volume was 2 µL with the run time of 5 min.

For faeces, kidney, and liver specimens, the analytical column used was Agilent Zorbax Eclipse XDB-Phenyl (2.1 mm I.D. × 50 mm, 3.5 µm). The mobile phase consisted of 5% methanol: 95% (0.1% formic acid). The flow rate was set at 0.2 mL/min and the injection volume was 2 µL with the run time of 6 min. The identification of eurycomanone and internal standard for plasma matrix were achieved by comparing the ion sets in selected ion monitoring (SIM) for eurycomanone with sodium adduct (m/z 431.0) and metronidazole (172.0 g/mol) in samples with the standard solution, at a similar retention time using LC-MS analysis. The concentration of the specimens analysed were determined by using an inverse prediction method for the best-fit regression curve using the weighted least-square (WLS) of $\frac{1}{x^2}$, obtained from the standard concentrations.

In the analytical run, each standard in the calibration curve for each matrix was checked for the accuracy to be in the range of 80–120% for the lower limit of quantification (LLOQ) concentration and 85–115% for the remaining standards. Each quality control (QC) concentration was also checked for the accuracy to be in the range of 80–120% for the LLOQ concentration and 85–115% for the remaining QC samples. Sample matrices from the control group (blank samples) were used in the preparation of the calibration curve for determining eurycomanone concentrations. The pharmacokinetic analysis was performed using the non-compartmental analysis of Phoenix™ WinNolin®software (version 1.3, Certara, L.P., Princeton, NJ, USA).

2.7. Aqueous Solubility, Lipophilicity, and Chemical Stability of Eurycomanone

The aqueous stability was estimated by adding 10 μL of eurycomanone stock solution (10 mM) to 490 μL of aqueous buffer at pH 5.4, pH 7.4 and DMSO in triplicates in deep-well plates. Three standards (propanolol, estriol, and tamoxifen) at the same concentration were also added in the deep-well plates. The plate was kept on a shaker (300 rpm) at room temperature for 16 h. The plate was then centrifuged at 25 °C, 4000 rpm for 25 min. The supernatant was transferred and analysed using LC-MS/MS. The aqueous solubility was calculated using the following formula:

$$\text{Aqueous stability} = \frac{200\ \mu\text{M} \times \text{Peak area 1}}{\text{Peak area 2}}$$

Peak area 1 = peak area of the compound in 2% DMSO at the different pH levels.
Peak area 2 = peak area of the compound in 100% DMSO.

The lipophilicity of eurycomanone was estimated using the shake flask method with octanol and buffer (pH 7.4). Eurycomanone (5 μL) at 5 mM concentration is added to octanol (495 μL) and DMSO (495 μL) and also into the aqueous and octanol phase in a 1:1 ratio (247.4 μL of octanol phase and 247.5 μL of aqueous phase). The octanol and aqueous phases were prepared using a saturation process, where equal amounts of D-PBS (pH 7.4) and octanol were saturated (300 rpm, room temperature) for 24 h before being separated and kept at room temperature. The prepared mixtures were vortexed and kept on the shaker (300 rpm) at room temperature for 16 h. The mixtures were allowed to stand for 30 min, and 200 μL of solution was transferred and sent for HPLC analysis. The analyses were conducted along with propranolol, estriol, metoprolol tartrate, and diethylstil bestrol (5 mM) as standards and were conducted in triplicates.

The chemical stability of eurycomanone was estimated in gastric simulated fluid (GSF), pH 2; fasted simulated intestinal fluid (FASSIF), pH 6.5; fed simulated intestinal fluid (FESSIF), pH 5.0; and in 150 mM NaHCO$_3$ at pH 9.2. Eurycomanone (3 μL) at 5 mM was added to 297 μL of the respective buffers. The mixture (100 μL) was added to 100 μL of ACN at time points 1 and 3 h and sent for LC-MS/MS analysis. The test was done in triplicates with propranolol and erythromycin (5 mM) as standards.

2.8. Permeability Assay

2.8.1. Parallel Artificial Membrane Permeability Assay (PAMPA)

Eurycomanone was added to Pion buffer (Pion Inc., Billerica, MA, USA) pH 7.4 to make a 10 μM working solution. Five microlitres of the lipid mix was applied on the membrane and allowed to dry for 10 min. The working solution (200 μL) was added to the donor plate and Pion buffer (200 μL) were added to the receiver plate. The plate was kept in a moist chamber and left for 18 h at room temperature. The solution from both the donor and receiver plate and the working solution was analysed using LC-MS/MS. This test was carried out in triplicates using propranolol, atenolol, and carbamazepine as standards. The test concentration for eurycomanone is 25 μM.

2.8.2. Caco-2 Cell Permeability Assay

The Caco-2 assay was carried out after seeding the cells onto the membrane to form a confluent monolayer in 21 days. The media is removed from apical (A) and basolateral (B) chambers and the membrane is washed with HBSS buffer. Eurycomanone (10 μM, 200 μL) was added to the A compartment (which represents the intestinal lumen), and buffer (300 μL) was added to the B compartment (representing the blood), and vice versa. The plate was kept in a shaking incubator (37 °C) for 1 h. The amount of eurycomanone that had permeated across the cells was measured by LC-MS/MS, and the apparent permeability (P_{app}) values and efflux ratio were calculated. The expression of P-glycoprotein (P-gp) by differentiated Caco-2 cells was confirmed by measuring the P_{app} value and efflux ratio of vinblastine with and without the presence of a competing P-gp substrate, cyclosporine A. Eurycomanone was also measured with the presence of cyclosporine A to investigate whether eurycomanone may be transported via P-gp transporters.

2.9. Liver Microsome Metabolic Stability Assay

The liver microsome stability assay of eurycomanone was estimated using phase I and phase II enzymes in five types of microsomes (mice, rat, dog, monkey, and human). Eurycomanone at 1 mM (20 μL), microsomes at 0.3 mg/mL (20 μL), and 10 mg/mL of alamethicin in 1:1 DMSO and methanol (20 μL) were preincubated at 37 °C for 10 min. The cofactor, 5 mM UDPGA (20 μL), and 1 mM NADPH (20 μL) were added to make the final assay volume of 100 μL. At timepoints 0, 15, 30, 45, 60, and 90 min, 100 μL of the reaction mixture is taken out and added to the stop solution. The supernatants (10,000 rpm, 10 min, 4 °C) were collected and analysed using LC-MS/MS. The standards used for mice and rat liver microsomes were propranolol and dasatinib. The standards used with the dog and monkey liver microsomes were propranolol and midazolam, while the standards used with the human liver microsomes were propranolol and terfinadine.

2.10. Plasma Stability

The plasma stability was estimated by preparing 5 μM of eurycomanone in 600 μL plasma in triplicates. The plasma stability of eurycomanone was determined in five types of plasma (mice, rat, dog, monkey, and human). The reaction was kept at 37 °C and ACN (100 μL) was added at timepoints 0, 30 min, and 1, 2, and 4 h to the reaction mixture (100 μL). The supernatant (10,000 rpm, 10 min, 4 °C) was collected and analysed by LC-MS/MS. The standards (propantheline bromide and enalapril) were analysed in triplicates.

2.11. Plasma Protein Binding Assay

The ability of eurycomanone to bind plasma protein was analysed in five types of plasma (mice, rat, dog, monkey, and human). Each type of plasma was spiked with eurycomanone (1 mM) to make the 10 μM test concentration of eurycomanone in the plasma. Equilibrium dialysis buffer (500 μL) at pH 7.4 was added to the right chamber in rapid equilibrium dialysis (RED), while the spiked plasma (300 μL) was added to the left chamber. The Teflon base plate was covered with aluminium foil and left on the shaking incubator at 37 °C for 4 h. The matrix was balanced by mixing 100 μL of the equilibrium buffer with the spiked plasma from the left chamber in RED before adding the stop solution (350 μL) to precipitate out the protein. The supernatant (10,000 rpm, 10 min, 4 °C) was collected and analysed using LC-MS/MS. The standards (propranolol, warfarin, and acebutalol) were analysed in duplicates.

2.12. Statistical Analysis

The statistical analysis was performed using one-way or two-way ANOVA with either Dunnett or Tukey analysis chosen as the post-hoc analysis (GraphPad Prism, version 7.00 for Windows, GraphPad Software, La Jolla, CA, USA). Statistical significant differences were recognised at $p \leq 0.05$.

3. Results

3.1. Pharmacokinetics of Eurycomanone in Mice

A summary of the PK parameters in mice obtained following an intravenous and oral dose of eurycomanone is shown in Table 1. The plots for the mean plasma concentration of eurycomanone over time are shown in Figure 1. Following intravenous administration to mice, plasma clearance was moderate (3.85 L/h/kg) for eurycomanone. The volume of distribution was small (1.51 L/kg) for eurycomanone, with the elimination half-life of 0.30 h. Following oral administration, the absorption was moderate, where the T_{max} was observed at 2 h post-dose for the eurycomanone (C_{max} 334.7 ng/mL). The bioavailability of eurycomanone in mice was moderately high at 54.9% compared to rats. At 8 h post-dosing, the concentration of eurycomanone increased slightly in mice for both administration routes (Figure 1), which may be an indication of the enterohepatic circulation of eurycomanone in its administered form.

Table 1. Summary of pharmacokinetic parameters following an intravenous and oral dose of eurycomanone to mice.

Parameters (Mice)	Units	Eurycomanone	
		1 mg/kg	10 mg/kg
		Intravenous	Oral
AUC_{0-8}	h·ng/mL	221.0	1213
Plasma Clearance (CL)	L/h/kg	3.85	NA
Volume of Distribution at Steady State (V_{ss})	L/kg	1.51	NA
Half-life ($t_{1/2}$)	h	0.30	NA
Observed T_{max}	h	NA	2.0
Observed C_{max}	ng/mL	NA	334.7
Bioavailability (F)	%	NA	54.9

NA: Not applicable, AUC: Area under the curve, T_{max}: time taken to reach the maximum concentration, C_{max}: maximum concentration of the compound achieved in the plasma.

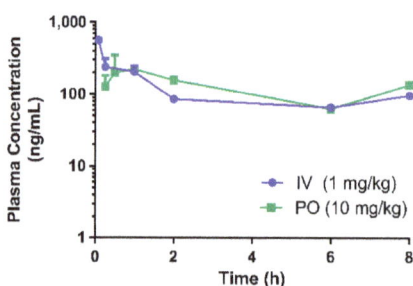

Figure 1. Pharmacokinetic profile of eurycomanone when administered as its pure compound in mice. (IV = intravenous route, PO = oral route)

3.2. Pharmacokinetics of Eurycomanone and SWE in Rats

A summary of the PK parameters in rats obtained following an intravenous and oral dose of eurycomanone and the SWE is shown in Table 2. The plots for the mean plasma concentration of eurycomanone over time are shown in Figure 2a,b. Following intravenous administration to rats, the plasma clearance was moderate (2.74 L/h/kg) for eurycomanone in the compound form and low (0.76 L/h/kg) for eurycomanone in the SWE. The volume of distribution was low (0.95 L/kg) for eurycomanone and lower (0.12 L/kg) for the SWE, while their elimination half-lives were 0.30 and 0.12 h, respectively. Following oral administration, the absorption was moderate, where the

T_{max} was observed at 2 h post-dose for the eurycomanone (C_{max} 238.3 ng/mL). The bioavailability of eurycomanone in rats was calculated to be low at 11.8%. At 6 and 8 h post-dosing of eurycomanone in the compound form, the concentration of eurycomanone increased slightly for the oral and intravenous routes, respectively (Figure 2). This may indicate that eurycomanone is recirculated via enterohepatic circulation in its unchanged administered form.

Table 2. Summary of pharmacokinetic parameters following an intravenous and oral dose of eurycomanone and SWE to rats.

Parameters (Rats)	Units	Eurycomanone		SWE	
		3 mg/kg	30 mg/kg	10 mg/kg	100 mg/kg
		Intravenous	Oral	Intravenous	Oral
AUC_{0-8}	h·ng/mL	970.0	1149.0	100.8	ND
Plasma Clearance (CL)	L/h/kg	2.74	NA	0.76	NA
Volume of Distribution at Steady State (V_{ss})	L/kg	0.95	NA	0.12	NA
Half-life ($t_{1/2}$)	h	0.30	NA	0.11	NA
Observed T_{max}	h	NA	2.0	NA	ND
Observed C_{max}	ng/mL	NA	238.3	NA	ND
Bioavailability (F)	%	NA	11.8	NA	NC
Urinary excretion 24 h post-dose	%	NA	NA	22.52	5.02
Fecal excretion 24 h post-dose	%	NA	NA	0.56	33.02
Liver accumulation	ng/mL	NA	NA	47.6	104.7
Kidney accumulation	ng/mL	NA	NA	NA	NA

NA: Not applicable, ND: Not detected, NC: Not calculated, AUC: Area under the curve, T_{max}: time taken to reach the maximum concentration, C_{max}: maximum concentration of the compound achieved in the plasma.

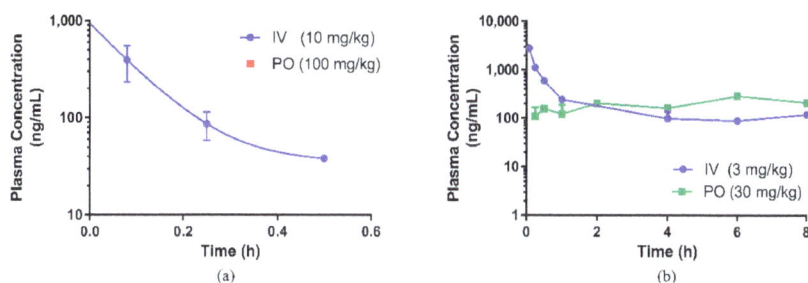

Figure 2. Pharmacokinetic profile of (**a**) standardized water extract (SWE) of *E. longifolia* and (**b**) eurycomanone compound, respectively, in rats. (IV = intravenous route, PO = oral route).

When SWE was orally administered, the plasma concentration of eurycomanone was undetectable in the plasma and it was mainly eliminated via faecal excretion. However, eurycomanone was detected in the liver samples at 47.6 ng/mL (intravenous) and 104.7 ng/mL (oral) at 24 h post-administration of SWE, indicating that a minimal amount of eurycomanone may have been absorbed, though not detectable. Intravenous administration of SWE showed that eurycomanone remains in the plasma up until 30 min and is mainly eliminated via urinary excretion.

3.3. Eurycomanone Aqueous Solubility, Lipophilicity, and Chemical Stability

Eurycomanone was highly soluble at pH 5.4 (205.5 µM) and 7.4 (205.4 µM) and was comparable to propranolol (Figure 3). Estriol, which has moderate solubility at both pHs, and tamoxifen, which was insoluble at pH 7.4 and highly soluble in pH 5.4, were used as internal controls. Due to this highly aqueous nature of eurycomanone, it is expected that its distribution coefficient log D at pH 7.4 is low (−0.35). Propranolol (0.82), estriol (2.82), metoprolol (−0.29), and diethylstilbestrol (3.18) were assayed together as internal controls as they have a wide range of log D values (Figure 4). The chemical stability of eurycomanone at the varying pH levels, mimicking changing pH environments in physiological conditions, i.e., using GSF (pH 2), FESIIF (pH 5.0), and FASSIF (pH 6.5), were also carried out. The percentage of eurycomanone remaining after 3 h of incubation showed that eurycomanone is chemically stable across all pH values tested (Figure 5).

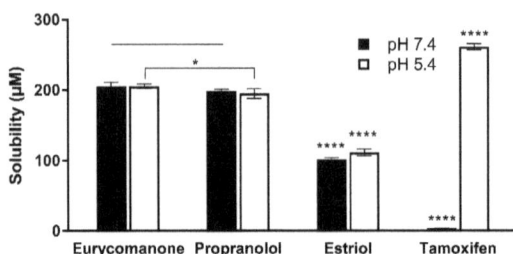

Figure 3. Aqueous solubility of eurycomanone, propranolol, estriol, and tamoxifen at pH 7.4 and pH 5.4. The values were plotted based on the mean ± standard deviation. **** denotes significant difference when compared to eurycomanone ($p \leq 0.0001$) at the two pH values. * denotes significance difference between propranolol and eurycomanone at pH 5.4 ($p \leq 0.05$). Line over bars indicates no significant difference when compared to eurycomanone ($p \geq 0.05$).

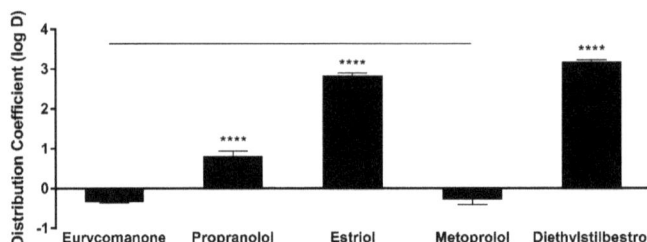

Figure 4. Lipophilicity properties of eurycomanone, propranolol, estriol, metoprolol, and diesthylstilbestrol. The distribution coefficient (log D) value for eurycomanone was −0.35. All standards showed acceptable log D values, respectively. The values were plotted based on the mean ± standard deviation. **** denotes significant difference when compared to eurycomanone ($p \leq 0.0001$). The log D value of eurycomanone is comparable to that of metoprolol. Line over bars indicates no significant difference between metoprolol and eurycomanone ($p \geq 0.05$).

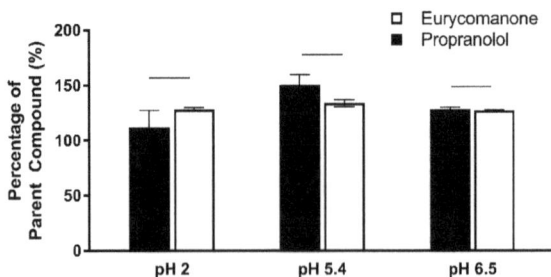

Figure 5. Eurycomanone showed high stability at pH 2, pH 5, and pH 6.5 and is comparable to the stability of propranolol. The values were plotted based on the mean ± standard deviation. There were no significant differences between propranolol and eurycomanone at all the pH levels tested. Line over bars indicates no significant difference when compared to eurycomanone ($p \geq 0.05$).

3.4. Eurycomanone Permeability

The rapid assessment of the absorption ability of eurycomanone was conducted via the PAMPA. Eurycomanone's permeation through this artificial membrane is low at 0.78×10^{-6} cm/s (Figure 6). As the PAMPA system lacks some similarity to natural membranes, i.e., lack of pores and proteins responsible for active transport such as P-gp protein, eurycomanone was also evaluated in a Caco-2 cell monolayer (Table 3). However, eurycomanone showed low permeability in Caco-2 cells at 0.45×10^{-6} cm/s (A to B direction) and 0.73×10^{-6} cm/s (B to A direction), similar to its permeation in the artificial membrane. Eurycomanone was not a substrate for efflux transporter as the efflux ratio is less than 2. Incubation of eurycomanone with cyclosporine A (a P-gp substrate) showed no changes and no competition with eurycomanone. Alongside eurycomanone, vinblastine, which is also a P-gp substrate, was also tested to ensure the Caco-2 cells were expressing P-gp transporters.

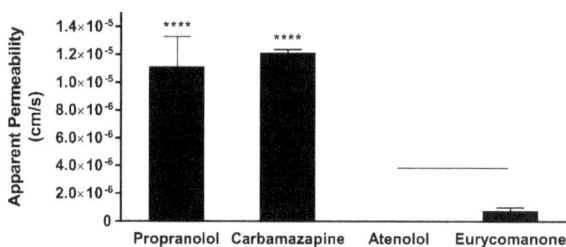

Figure 6. Eurycomanone showed low permeability as compared to propranolol and carbamazepine when assayed using the parallel artificial membrane permeability assay (PAMPA). The values were plotted based on the mean ± standard deviation. **** denotes significant difference when compared to eurycomanone ($p \leq 0.0001$). Line over bars indicates no significant difference between atenolol and eurycomanone ($p \geq 0.05$).

Table 3. Apparent permeability of eurycomanone assayed via the Caco-2 permeability assay.

Tested Compounds	Direction	P_{app} ($\times 10^{-6}$ cm/s)	Efflux Ratio
Eurycomanone	A to B	0.45	1.62
	B to A	0.73	
Eurycomanone + Cyclosporine A	A to B	1.20	1.13
	B to A	1.35	
Vinblastine	A to B	3.76	14.72
	B to A	55.34	
Vinblastine + Cyclosporine A	A to B	16.71	2.39
	B to A	40.00	

P_{app}: Apparent permeability.

3.5. Liver Microsome Metabolic Stability

Eurycomanone was relatively stable in rat liver microsomes and hepatocytes and in human liver microsomes, with the half-life of more than 90 min (Table 4). The intrinsic clearances (Cl_{int}) calculated from the rate of metabolism of eurycomanone in the liver microsomal incubations were high for rat (83.16 mL/min/kg) and slightly lower in human microsomes (52.39 mL/min/kg). Intrinsic clearance in the rat liver hepatocytes was also slow at 0.67 µL/min/million cells. These results suggest that eurycomanone is not a species-specific substrate and that is may be highly metabolised in the liver.

Table 4. Rat liver microsomes and hepatocytes and human liver microsome stability of eurycomanone.

Parameters	Units	Rat Liver Microsomes	Rat Liver Hepatocytes	Human Liver Microsomes
Half-life ($t_{1/2}$)	h	>1.5	>1.5	>1.5
Intrinsic clearance (Cl_{int})	mL/min/kg	83.16	NA	52.39
Intrinsic clearance (Cl_{int})	µL/min/million cells	NA	0.67	NA

NA: Not applicable.

3.6. Plasma Stability and Plasma Protein Binding

Eurycomanone was highly stable in the human, rat, and dog plasma, while stability was slightly lower in the monkey and mice plasma (Figure 7). The varied species used in the plasma profiling were used to assess possible differences in eurycomanone's stability as exhibited by other compounds such as propantheline bromide and enalapril. However, eurycomanone were shown to be stable in all the species tested. From the plasma protein binding study (Figure 8), it was found that the percentages of bound eurycomanone were 30.1% (rat), 35.4% (monkey), 21.6% (mice), 38.9% (human), and 67.8% (dog). Apart from in the dog plasma, eurycomanone exhibited a low plasma binding ability in all the other species' plasma, with a high fraction of unbound eurycomanone (61.1–78.4%) with free access to its target sites.

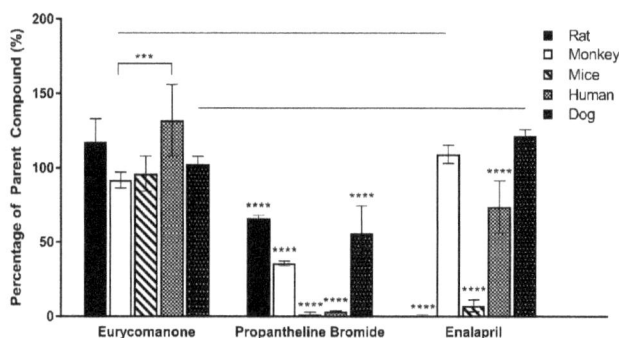

Figure 7. Eurycomanone's stability in rat, monkey, mice, human, and dog plasma as compared to propantheline bromide and enalapril. The values were plotted based on the mean ± standard deviation. **** denotes significant difference when compared to eurycomanone ($p \leq 0.0001$) in the five species tested. *** denotes significance difference ($p \leq 0.001$) in eurycomanone's stability between species monkey and human. Line over bars indicates no significant difference when compared to eurycomanone in species monkey and dog for enalapril ($p \geq 0.05$).

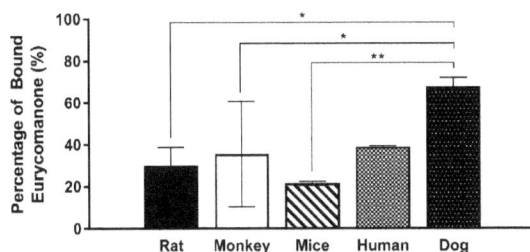

Figure 8. Eurycomanone plasma protein binding in rat, monkey, mice, human, and dog plasma. The values were plotted based on the mean ± standard deviation. ** and * denote significant difference when compared to across species ($p \leq 0.01$) and ($p \leq 0.05$) respectively. No significant difference was found between the rest of the species tested ($p \geq 0.05$) (not indicated on graph).

4. Discussion

Eurycomanone has been evaluated for its biological activities via various in vitro methods [17,20,24–27], while the extract form was mainly used in various in vivo tests [28–32]. From this study, the concentration of the pure eurycomanone in rat plasma was at its maximum (C_{max} 238.3 ng/mL) at 2 h post oral administration, and the bioavailability for the eurycomanone compound was low (11.8%). The findings in this study with regard to eurycomanone's bioavailability was similar to findings by Low et al. [22], where it was reported that the bioavailability of the orally administered fortified eurycomanone in *E. longifolia* extract was 10.5% and the C_{max} was found to be 330 ng/mL. There was no notable difference in terms of eurycomanone's bioavailability and maximum concentration when using a pure compound as in the current study and when compared to using a fortified extract as used by Low et al. [22]. Rehman and his coworkers, in their investigation, found the C_{max} to be lower at 40.43 ng/mL for the pure eurycomanone and 9.90 ng/mL for eurycomanone in *E. longifolia* extract [7]. In this study, interspecies variation in the bioavailability of eurycomanone was noted. The pure compound was found to be more bioavailable (higher absorption) in mice (54.9%) than in rats, and the C_{max} (335 ng/mL) in mice was slightly higher than the levels found in rats. This also indicates that eurycomanone may behave differently in different species and the PK values may not be able to be directly extrapolated from rodents to humans. This species-dependent characteristic of eurycomanone behaviour in rodents may be due to species differences in the metabolism and disposition of eurycomanone, as there was a variation in the absorption, distribution, and metabolism of eurycomanone, in which they were faster in mice than in rats. Two peaks were observed in the PK profiles in both the oral and intravenous profiles. The presence of these secondary peaks may indicate the occurrence of enterohepatic circulation of eurycomanone [33]; however, this must be further investigated in a separate study. Ma et al. suggest that the secondary peak of eurycomanone may be caused by eurycomanone's activity as a muscle relaxant, which caused delayed gastric emptying and hence delayed intestinal absorption, resulting in the secondary peak in the profile [23]. In the present study, the plasma concentration–time profile was only conducted for 8 h, which limits the window of analysis to confirm the second peak.

Previously, Zakaria et al. reported eurycomanone activity in vivo, where eurycomanone was orally administered at 6 mg/kg and 17 mg/kg to mice. At the dose of 17 mg/kg, tumour suppression ability was demonstrated in nude mice with HepG2 cell-induced tumours, which showed that there was sufficient or better bioavailability to exert the reported efficacy [32]. However, in relation to previous in vitro studies, the C_{max} value obtained in the current study was much lower than those shown in previous studies of eurycomanone and *E. longifolia* extracts (in the range of micrograms to miligrams) [17,20,24–27]. The reported efficacy via in vitro models may not accurately represent eurycomanone's level in vivo. Stability in plasma was measured via predetermined time incubation (0 and 30 min and 1, 2, 4 h) of eurycomanone and it was found to be highly stable; nevertheless, eurycomanone's ability to bind to proteins present in the plasma may affect its availability to its target site of action. However, the plasma protein binding in rats indicates that a low percentage of eurycomanone (30%) is bound to plasma proteins. In other words, the remaining 70% unbound fraction of eurycomanone is freely available and can possibly access the target sites [34].

The low absorption of eurycomanone in vivo correlates with findings from in vitro studies, namely the lipophilicity, solubility, and permeability assessment of eurycomanone. The lipophilicity of eurycomanone was very low and its solubility was high, which influences its permeation rate via lipid membranes as well as cell membranes such as of Caco-2 cells. The low log D value determined in this study indicates the extent to which eurycomanone was likely to stay in the aqueous environment instead of dissociating into the hydrophobic octanol. This relates to eurycomanone being highly soluble and its low permeation when assayed using the PAMPA method. When eurycomanone's permeability was assessed using the Caco-2 cells, the results also indicated that a low amount of eurycomanone permeated the cell monolayer. However, this may be due to the condition where eurycomanone, which was not lipophilic enough to be absorbed, accumulates on the cell monolayer, introducing a sink condition [35]. This accumulation then draws the compound to cross the membrane, which may not be due to the compound's innate ability to cross the membrane freely.

The ability of the compound to cross the biological membrane without the use of transporters is possible when the compound of interest is in its uncharged state. Eurycomanone is predicted to have an acid dissociation constant (pK_a) value of 11 [36]. The pH values of the environments in the stomach and small intestine vary in the different sections and depending on the fasted or fed state. The pH range in the stomach in its fasted state is between 1.4 and 2.1; while in its fed state, it is in between 4.3 and 5.4. In the small intestine, the pH values of the different segments in their fasted state are 4.9–6.4 (duodenum); 4.4–6.6 (jejunum), and 6.5–7.4 (ileum); while in their fed state, the pH values are 4.2–6.1 (duodenum); 5.2–6.2 (jejunum), and 6.8–7.5 (ileum) [37]. The changing pH values then affect the ionic state of eurycomanone. The predicted pK_a for eurycomanone was high, which means that in a lower pH environment, eurycomanone exists in its ionised form. This then prevents eurycomanone from crossing the membrane barriers passively.

As determined in the Caco-2 permeability assessment, eurycomanone was not an active transporter P-gp substrate. The chemical stability assay conducted using the fasted and fed state simulative buffer system indicates that eurycomanone was stable; however, its ionic state could not be confirmed. The plasma stability and liver metabolic stability study also showed eurycomanone to be stable in the different matrices, indicating that eurycomanone may stay intact and survive first-pass metabolism in vivo. This study hypothesised that when eurycomanone was administered orally, only a small amount crosses the membrane to enter the blood stream, while when it was administered intravenously, only a small amount of eurycomanone permeates into tissues, while most remained in the blood in its ionised form. The small amount of eurycomanone which may have been absorbed (as a low amount was detected in liver tissues) could still potentially exert the desired effects of eurycomanone or *E. longifolia* extract in general.

5. Conclusions

In conclusion, the results indicate that eurycomanone was a very polar compound with high stability at different pHs, in the plasma and in liver microsome. No major degradation of the compound in the gastrointestinal tract and blood plasma was noted and eurycomanone also exhibited low plasma protein binding ability. Despite the favourable properties of eurycomanone, its low permeability hinders its absorption, hence its bioavailability in in vivo models. The low absorptive value of eurycomanone may indicate the need to use eurycomanone at lower concentrations in assays aimed at finding its efficacy. The adoption of eurycomanone as the bioactive marker for *E. longifolia* may be considered with further evaluations of eurycomanone in in vivo models.

Author Contributions: Conceptualization, N.A. and D.S.S.; Methodology, N.A. and D.S.S.; Software, N.A. and D.S.S.; Validation, N.A. and D.S.S.; Formal Analysis, N.A. and D.S.S.; Investigation, N.A., D.S.S., B.P.T., N.A.Z., A.M., E.M. and A.Z.; Resources, N.A., D.S.S., B.P.T. and A.Z.; Data Curation, N.A. and D.S.S.; Writing–Original Draft Preparation, N.A.; Writing–Review & Editing, N.A., T.B.P., M.Z. and A.F.S.M.; Visualization, N.A. and D.S.S.; Supervision, N.R.A., Z.I. and A.F.S.M.; Project Administration, N.A. and D.S.S.; Funding Acquisition, N.A., M.Z., N.R.A, Z.I. and A.F.S.M.

Funding: This research received no external funding.

Acknowledgments: This study was funded by the Ministry of Agriculture, Malaysia, under project number NH0712PC001 and the Ministry of Health, Malaysia, under project number NMRR-12-1033-13911 (JPP-IMR 12-032). We would like to thank the Director General of Health Malaysia for his permission to publish this article. The authors also would like to acknowledge those who contributed directly or indirectly to this study's accomplishment. There are no competing financial interests in this study.

Conflicts of Interest: The authors declare no conflict of interest.

References

1. Chan, K.L.; Choo, C.Y.; Morita, H.; Itokawa, H. High performance liquid chromatography in phytochemical analysis of *Eurycoma longifolia*. *Planta Med.* **1998**, *64*, 741–745. [CrossRef] [PubMed]
2. Chua, L.S.; Amin, N.A.M.; Neo, J.C.H.; Lee, T.H.; Lee, C.T.; Sarmidi, M.R.; Aziz, R.A. LC-MS/MS-based metabolites of *Eurycoma longifolia* (Tongkat Ali) in malaysia (perak and pahang). *J. Chromatogr. B* **2011**, *879*, 3909–3919. [CrossRef] [PubMed]
3. Han, Y.M.; Jang, M.; Kim, I.S.; Kim, S.H.; Yoo, H.H. Simultaneous quantitation of six major quassinoids in Tongkat Ali dietary supplements by liquid chromatography with tandem mass spectrometry. *J. Sep. Sci.* **2015**, *38*, 2260–2266. [CrossRef] [PubMed]
4. Low, B.S.; Choi, S.B.; Wahab, H.A.; Das, P.K.; Chan, K.L. Eurycomanone, the major quassinoid in *Eurycoma longifolia* root extract increases spermatogenesis by inhibiting the activity of phosphodiesterase and aromatase in steroidogenesis. *J. Ethnopharmacol.* **2013**, *149*, 201–207. [CrossRef] [PubMed]
5. Miyake, K.; Tezuka, Y.; Awale, S.; Li, F.; Kadota, S. Quassinoids from *Eurycoma longifolia*. *J. Nat. Prod.* **2009**, *72*, 2135–2140. [CrossRef] [PubMed]
6. Morita, H.; Kishi, E.; Takeya, K.; Itokawa, H.; Tanaka, O. New quassinoids from the roots of *Eurycoma longifolia*. *Chem. Lett.* **1990**, *44*, 749–752. [CrossRef]
7. Rehman, S.U.; Choi, M.S.; Han, Y.M.; Kim, I.S.; Kim, S.H.; Piao, X.L.; Yoo, H.H. Determination of eurycomanone in rat plasma using hydrophilic interaction liquid chromatography-tandem mass spectrometry for pharmacokinetic study. *Biomed. Chromatogr.* **2017**, *31*. [CrossRef] [PubMed]
8. Teh, C.H.; Murugaiyah, V.; Chan, K.L. Developing a validated liquid chromatography-mass spectrometric method for the simultaneous analysis of five bioactive quassinoid markers for the standardization of manufactures batches of *Eurycoma longifolia* Jack extract as antimalarial medicaments. *J. Chromatogr. A* **2011**, *1218*, 1861–1877. [CrossRef] [PubMed]
9. Gimlette, J.D.; Burkhill, I.H. *The Medical Book of Malayan Medicine*; The Gardens Buletin Straits Settlements: Singapore, Singapore, 1930; Volume 6, p. 329.
10. Burkill, I.H.; Haniff, M. *Malay Village Medicine*; The Gardens Bulletin Straits Settlements: Singapore, Singapore, 1930; Volume 2, p. 182.
11. Low, B.S.; Das, P.K.; Chan, K.L. Standardized quassinoid-rich *Eurycoma longifolia* extract improved spermatogenesis and fertility in male rats via the hypothalamic-pituitary-gonadal axis. *J. Ethnopharmacol.* **2013**, *145*, 706–714. [CrossRef] [PubMed]
12. Ang, H.H.; Chan, K.L.; Mak, J.W. In vitro antimalarial activity of quassinoids from *Eurycoma longifolia* against malaysian chloroquine-resistant plasmodium falcifarum isolates. *Planta Med.* **1995**, *61*, 177–178. [CrossRef] [PubMed]
13. Chan, K.L.; O'Neill, M.J.; Phillipson, J.D.; Warhurst, D.C. Plants as sources of antimalarial drugs. Part 31 *Eurycoma longifolia*. *Planta Med.* **1986**, *52*, 105–107. [CrossRef]
14. Kardono, L.B.; Angerhofer, C.K.; Tsauri, S.; Padmawinata, K.; Pezzuto, J.M.; Kinghorn, A.D. Cytotoxic and antimalarial constituents of the roots of *Eurycoma longifolia*. *J. Nat. Prod.* **1991**, *54*, 1360–1367. [CrossRef] [PubMed]

15. Kuo, P.C.; Damu, A.G.; Lee, K.H.; Wu, T.S. Cytotoxic and antimalarial constituents from the roots of *Eurycoma longifolia*. *Bioorg. Med. Chem.* **2004**, *12*, 537–544. [CrossRef] [PubMed]

16. Low, B.S.; Teh, C.H.; Yuen, K.H.; Chan, K.L. Physico-chemical effects of the major quassinoids in a standardized *Eurycoma longifolia* extract (Fr 2) on the bioavailability and pharmacokinetic properties, and their implications for oral antimalarial activity. *Nat. Prod. Commun.* **2011**, *6*, 337–341. [PubMed]

17. Wernsdorfer, W.H.; Ismail, S.; Chan, K.L.; Congpuong, K.; Wernsdorfer, G. Activity of *Eurycoma longifolia* root extract against plasmodium falciparum in vitro. *Wien. Klinische Wochenschr.* **2009**, *121*, 23–26. [CrossRef] [PubMed]

18. Rehman, S.U.; Choe, K.; Yoo, H.H. Review on a traditional herbal medicine, *Eurycoma longifolia* Jack (Tongkat Ali). Its traditional uses, chemistry, evidence-based pharmacology and toxicology. *Molecules* **2016**, *21*, 331. [CrossRef] [PubMed]

19. Hajjouli, S.; Chateauvieux, S.; Teiten, M.H.; Orlikova, B.; Schumacher, M.; Dicato, M.; Choo, C.Y.; Diederich, M. Eurycomanone and eurycomanol from *Eurycoma longifolia* Jack as regulators of signalling pathways involved in proliferation, cell death and inflammation. *Molecules* **2014**, *19*, 14649–14666. [CrossRef] [PubMed]

20. Wong, P.F.; Cheong, W.F.; Shu, M.H.; Teh, C.H.; Chan, K.L.; AbuBakar, S. Eurycomanone suppress expression of lung cancer cell tumor markers, prohibitin, annexin 1 and endoplasmic reticulum protein 28. *Phytomedicine* **2012**, *19*, 138–144. [CrossRef] [PubMed]

21. Tada, H.; Yasuda, F.; Otani, K.; Doteuchi, M.; Ishihara, Y.; Shiro, M. New antiulcer quassinoids from *Eurycoma longifolia*. *Eur. J. Med. Chem.* **1991**, *26*, 345–349. [CrossRef]

22. Low, B.S.; Ng, B.H.; Choy, W.P.; Yuen, K.H.; Chan, K.L. Bioavailability and pharmacokinetic studies of eurycomanone from *Eurycoma longifolia*. *Planta Med.* **2005**, *71*, 803–807. [CrossRef] [PubMed]

23. Ma, H.Q.; Ebrahimi, F.; Khan, N.A.K.; Chan, K.L. Investigating the double-peak phenomenon in oral pharmacokinetics of *Eurycoma longifolia* quassinoids in lipid-based solid dispersion. *J. Bioequivalence Stud.* **2015**, *1*, 1–10.

24. Pan, Y.; Tiong, K.H.; Abd-Rashid, B.A.; Ismail, Z.; Ismail, R.; Mak, J.W. Effect of eurycomanone on cytochrome P450 isoforms CYP1A2, CYP2A6, CYP2C8, CYP2C9, CYP2C19, CYP2E1 and CYP3A4 in vitro. *J. Nat. Med.* **2014**, *68*, 402–406. [CrossRef] [PubMed]

25. Purwantiningsih; Hussin, A.H.; Chan, K.L. Phase 1 drug metabolism study of the standardised extract of *Eurycoma longifolia* (TAF-273) in rat hepatocytes. *Int. J. Pharm. Pharm. Sci.* **2010**, *2*, 147–152.

26. Purwantiningsih; Hussin, A.H.; Chan, K.L. Free radical scavenging activity of the standardized ethanolic extract of *Eurycoma longifolia* (TAF-273). *Int. J. Pharm. Pharm. Sci.* **2011**, *3*, 343–347.

27. Zakaria, Y.; Rahmat, A.; Pihie, A.H.L.; Abdullah, N.R.; Houghton, P.J. Eurycomanone induce apoptosis in HepG2 cells via up-regulation of p53. *Cancel Cell Int.* **2009**, *9*, 16. [CrossRef] [PubMed]

28. Ang, H.H.; Ikeda, S.; Gan, E.K. Evaluation of the potency activity of aphrodisiac in *Eurycoma longifolia* Jack. *Phytother. Res.* **2001**, *15*, 435–436. [CrossRef] [PubMed]

29. Ang, H.H.; Ngai, T.H. Aphrodisiac evaluation in non-copulator male rats after chronic administration of *Eurycoma longifolia* Jack. *Fundam. Clin. Pharmacol.* **2001**, *15*, 265–268. [CrossRef] [PubMed]

30. Solomon, M.C.; Erasmus, N.; Henkel, R.R. In vivo effects of *Eurycoma longifolia* Jack (Tongkat Ali) extract on reproductive functions in the rat. *Andrologia* **2014**, *46*, 339–348. [CrossRef] [PubMed]

31. Teh, C.H.; Abdulghani, M.; Morita, H.; Shiro, M.; Hussin, A.H.; Chan, K.L. Comparative X-ray and conformational analysis of a new crystal of 13-alpha, 21-dihydroeurycomanone with eurycomanone from *Eurycoma longifolia* and their anti-estrogenic activity using the uterotrophic assay. *Planta Med.* **2011**, *77*, 128–132. [CrossRef] [PubMed]

32. Zakaria, Y.; Rain, A.N.; Hawariah, L.P.A. Suppression effect of eurycomanone on the growth of HepG2 tumor transplanted in mice. In Proceedings of the 1st International Congress on Natural Products, Putrajaya, Malaysia, 14–16 November 2011; pp. 51–57.

33. Roberts, M.S.; Magnusson, B.M.; Burczynski, F.J.; Weiss, M. Enterohepatic circulation: Physiological, pharmacokinetic and clinical implications. *Clin. Pharm.* **2002**, *41*, 751–790. [CrossRef] [PubMed]

34. Stern, S.T.; Martinez, M.N.; Stevens, D.M. When is it important to measure unbound drug in evaluating nanomedicine pharmacokinetics? *Drug Metab. Dispos.* **2016**, *44*, 1934–1939. [CrossRef] [PubMed]

35. Valko, K. *Physicochemical and Biomimetic Properties in Drug Discovery. Chromatographic Techniques for Lead Optimization*; John Wiley & Sons, Inc.: Hoboken, NJ, USA, 2014; pp. 150–181.

36.   JChem. Chemaxon Version 17.29.0. Available online: https://chemaxon.com/ (accessed on 1 March 2018).
37.   Mudie, D.M.; Amidon, G.L.; Amidon, G.E. Physiological parameters for oral delivery and in vitro testing. *Mol. Pharm.* **2010**, *7*, 1388–1405. [CrossRef] [PubMed]

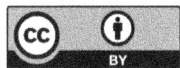

pharmaceutics

MDPI

Article

Development of a Column-Switching HPLC-MS/MS Method and Clinical Application for Determination of Ethyl Glucuronide in Hair in Conjunction with AUDIT for Detecting High-Risk Alcohol Consumption

Yeon Gyeong Kim [1,†], Jihye Hwang [1,†], Hwakyung Choi [2] and Sooyeun Lee [1,*]

[1] College of Pharmacy, Keimyung University, 1095 Dalgubeoldaero, Dalseo-gu, Daegu 42601, Korea; dusrud2307@naver.com (Y.G.K.); goldwise@postech.ac.kr (J.H.)
[2] Bugok National Hospital, 145 Bugok-ro, Bugok-myeon, Changnyeong-gun, Gyeongsangnam-do 50365, Korea; chk321@korea.kr
* Correspondence: sylee21@kmu.ac.kr; Tel.: +82-53-580-6651; Fax: +82-53-580-5164
† These authors contributed equally.

Received: 17 May 2018; Accepted: 28 June 2018; Published: 4 July 2018

Abstract: It is critical to assess the severity of alcohol consumption in certain diseases such as alcohol liver disease and alcohol addiction. Ethyl glucuronide (EtG) is a highly stable metabolite of ethanol in hair; thus, it was proposed as a long-term monitoring marker for alcohol consumption. Therefore, an HPLC-MS/MS method for EtG in hair was developed and applied to a clinical setting to assess the relevance of the EtG concentration and/or the Alcohol Use Disorders Identification Test (AUDIT) score to high-risk alcohol consumption. EtG was extracted from 10 mg of hair using water and analyzed using on-line sample purification coupled to HPLC-MS/MS. The diagnostic performances of the EtG concentration and/or the AUDIT score for detecting high-risk alcohol consumption were statistically evaluated between alcohol addicts ($n = 44$) and average alcohol users ($n = 19$). The on-line sample purification resulted in labor-saving with smaller sample amount. Both the EtG concentrations (4.0–587.4 pg/mg vs. 12.9–74.9 pg/mg) and the AUDIT scores (4–40 vs. 5–28) obtained from the alcohol addicts were significantly higher than those from the average alcohol users. The performance evaluation demonstrated that the integration score of the EtG concentration and the AUDIT score increased diagnostic performance for high-risk alcohol consumption.

Keywords: ethyl glucuronide; hair; HPLC-MS/MS; AUDIT score; alcohol addiction

1. Introduction

Alcohol is one of the most consumed and easily accessible drugs globally. In particular, certain alcohol consumption patterns such as binge drinking tend to increase among young people around the world [1]. Chronic and binge drinking was mentioned as the main determinant of the risk of alcoholic liver disease (ALD) [2]. The close relationship between the risk of worsening health conditions, such as dementia, and alcohol dependence has been also reported [3]. Alcoholism is one of the most frequent addictions and attracts great interest in clinical and forensic medicine [4]. In 2004, the World Health Organization reported that around 276.3 million people showed alcohol use disorders [5].

Ethanol rapidly undergoes both oxidative and non-oxidative metabolic processes and is converted to multiple metabolites. Among the non-oxidative metabolites, ethyl glucuronide (EtG) was firstly found in urine of a rabbit in 1952, and 15 years later it was also detected in human urine [6,7]. In 1994,

EtG was found to be a stable metabolite in hair after repeated consumption of alcohol, and many studies on the quantification of EtG in hair have thus far been conducted [6,8–11]. Since EtG in hair is significantly more stable than ethanol and other oxidative metabolites, it was proposed as a long-term monitoring marker to measure alcohol consumption [11,12]. Nevertheless, previous studies did not report the actual amount of alcohol consumed by alcohol drinkers, based on hair EtG concentrations, due to individual differences among the degrees to which EtG was taken up from the blood into hair [13]. According to the criteria set by the Society of Hair Testing (SoHT), the EtG concentrations in hair less than 7 pg/mg do not contradict self-reported abstinence and those above 7 pg/mg and 30 pg/mg are considered as indicators of repeated alcohol consumption and chronic excessive alcohol consumption, respectively [14].

From a clinical point of view, accurate monitoring of alcohol abstinence can significantly improve the therapeutic effect in alcohol-dependent patients [6]. Moreover, it is critical to assess alcohol intake and severity of alcohol abuse for subjects with certain diseases, such as ALD. For this, suitable markers are needed to objectively evaluate high-risk alcohol consumption. Since EtG is a hydrophilic compound that is detected in trace amounts in hair, its analysis in hair is not straightforward. Previous studies used aqueous incubation following either long-term sonication treatments or solid-phase extraction with large amounts of hair for sample preparation [15]. For the clinical application of the EtG analysis of hair, a highly sensitive analytical method with simple sample preprocessing is required.

We assessed the relevance of hair EtG concentration and/or the Alcohol Use Disorders Identification Test (AUDIT) score to high-risk alcohol consumption in well-characterized study participants of authentic alcohol addicts and average alcohol users. For this, a simple and sensitive high-performance liquid chromatography (HPLC)-tandem mass spectrometry (MS/MS) was developed using a column-switching technique was employed. We furthermore proposed an improved diagnostic approach to detect high-risk alcohol consumption, by combining the hair EtG concentration with the AUDIT score.

2. Materials and Methods

2.1. Chemicals

EtG and deuterium-labeled EtG (EtG-d_5) were obtained from Sigma-Aldrich (St. Louis, MO, USA). The stock solutions of EtG and EtG-d_5 were prepared at a concentration of 1 mg/mL in methanol for each. The working standard solutions of EtG (100 µg/mL, 10 µg/mL and 1 µg/mL) were prepared by serial dilution with deionized water from stock solutions. The working internal standard (IS) solution of EtG-d_5 (1 µg/mL) was also prepared using deionized water from the stock IS solution. All solvents were of HPLC grade.

2.2. Hair Sample Preparation

All hair samples were washed using methanol, deionized water and methanol in sequence and then dried at laboratory temperature. Each sample was cut into small pieces (1–2 mm length) and weighted. Each analysis was performed using approximately 10 mg of hair, to which 5 µL of 1 µg/mL EtG-d_5 and 95 µL deionized water were added. Then, the samples were quickly spun down and incubated at 4 °C for 15 h. After incubation, the samples were briefly vortexed and centrifuged (10,000 rpm, 30 min, 4 °C). The supernatants were filtered with a 0.45-µm polyvinylidenefluoride syringe filter (4 mm, Millipore, Molsheim, France) and 30 µL was injected into the HPLC-MS/MS system.

2.3. HPLC-MS/MS Analysis

The HPLC-MS/MS system consisted of an Agilent 1260 Infinity LC and 6460 triple quadrupole MS/MS system (Agilent Technologies, Santa Clara, CA, USA). The separation mode was optimized over four different conditions, using the non-polar C18 and/or HILIC column, as shown in Figure 1A.

Finally, a Poroshell C18 (3.0 × 50 mm, 2.7 μm, Agilent Technologies, Santa Clara, CA, USA) column and an XBridge HILIC (4.6 × 30 mm, 3.5 μm, Waters, Worchester, MA, USA) column were chosen for the on-line sample purification column and the analytical column, respectively. The prepared hair sample was loaded onto the purification column on valve position 1 for 0.3 min, during which the interfering matrix was enabled to be wasted from the column. At 0.3 min, the valve position was switched to position 2 and the analyte was then eluted to the analytical column (Figure 1B). The mobile phase consisted of 20 mM ammonium formate and 0.05% ammonium hydroxide in water (A) and 100% acetonitrile (B). The gradient condition for both columns was as follows: 0–10 min, 7–95% (B); 10–11.5 min, 95–95% (B); 11.5–12 min, 95–7% (B) and 12–13 min, 7–7% (B) at a flow rate of 300 μL/min. The autosampler and the column oven temperature were set at 4 °C and 20 °C, respectively.

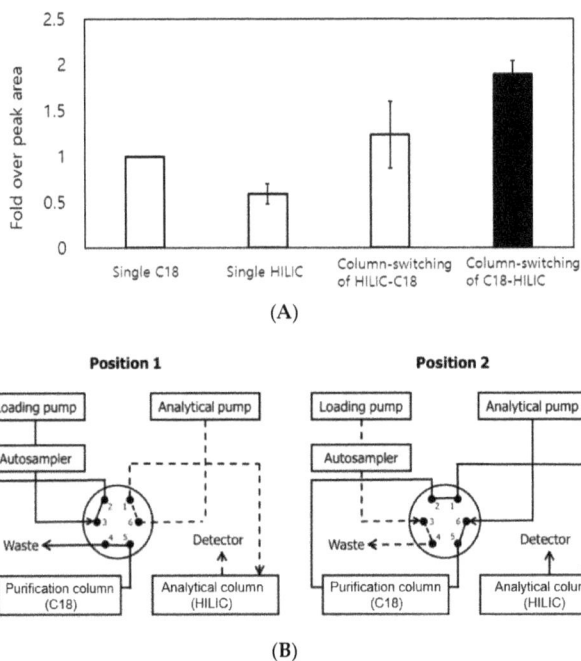

Figure 1. Comparison of peak areas of EtG by different modes of separation ((**A**), $n = 3$; mean ± standard deviation) and the schematic of the column-switching HPLC system used in the current study (**B**).

The MS system was operated using electrospray ionization in the negative mode. The optimum conditions were capillary voltage, 5.5 kV; nebulization pressure, 55 psi; temperature of drying gas, 300 °C; drying gas flow, 5 L/min; sheath gas temperature, 380 °C; sheath gas flow, 12 L/min and nozzle voltage, 0.5 V. EtG and EtG-d$_5$ were identified using selected reaction monitoring as follows: EtG, m/z 221.0 → 84.9 (quantitation ion, collision energy; 10 V); EtG-d$_5$, m/z 226.0 → 84.9 (collision energy; 10 V). Data were processed using the MassHunter software (B. 04. 00; Agilent Technologies).

2.4. Method Validation

Method validation parameters including selectivity, matrix effect, sensitivity, linearity, precision, accuracy and stability were determined as per criteria described in previous studies [15–17]. EtG-free human hair pooled from five different volunteers was used, except for the evaluation of selectivity and matrix effect, for which each hair sample was separately analyzed. To compensate for matrix effects, EtG-d$_5$ was used as an IS.

To investigate the selectivity of the method, five different sources of blank hair were analyzed to check the absence of responses interfering with the signals of EtG and EtG-d$_5$. The matrix effect was investigated with five sets of the regression lines prepared from five different hair matrices, for each. The calibration curves consisted of 8 points ranging from 5–5000 pg/mg. The coefficient of variation (CV) of the matrix effect was calculated using the slopes of the regression lines [15]. The sensitivity was expressed as limit of detection (LOD) and limit of quantification (LOQ). The analyte concentration at which the signal-to-noise ratio was greater than 3 was chosen for the LOD and that with less than 20% CV for precision and less than ±20% for bias for the LOQ. The linearity was established by a regression model, using 1/x as the weight factor, from five sets of the calibration curves. The precision and accuracy were examined using five replicates of EtG-spiked quality control (QC) samples for five days at 5, 100 and 5000 pg/mg. Repeatability and intermediate precision were evaluated using a one-way analysis of variance (ANOVA) with the grouping variable 'day' at the respective concentration level. The accuracy (bias, %) was calculated by comparing an experimentally determined mean concentration with each nominal concentration. Values of repeatability and intermediate precision that were lower than 20% CV at 5 pg/mg and lower than 15% CV at 100 and 5000 pg/mg were considered acceptable. The accuracy results that were within a range ±20% bias at the 5 pg/mg and ±15% bias at 100 and 5000 pg/mg were considered as satisfactory ranges [16,17]. As hair is considered a stable sample, only the in-process stability and processed stability were evaluated using the QC samples of 5, 100 and 5000 pg/mg. The QC samples were prepared for 6 and 15 h at 4 °C for investigation of the in-process stability. The processed sample stability was checked after keeping the samples for 8 h and 16 h in the autosampler (4 °C). The range from 90% to 110% of their nominal concentrations was suggested to be stable.

2.5. Clinical Study

The clinical study was approved by the Institutional Review Board of Bugok National Hospital (Gyeongsangnam-do, Republic of Korea, approval number: 5-018, approval date: 4 December 2015). Two groups of alcohol addicts ($n = 44$) and average alcohol users ($n = 19$) were included in this study. The age and body mass indices of the two groups were 53.2 ± 9.4 and 27.5 ± 4.8 years and 22.7 ± 2.6 and 23.6 ± 2.8 kg/m^2, respectively (mean ± standard deviation, Table 1). The alcohol addicts were known patients who were initially diagnosed by medical professionals and had less than five days of alcohol abstinence at the time of hair sampling. Average alcohol users were recruited and participated in a survey of drinking patterns as recording the amount of ethanol consumed for two months. Their hair samples were taken on the last day of recording. Hair samples were collected, as close to the scalp as possible, from three separate areas of the back of the head. The first 2-cm hair segment from the root was cut into small pieces and homogenized and approximately 10 mg of the finely cut hair was used for analysis. In addition, both the alcohol addicts and the average alcohol users answered 10 questions of the self-report version of the Alcohol Use Disorders Identification Test (AUDIT) [18] and their answers were scored. Since EtG levels in hair are known not to be significantly influenced by gender, BMI, or age [6,19], the statistical analysis for the concentrations of EtG in hair were performed based on those from the two groups with different ages, regardless of gender.

Table 1. Characteristics of alcohol addicts and alcohol users.

	Alcohol Addicts			Alcohol Users		
	Male ($n = 41$)	Female ($n = 3$)	Total ($n = 44$)	Male ($n = 11$)	Female ($n = 8$)	Total ($n = 19$)
Age (year)	53.0 ± 9.5	56.0 ± 10.1	53.2 ± 9.4	28.4 ± 5.5	26.2 ± 3.6	27.5 ± 4.8
BMI (kg/m^2)	23.0 ± 3.3	17.1 ± 1.5	22.7 ± 3.5	25.0 ± 2.5	21.6 ± 1.7	23.6 ± 2.8

Data are presented as mean ± standard deviation; BMI, body mass index.t.

2.6. Statistical Analysis

Statistical evaluations of the comparison of the EtG concentrations in hair and the AUDIT scores were performed by Mann–Whitney *U* test and Student *t*-test, respectively. The relationship among the hair EtG concentration, the AUDIT score and alcohol intake were evaluated using the Pearson correlation coefficient. The diagnostic performance of the hair EtG concentration and/or the AUDIT scores for detecting high-risk alcohol consumption was determined with the receiver operating characteristic (ROC) curve analysis. Toward this end, the integration score was first devised by combining the EtG concentration with the AUDIT score, using the machine-learning algorithm, support vector machine, which was used for classification. For data that cannot be perfectly classified, the support vectors lie on the margin boundaries. Thus, when classifying a new sample, its EtG concentration and AUDIT score are compared with those of the support vectors of the training sample that is most similar to the new sample. The linear support vector classification approach was applied in the current study. As a result, the summation of 0.095-fold of the EtG concentration and the original value of the AUDIT score were used to generate the integration score. To to compare the diagnostic performance of the EtG concentration, AUDIT score and integration score, the areas under the ROC curve (AUC) were calculated. Intuitively, the AUC reflects the false-positive rate needed to achieve various levels of sensitivity, with a perfect classifier having an AUC of 1.0 and a random classifier having an AUC of 0.5.

3. Results

3.1. Method Validation

The column-switching method from the C18 column for purification to the hydrophilic interaction liquid chromatography (HILIC) column for separation generated the best performance with the highest peak area and reproducibility (Figure 1A). The chosen method produced both EtG and EtG-d_5 at 2.4 min in chromatograms, where minor interference was observed in Figure 2A. However, it was possible to carry out the experiment because no difference in pattern and no significant effects on method accuracy and precision were observed. Figure 2B shows the chromatograms obtained for EtG and EtG-d_5 in a spiked hair sample at the LOQ level (5 pg/mg) and Figure 2C displays those in an EtG positive hair sample. Any significant variation due to different matrices was not observed as the CV of the slopes of five regression lines prepared from five different hair matrices, for each, was 1.6% (Figure 3). The LOD and the LOQ were 5 pg/mg for both. Moreover, EtG produced effective linearity within the wide calibration range (5–5000 pg/mg) with the r value of 0.997 (*n* = 5).

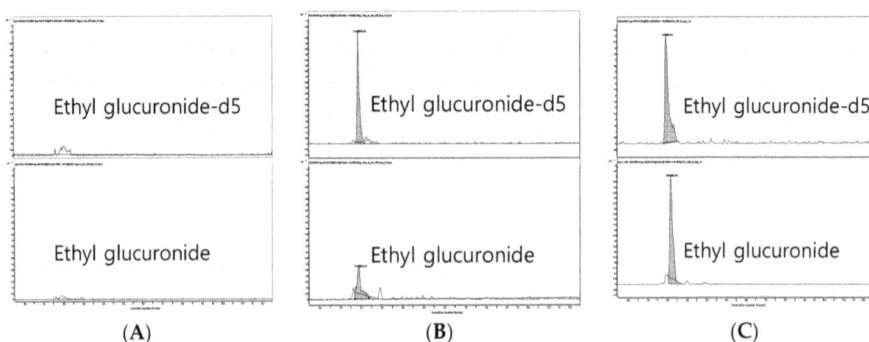

Figure 2. Representative chromatograms of EtG and EtG-d_5. (**A**) A blank hair sample. (**B**) A fortified hair sample (spiked with the limit of quantification level). (**C**) An EtG-positive sample collected from an alcohol user.

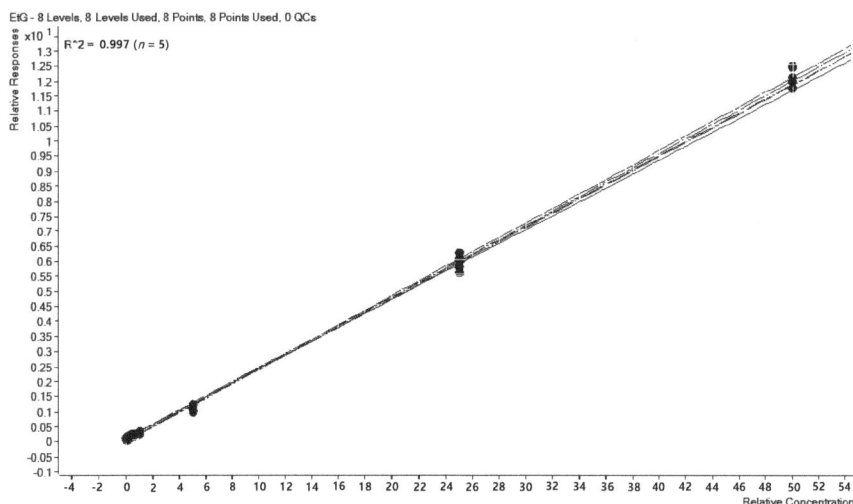

Figure 3. Overlay of regression lines prepared from different hair matrices (n = 5).

As shown in Table 2, the repeatability and intermediate precision were lower than 10% at 5, 100 and 5000 pg/mg. The worst accuracy value obtained was −10.7% at 100 pg/mg. These results were regarded acceptable, as the guidelines of analytical method validation (precision, less than 20% CV near lower limit of quantification (LLOQ) and less than 15% for higher levels; accuracy, within ±20% bias near LLOQ and less than ±15% bias for the higher level) [17]. The in-process stability was investigated under the conditions used to extract EtG from hair, up to 15 h at 4 °C. The processed stability was checked as keeping the prepared samples for 8 h and 16 h in the autosampler (4 °C). The mean values of the in-process stability ranged from 90% to 101% and those of the processed stability ranged from 92% to 103%, which was acceptable based on the criteria (90–110% of nominal concentrations) [17] (Table 2). Therefore, the analytical process was conducted under the stated conditions.

Table 2. Summary of validation data.

Concentration (pg/mg)	Repeatability [a] (CV [b], %)	Intermediate Precision [c] (CV, %)	Accuracy (Bias, %)	In-Process Stability (Mean, %)		Processed Stability (Mean, %)	
				6 h	15 h	8 h	16 h
5	3.6	3.8	−3.5	96	90	97	100
100	8.3	9.1	−10.7	93	99	92	92
5000	9.3	4.0	−4.0	98	101	103	99

[a] Within-day variation; [b] Coefficient of variation; [c] Combination of within- and between-day variation.

3.2. Evaluation of the Diagnostic Performance of the Hair EtG Concentrations

The concentrations of EtG in hair samples obtained from the alcohol addicts (n = 44) were significantly higher than those from the average alcohol users (p = 0.008). The hair EtG concentrations did not follow a Gaussian distribution; thus, the non-parametric Mannwhitney U test was used to investigate the significance of differences in EtG concentrations between alcohol addicts and average users. The concentrations of EtG in hair from the alcohol addicts and the average alcohol users ranged from 4.0 to 587.4 pg/mg (mean, 99.0 pg/mg; median, 59.9 pg/mg; standard deviation, 111.5 pg/mg) and from 12.9 to 74.9 pg/mg (mean, 41.2 pg/mg; median, 42.5 pg/mg; standard deviation, 19.4 pg/mg), respectively. Moreover, the AUDIT scores of the formal group were even more significantly higher than those of the latter group (p = 1.09E-7). The AUDIT scores of the alcohol addicts were between 4 and 40 (mean, 26.9; median, 29.5; standard deviation, 9.6) and those of the average alcohol users were between 5 and 28 (mean, 12.7; median, 11.0; standard deviation, 5.4) (Figure 4).

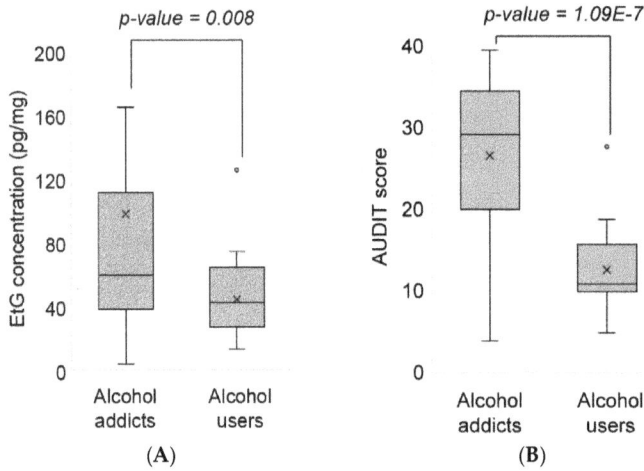

Figure 4. Distribution of the hair EtG concentrations (**A**) and the AUDIT scores (**B**) in alcohol addicts (n = 44) and average alcohol users (n = 19).

The correlation analysis demonstrated that EtG concentrations from the hair of alcohol addicts were not associated with their AUDIT scores (r = 0.2284, Figure 5A), while the EtG concentrations from the hair of the average alcohol users were moderately correlated with their AUDIT scores (r = 0.534, Figure 5B). For the average alcohol users, moderate correlations were shown between the self-reported alcohol intake and the hair EtG concentrations (r = 0.440, Figure 6A) and between the self-reported alcohol intake and the AUDIT scores (r = 0.615, Figure 6B). The self-reported alcohol intake was more strongly correlated with the AUDIT scores than with the hair EtG concentrations.

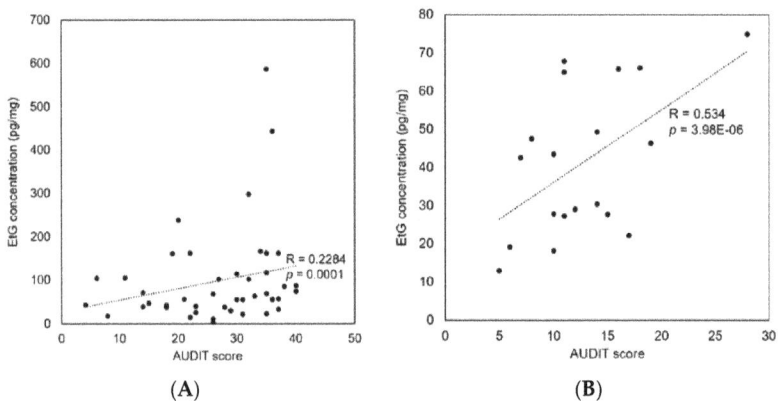

Figure 5. Correlation between the AUDIT scores and the hair EtG concentrations in alcohol addicts (n = 44, (**A**)) and average alcohol users (n = 19, (**B**)).

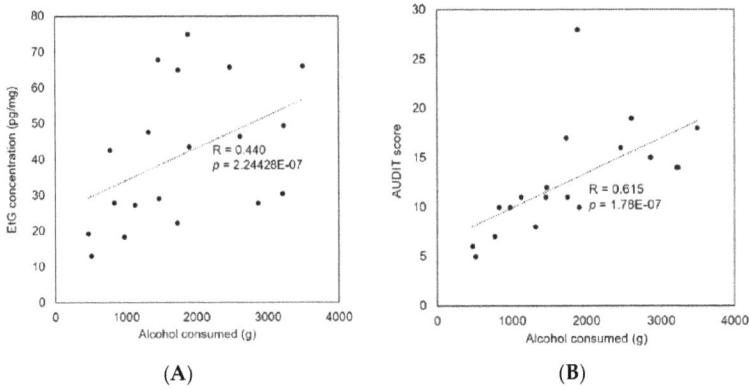

Figure 6. Correlation between alcohol consumed and the hair EtG concentrations (**A**) and between alcohol consumed and the AUDIT scores (**B**) in average alcohol users (n = 19).

In the scatter plot of the EtG concentrations in hair and the AUDIT scores from the both groups (Figure 7A), the training data are linearly separable. The best separating hyperplane was generated by a linear equation of $0.095x + y - 20.274 = 0$ (x, hair EtG concentration; y, AUDIT score), from which the distance to the nearest data point on each side was maximized. With this hyperplane equation, the integration scores were generated using $0.095x + y$. The results of the ROC analysis to compare the AUC of the hair EtG concentration, the AUDIT score and the integration score are shown in Figure 7B. The highest AUC was shown for the integration score with 0.90. The hair EtG concentration and the AUDIT score achieved AUCs of 0.69 and 0.88, respectively. For the diagnosis of high-risk alcohol consumption, the score cutoffs for the hair EtG concentration, the AUDIT score and the integration score were optimized. The thresholds were determined by examining the lowest false-positive rate (FPR) and the highest true-positive rate (TPR) at each given score. The resultant cutoff scores of the hair EtG concentration, the AUDIT score and the integration score were 55 pg/mg, 20 and 21 (x = 50 pg/mg, y = 16), respectively. The integration score of 21 was the best diagnostic cutoff with 19% FPR rate and 89% TPR.

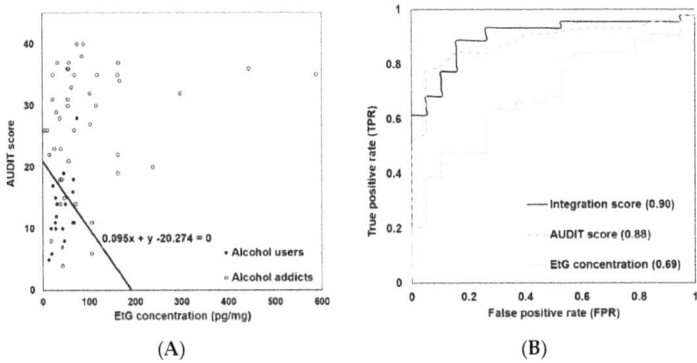

Figure 7. Performance evaluation of the hair EtG concentration, the AUDIT score and the integration score. (**A**) Scatter plot of the hair EtG concentrations and the AUDIT scores in alcohol addicts (n = 44, closed circle) and average alcohol users (n = 19, open circle). The optimal dividing line is presented as a black line with its equation. (**B**) ROC of the hair EtG concentration, the AUDIT score and the integration score. The AUC values are in parentheses.

4. Discussion

Hair has many advantages as a diagnostic sample for assessing substance use, including long detection window, easy sample collection, convenient sample transport and storage and facilitates repeated sampling, if necessary. In Switzerland, EtG in hair was used as a direct marker for abstinence monitoring in driving aptitude assessment [20]. In another previous study, the EtG concentrations in hair from cadavers improved the diagnosis of alcoholism in the forensic domain [21]. The usage of hair care products, including products containing ethanol, does not significantly affect EtG in hair [4,22]. In addition, the correlation between EtG concentrations in hair and alcohol consumption was not affected by the differences of gender and age [6]. Since the analysis of EtG in hair can provide reliable data on the history of individual alcohol use, it can be used as a diagnostic tool for high-risk alcohol consumption.

Previous studies employed GC-MS/MS [23] or LC-MS/MS [24–29] for the quantitative analysis of EtG in hair samples. For hair sample preparation, aqueous incubation following sonication for 1.5–3 h and/or solid phase extraction with 20–100 mg of hair was often performed in those studies [15,24,26]. For more effective clinical application of the hair EtG analysis, a time and labor-saving method with smaller sample amount was devised as employing on-line sample purification using the C18 column in the present study. This technique enabled the hair EtG analysis with 10 mg of hair, as the C18 stationary phase could remove some hydrophilic interference and concentrate EtG. The validation results proved that the developed method was sensitive enough to determine the cut-off (7 pg/mg) proposed by SoHT and highly accurate and precise in the wide calibration range.

The hair EtG concentrations in this study were within the concentration ranges reported in other previous studies. In the study of Crunelle et al., the concentrations of EtG ranged from 32 to 662 pg/mg for the subjects (male, $n = 25$; female, $n = 11$) whose total alcohol consumption dose for 3 months was 60–650 g/day. There were no gender and age-related effects on the correlation between hair EtG and alcohol consumption [6]. In another previous study, only 4 out of 7 people who consumed 32 g of alcohol per day for 3 months showed measurable EtG levels in hair and 16 g of alcohol per day for 3 months did not result in detectable EtG levels (LOQ; 2 pg/mg using 30 mg hair) [30].

The hair EtG concentration proved to be a more reliable diagnostic marker in identifying heavy alcohol consumption when compared with traditional biomarkers such as alanine aminotransferase, aspartate aminotransferase, carbohydrate-deficient transferrin and gamma-glutamyltransferase [31]. However, the AUC of the hair EtG concentration, 0.69, in the current study implies that the use of the EtG concentration alone does not have a strong potential to detect alcohol addiction. Both environmental and genetic factors play important roles in the initiation of alcohol drinking and progression to alcoholism [32]. Therefore, alcohol addiction could not be reliably detected based only on the EtG concentration or alcohol consumption dose. The integration score demonstrated the performance advantage, compared with either the hair EtG concentration or the AUDIT score, in diagnosing high-risk alcohol consumption. In a previous study on the analyses of meconium fatty acid ethyl esters, EtG and ethyl sulfate for detecting maternal drinking during pregnancy, the combination of the markers including EtG increased the agreement of self-reported prenatal alcohol exposure [33]. By integrating the AUDIT score and the hair EtG concentration, the highest performance was obtained for the diagnosis of high-risk alcohol consumption, with a cutoff value 21 and the best combination of sensitivity (0.89, TPR) and specificity (0.81, 1-FPR). In a previous study, 27 pg/mg of hair EtG was suggested to identify heavy drinkers and the sensitivity and specificity were 0.92 and 0.96, respectively [34]. Compared with the cutoff of 30 pg/mg of the hair EtG level recommended by the SoHT [35], a higher EtG concentration (x = 50 pg/mg) was obtained using the current optimal integration score. To the best of our knowledge, this is the first study investigating the usefulness of the combination of the hair EtG concentration and the AUDIT score in diagnosing alcohol addiction, which is often a significant consequence of chronic and excessive alcohol consumption. As many factors, including the amount of alcohol consumption, behavior and psychiatric state, influence alcohol addiction, the integration of multiple markers could show stronger performance and would be useful in clinical diagnosis.

Author Contributions: Conceptualization, S.L. and H.C.; Methodology, Y.G.K. and H.C.; Validation, Y.G.K.; Data Curation, J.H.; Writing—Original Draft Preparation, Y.G.K. and S.L.; Writing—Review and Editing, S.L.; Visualization, J.H.; Supervision, S.L.; Funding Acquisition, S.L.

Funding: This research was funded by the Research Program to Solve Social Issues (NRF-2015M3C8A8074697) and the Bio and Medical Technology Development Program (NRF-2015M3A9E1028327) of the National Research Foundation of Korea (NRF) funded by the Ministry of Science and ICT and by the Basic Science Research Program of the NRF funded by the Ministry of Education (NRF-2016R1A6A1A03011325).

Conflicts of Interest: The authors declare that they have no conflict of interest.

References

1. Gomez, P.; Moure-Rodriguez, L.; Lopez-Caneda, E.; Rial, A.; Cadaveira, F.; Caamano-Isorna, F. Patterns of alcohol consumption in spanish university alumni: Nine years of follow-up. *Front. Psychol.* **2017**, *8*, 756. [CrossRef] [PubMed]

2. Liangpunsakul, S.; Puri, P.; Shah, V.H.; Kamath, P.; Sanyal, A.; Urban, T.; Ren, X.; Katz, B.; Radaeva, S.; Chalasani, N.; et al. Effects of age, sex, body weight, and quantity of alcohol consumption on occurrence and severity of alcoholic hepatitis. *Clin. Gastroenterol. Hepatol.* **2016**, *14*, 1831–1838e3. [CrossRef] [PubMed]

3. Li, T.K. Quantifying the risk for alcohol-use and alcohol-attributable health disorders: Present findings and future research needs. *J. Gastroenterol. Hepatol.* **2008**, *23* (Suppl. S1), S2–S8. [CrossRef] [PubMed]

4. Martins Ferreira, L.; Binz, T.; Yegles, M. The influence of ethanol containing cosmetics on ethyl glucuronide concentration in hair. *Forensic Sci. Int.* **2012**, *218*, 123–125. [CrossRef] [PubMed]

5. Global Ststus Report on Alcohol and Health 2014. Available online: http://apps.who.int/iris/bitstream/ 10665/112736/1/9789240692763_eng.pdf?ua=1 (accessed on 15 November 2016).

6. Crunelle, C.L.; Cappelle, D.; Covaci, A.; van Nuijs, A.L.; Maudens, K.E.; Sabbe, B.; Dom, G.; Michielsen, P.; Yegles, M.; Neels, H. Hair ethyl glucuronide as a biomarker of alcohol consumption in alcohol-dependent patients: Role of gender differences. *Drug Alcohol Depend.* **2014**, *141*, 163–166. [CrossRef] [PubMed]

7. Sutker, P.B.; Tabakoff, B.; Goist, K.C., Jr.; Randall, C.L. Acute alcohol intoxication, mood states and alcohol metabolism in women and men. *Pharmacol. Biochem. Behav.* **1983**, *18* (Suppl. S1), 349–354. [CrossRef]

8. Gomez-Roig, M.D.; Marchei, E.; Sabra, S.; Busardo, F.P.; Mastrobattista, L.; Pichini, S.; Gratacos, E.; Garcia-Algar, O. Maternal hair testing to disclose self-misreporting in drinking and smoking behavior during pregnancy. *Alcohol* **2018**, *67*, 1–6. [CrossRef] [PubMed]

9. Joya, X.; Mazarico, E.; Ramis, J.; Pacifici, R.; Salat-Batlle, J.; Mortali, C.; Garcia-Algar, O.; Pichini, S. Segmental hair analysis to assess effectiveness of single-session motivational intervention to stop ethanol use during pregnancy. *Drug Alcohol Depend.* **2016**, *158*, 45–51. [CrossRef] [PubMed]

10. Morini, L.; Marchei, E.; Vagnarelli, F.; Garcia Algar, O.; Groppi, A.; Mastrobattista, L.; Pichini, S. Ethyl glucuronide and ethyl sulfate in meconium and hair-potential biomarkers of intrauterine exposure to ethanol. *Forensic Sci. Int.* **2010**, *196*, 74–77. [CrossRef] [PubMed]

11. Hoiseth, G.; Bernard, J.P.; Karinen, R.; Johnsen, L.; Helander, A.; Christophersen, A.S.; Morland, J. A pharmacokinetic study of ethyl glucuronide in blood and urine: Applications to forensic toxicology. *Forensic Sci. Int.* **2007**, *172*, 119–124. [CrossRef] [PubMed]

12. Wurst, F.M.; Skipper, G.E.; Weinmann, W. Ethyl glucuronide—The direct ethanol metabolite on the threshold from science to routine use. *Addiction* **2003**, *98* (Suppl. S2), 51–61. [CrossRef] [PubMed]

13. Ferraguti, G.; Ciolli, P.; Carito, V.; Battagliese, G.; Mancinelli, R.; Ciafre, S.; Tirassa, P.; Ciccarelli, R.; Cipriani, A.; Messina, M.P.; et al. Ethylglucuronide in the urine as a marker of alcohol consumption during pregnancy: Comparison with four alcohol screening questionnaires. *Toxicol. Lett.* **2017**, *275*, 49–56. [CrossRef] [PubMed]

14. 2016 Consensus for the Use of Alcohol Markers in Hair for Assessment of both Abstinence and Chronic Excessive Alcohol Consumption. Available online: http://www.soht.org/consensus (accessed on 15 November 2016).

15. Pirro, V.; Di Corcia, D.; Seganti, F.; Salomone, A.; Vincenti, M. Determination of ethyl glucuronide levels in hair for the assessment of alcohol abstinence. *Forensic Sci. Int.* **2013**, *232*, 229–236. [CrossRef] [PubMed]

16. Peters, F.T.; Hartung, M.; Schmitt, M.H.G.; Daldrup, T.; Musshoff, F. Requirements for the Validation of Analytical Methods. Available online: https://www.gtfch.org/cms/images/stories/files/Appendix%20B% 20GTFCh%2020090601.pdf (accessed on 1 March 2016).

17.   Peters, F.T.; Drummer, O.H.; Musshoff, F. Validation of new methods. *Forensic Sci. Int.* **2007**, *165*, 216–224. [CrossRef] [PubMed]

18.   Alcohol Use Disorders Identification Test (Audit). Available online: https://www.drugabuse.gov/sites/default/files/files/AUDIT.pdf (accessed on 1 March 2016).

19.   Crunelle, C.L.; Neels, H.; Maudens, K.; De Doncker, M.; Cappelle, D.; Matthys, F.; Dom, G.; Fransen, E.; Michielsen, P.; De Keukeleire, S.; et al. Influence of body mass index on hair ethyl glucuronide concentrations. *Alcohol Alcohol.* **2017**, *52*, 19–23. [CrossRef] [PubMed]

20.   Schrock, A.; Pfaffli, M.; Konig, S.; Weinmann, W. Application of phosphatidylethanol (peth) in whole blood in comparison to ethyl glucuronide in hair (hetg) in driving aptitude assessment (daa). *Int. J. Leg. Med.* **2016**, *130*, 1527–1533. [CrossRef] [PubMed]

21.   Bendroth, P.; Kronstrand, R.; Helander, A.; Greby, J.; Stephanson, N.; Krantz, P. Comparison of ethyl glucuronide in hair with phosphatidylethanol in whole blood as post-mortem markers of alcohol abuse. *Forensic Sci. Int.* **2008**, *176*, 76–81. [CrossRef] [PubMed]

22.   Hartwig, S.; Auwarter, V.; Pragst, F. Effect of hair care and hair cosmetics on the concentrations of fatty acid ethyl esters in hair as markers of chronically elevated alcohol consumption. *Forensic Sci. Int.* **2003**, *131*, 90–97. [CrossRef]

23.   Shi, Y.; Shen, B.; Xiang, P.; Yan, H.; Shen, M. Determination of ethyl glucuronide in hair samples of chinese people by protein precipitation (ppt) and large volume injection-gas chromatography-tandem mass spectrometry (lvi-gc/ms/ms). *J. Chromatogr. B* **2010**, *878*, 3161–3166. [CrossRef] [PubMed]

24.   Binz, T.M.; Baumgartner, M.R.; Kraemer, T. The influence of cleansing shampoos on ethyl glucuronide concentration in hair analyzed with an optimized and validated lc-ms/ms method. *Forensic Sci. Int.* **2014**, *244*, 20–24. [CrossRef] [PubMed]

25.   Hegstad, S.; Kristoffersen, L.; Liane, V.H.; Spigset, O. Etg and ets in autopsy blood samples with and without putrefaction using uplc-ms-ms. *J. Anal. Toxicol.* **2017**, *41*, 107–113. [CrossRef] [PubMed]

26.   Janda, I.; Weinmann, W.; Kuehnle, T.; Lahode, M.; Alt, A. Determination of ethyl glucuronide in human hair by spe and lc-ms/ms. *Forensic Sci. Int.* **2002**, *128*, 59–65. [CrossRef]

27.   Kummer, N.; Wille, S.; Di Fazio, V.; Lambert, W.; Samyn, N. A fully validated method for the quantification of ethyl glucuronide and ethyl sulphate in urine by uplc-esi-ms/ms applied in a prospective alcohol self-monitoring study. *J. Chromatogr. B* **2013**, *929*, 149–154. [CrossRef] [PubMed]

28.   Madry, M.M.; Spycher, B.S.; Kupper, J.; Fuerst, A.; Baumgartner, M.R.; Kraemer, T.; Naegeli, H. Long-term monitoring of opioid, sedative and anti-inflammatory drugs in horse hair using a selective and sensitive lc-ms/ms procedure. *BMC Vet. Res.* **2016**, *12*, 84.

29.   Slawson, M.H.; Johnson-Davis, K.L. Quantitation of ethyl glucuronide and ethyl sulfate in urine using liquid chromatography-tandem mass spectrometry (lc-ms/ms). *Methods Mol. Biol.* **2016**, *1383*, 167–175. [PubMed]

30.   Kronstrand, R.; Brinkhagen, L.; Nystrom, F.H. Ethyl glucuronide in human hair after daily consumption of 16 or 32 g of ethanol for 3 months. *Forensic Sci. Int.* **2012**, *215*, 51–55. [CrossRef] [PubMed]

31.   Kharbouche, H.; Faouzi, M.; Sanchez, N.; Daeppen, J.B.; Augsburger, M.; Mangin, P.; Staub, C.; Sporkert, F. Diagnostic performance of ethyl glucuronide in hair for the investigation of alcohol drinking behavior: A comparison with traditional biomarkers. *Int. J. Leg. Med.* **2012**, *126*, 243–250. [CrossRef] [PubMed]

32.   Tabakoff, B.; Hoffman, P.L. The neurobiology of alcohol consumption and alcoholism: An integrative history. *Pharmacol. Biochem. Behav.* **2013**, *113*, 20–37. [CrossRef] [PubMed]

33.   Himes, S.K.; Dukes, K.A.; Tripp, T.; Petersen, J.M.; Raffo, C.; Burd, L.; Odendaal, H.; Elliott, A.J.; Hereld, D.; Signore, C.; et al. Clinical sensitivity and specificity of meconium fatty acid ethyl ester, ethyl glucuronide, and ethyl sulfate for detecting maternal drinking during pregnancy. *Clin. Chem.* **2015**, *61*, 523–532. [CrossRef] [PubMed]

34.   Morini, L.; Politi, L.; Polettini, A. Ethyl glucuronide in hair. A sensitive and specific marker of chronic heavy drinking. *Addiction* **2009**, *104*, 915–920. [CrossRef] [PubMed]

35.   Kintz, P. Consensus of the society of hair testing on hair testing for chronic excessive alcohol consumption 2009. *Forensic Sci. Int.* **2010**, *196*, 2. [CrossRef] [PubMed]

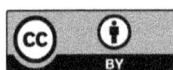

pharmaceutics

MDPI

Article

Effect of Red Ginseng Extract on the Pharmacokinetics and Efficacy of Metformin in Streptozotocin-Induced Diabetic Rats

So Jeong Nam [1], You Jin Han [1], Wonpyo Lee [2], Bitna Kang [2], Min-Koo Choi [2], Yong-Hae Han [3] and Im-Sook Song [1,*]

[1] College of Pharmacy and Research Institute of Pharmaceutical Sciences, Kyungpook National University, Daegu 41566, Korea; goddns159@nate.com (S.J.N.); gksdbwls2@nate.com (Y.J.H.)
[2] College of Pharmacy, Dankook University, Cheon 31116, Korea; dldjsvy93@naver.com (W.L.); qlcska@gmail.com (B.K.); minkoochoi@dankook.ac.kr (M.-K.C.)
[3] Life Science Institute, Daewoong Pharmaceutical, Yongin 17028, Korea; yonghae.han@gmail.com
* Correspondence: isssong@knu.ac.kr; Tel.: +82-53-950-8575

Received: 8 June 2018; Accepted: 2 July 2018; Published: 3 July 2018

Abstract: The purpose of this study was to investigate the effect of red ginseng extract on the pharmacokinetics (PK) and efficacy of metformin in streptozotocin-induced diabetic rats. The diabetes mellitus rat model was established by intraperitoneally administering multiple doses of streptozotocin (30 mg/kg, twice on day 1 and 8), and diabetic rats received metformin 50 mg/kg with or without single or multiple administration of Korean red ginseng extract (RGE, 2 g/kg/day, once or for 1 week). RGE administration did not affect the plasma concentration and renal excretion of metformin. Further, diabetic rats were administered metformin (50 mg/kg) and RGE (2 g/kg) alone or concomitantly for 5 weeks, and both regimens decreased the fasting blood glucose and glycated hemoglobin (Hb-A1c) levels. Furthermore, fasting blood glucose levels were reduced by metformin or RGE administered alone but recovered to the control level following co-administration, suggesting that the effect was additive. However, triglyceride and free fatty acid levels were not different with metformin and RGE treatment alone or in combination. Biochemical parameters such as alanine aminotransferase (ALT), aspartate aminotransferase (AST), triglycerides, total cholesterol, high-density lipoprotein (HDL) cholesterol, low-density lipoprotein (LDL) cholesterol levels were not different among the three treatment groups. In conclusion, RGE and metformin showed an additive effect in glycemic control. However, the co-administration of RGE and metformin did not cause PK interactions or affect biochemical parameters including the free fatty acid, triglyceride, AST, ALT, or cholesterol levels.

Keywords: Korean red ginseng extract; metformin; diabetes; drug interaction; pharmacokinetics; efficacy

---

1. Introduction

Diabetes mellitus (DM) is a common chronic disease worldwide and is major health problem [1,2]. Type 2 DM accounts for approximately 90% of all incidences of DM and is characterized by insulin resistance and pancreatic β-cell dysfunction [2–5]. In patients with type 2 DM, metformin has been recommended as a first-line treatment. Metformin lowers blood glucose concentration without increasing insulin secretion [6–8]. However, metformin alone is thought to be insufficient for glycemic control and, therefore, often requires co-therapy with other agents. Thus, drug–drug interactions between co-therapy drugs in patients with type 2 DM should be carefully considered and monitored. Red ginseng is obtained from fresh ginseng grown for 6 years through the process of steaming and drying, and has been reported to provide various therapeutic effects for diseases including cardiovascular disease, diabetes, allergies, insomnia, gastritis, hepatotoxicity, and sexual dysfunction [9–11]. Korean red ginseng was beneficial in a diabetic mouse model induced by streptozotocin (STZ) administration, not only for its hypoglycemic effects but also for its immunomodulation [12]. Supplementation with Korean red ginseng or Korean red ginseng extract (RGE) has been shown to improve DM in STZ-induced diabetic animals as well as in humans [12–15]. Fermented red ginseng also exhibited a strong antidiabetic effects in STZ-induced diabetic rats [12] and patients with type 2 DM [13]. STZ is most commonly used to establish experimental DM models because it damages pancreatic β-cells of the islets of Langerhans [16]. High-dose STZ severely impairs insulin secretion, similar to type 1 DM, but low-dose STZ causes some damage to insulin secretion, similar to type 2 DM. STZ can also be administered in multiple low doses to gradually achieve immune destruction of β-cells [3]. Consequently, we established the DM rat model used in this study with multiple low doses of STZ (two 30 mg/kg intraperitoneal injections administered 1 week apart) according to the method of Zhang et al. [2,3]. Using this STZ-induced DM rat model, therefore, the purpose of this study was to evaluate the possibility of drug–drug interactions between RGE and metformin based on their PK and efficacy.

2. Materials and Methods

2.1. Materials

Korean RGE was obtained from Punggi Ginseng Cooperative Association (Punggi, Korea), and was produced in the facilities following the current guidelines of the Korea Good Manufacturing Practice (Lot No. 1614-2). Furthermore, 2 g RGE contained 3.85 mg ginsenoside Rb1, 1.85 mg ginsenoside Rb2, 2.0 mg ginsenoside Rd, and 2.6 mg ginsenoside Rg3. Metformin and STZ were purchased from Sigma-Aldrich Corp. (St. Louis, MO, USA). All other reagents and solvents were of reagent grade.

2.2. Animals

Male Sprague–Dawley rats (7–8 weeks, 220–250 g) were purchased from Samtako Co. (Osan, Korea). On arrival, the rats were housed on a 12-h light/dark cycle and were provided food and water ad libitum for 1 week prior to the animal experiments. All animal procedures were approved by the Animal Care and Use Committee of Kyungpook National University (Approval No. 2017-0021) and carried out in accordance with the National Institutes of Health guidance for the care and the use of laboratory animals.

2.3. Induction of Diabetes Mellitus (DM) and Efficacy Monitoring

The rats were fasted overnight before the induction of DM with STZ. The rats were administered STZ 30 mg/kg (dissolved in 0.1 M citrate buffer, pH 4.5) intraperitoneally once and the treated was repeated 1 week later. Rats were fed for 4 h post STZ dose to avoid the anticipated hypoglycemic shock. Body weights, water intake, and urine output were closely monitored daily after STZ administration. Fasting blood glucose concentration was measured in tail vein blood using an Accu-Chek glucometer (Roche Korea, Seoul, Korea), every 2 or 3 days at 9 a.m. following overnight fasting for 35 days. Rats with fasting blood glucose >250 mg/dL were considered diabetes-induced and used in this study.

STZ-induced diabetic rats were divided into four groups: DM control (DC), DM with metformin (D + M), DM with RGE (D + RGE), and DM with metformin and RGE groups (D + RGE + M). Oral administration of water (vehicle), metformin, and red ginseng to rats were conducted daily via oral gavage.

Rats in the DC group were orally administered water as the vehicle for 5 weeks in addition to STZ administration. Rats in the D + M group received water as the vehicle and 2 h later they were orally administered metformin (50 mg/kg, dissolved in water). Rats in the D + RGE group received RGE (2 g/kg, dissolved in water) orally. Rats in the D + GRE + M group first received

RGE (2 g/kg, dissolved in water) and 2 h later, metformin (50 mg/kg, dissolved in water) orally. At the end of the experimental day, abdominal arterial blood and the liver and pancreatic tissues were collected from rats in all groups. The collected blood was centrifuged at 13,000 rpm for 10 min at 4 °C and the supernatant plasma samples were used to the biochemical parameters such as alanine aminotransferase (ALT), aspartate aminotransferase (AST), triglycerides, total cholesterol, high-density lipoprotein (HDL)-cholesterol, low-density lipoprotein (LDL)-cholesterol, free fatty acids, and hemoglobin A1c (Hb-A1c). These biochemical parameters were measured in Seoul Clinical Laboratories (Yongin, Korea).

2.4. Pharmacokinetic Interaction Study

STZ-induced diabetic rats were divided into three groups: control, single administration of RGE (SA), and repeated administrations of RGE for 1 week (1WRA). The rats were fasted for at least 12 h before the oral administration of metformin.

Rats in the SA group were administered RGE (2 g/kg, 2 mL/kg suspended in water) once and 2 h later, they received metformin (50 mg/kg, dissolved in water) or vehicle orally. Rats in the 1WRA group received RGE suspension (2 g/kg/day, 2 mL/kg suspended in water) orally at 9 a.m. for 7 days. Twenty four hours after the last dose of RGE, rats received metformin (50 mg/kg, dissolved in water) or vehicle orally. For the comparison (control group), rats in were administered water as the vehicle for 8 days and 2 h later, they received metformin (50 mg/kg, dissolved in water) orally. Rats were kept in a metabolic cage to collect the urine during the experimental procedure. Blood samples were collected at 0, 0.083, 0.25, 0.5, 1, 2, 3, 4, 8, and 24 h via the retro-orbital vein following oral administration of metformin. The blood was centrifuged at 13,200 rpm for 10 min to separate the plasma. Urine samples were collected for 24 h. Aliquots (50 µL) of plasma and urine samples were stored at −80 °C until the analysis.

2.5. LC-MS/MS Analysis of Metformin and Ginsenoside Rb1

The concentration of metformin was analyzed using a modified liquid chromatography-tandem mass spectrometry (LC-MS/MS) method as previously reported by Kwon et al. [17]. Briefly, plasma and urine samples (50 µL) were mixed with 100 µL propranolol (internal standard, IS) in acetonitrile using a vortex mixer for 2 min. After centrifugation at 13,200 rpm for 5 min, an aliquot (2 µL) was injected into the Agilent 6430 Triple Quad LC-MS/MS system (Agilent, Wilmington, DE, USA), which was coupled to an Agilent 1260 series high-performance liquid chromatography (HPLC) system. The separation was performed using a Synergy Polar reverse phase (RP) column (2.0 mm × 150 mm, 4 µm particle size, Phenomenex, Torrence, CA, USA) using a mobile phase that consisted of methanol and water (70:30, v/v) with 0.1% formic acid at a flow rate of 0.2 mL/min. The retention time was 2.09 and 3.03 min for metformin and propranolol (IS), respectively. The mass spectra were recorded using electrospray ionization in a positive mode. Quantification was carried out using selected reaction monitoring at m/z 130.2 → 71.4 for metformin, and m/z 260.0 → 116.0 for propranolol (IS). Plasma and urine calibration standards were 0.1–15 µg/mL. The interday precision and accuracy were within the acceptance criteria for assay validation.

The plasma Rb1 concentration was analyzed using an Agilent 6470 Triple Quadrupole LC MS/MS system with a modified method of Choi et al. [18]. Briefly, plasma samples (50 µL) were mixed with 200 µL of methanol containing berberine (0.5 ng/mL; IS) for 10 min and centrifuged. An aliquot (10 µL) of the supernatant was injected into the LC-MS/MS system. Separation was performed on a Synergi Polar RP column using a mobile phase consisting of water and methanol (24:76, v/v) with 0.1% formic acid at a flow rate of 0.2 mL/min. Quantification was carried out at m/z 1131.6 → 365.1 for Rb1 and m/z 336.1 → 320.0 for berberine (IS) in the positive ionization mode. For the analytical validation of Rb1 in plasma samples, the standard curve range was 0.5–100 ng/mL.

2.6. Data Analysis

PK parameters were calculated using the WinNonlin (version 2.0, Pharsight Corporation, Mountain View, CA, USA) using non-compartmental analysis. The data are expressed as the means ± standard deviation (SD) for the groups.

Statistical analysis was performed using the Student *t*-test (between two groups), one-way ANOVA test (among three groups), or two-way ANOVA test (differences between time period and treatment groups in fasting blood glucose level). In all cases, a difference was considered significant when $p < 0.05$.

3. Results

3.1. Pharmacokinetics (PK) Interaction between Metformin and Red Ginseng Extract (RGE) in Diabetic Rats

The PK profiles of metformin after a single oral administration of metformin (50 mg/kg) in the presence or absence of single or multiple administration of RGE (2 g/kg) are shown in Figure 1, and the PK parameters calculated from the plasma concentration-time profile are presented in Table 1. There was no significant difference in any PK parameters of metformin among the three groups. Moreover, the urinary recovery of metformin was not changed by the single or multiple administration of RGE. The results suggested that RGE pretreatment did not affect the absorption or disposition of metformin and, consequently, the plasma concentrations of metformin were not changed by co-administration of RGE.

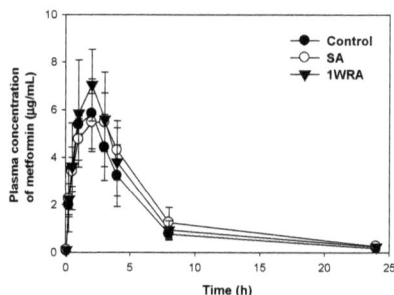

Figure 1. Plasma concentration-time profile of metformin after single oral administration (50 mg/kg) alone (●, control) and following single (○, SA) or multiple administration (▼, 1WRA) of red ginseng extract (RGE, 2 g/kg/day) in streptozotocin (STZ)-induced diabetic rats. Data points are means ± SD of five rats.

Table 1. Pharmacokinetic parameters of metformin after single oral administration (50 mg/kg) alone and following single (SA) or multiple administration (1WRA) of red ginseng extract (RGE, 2 g/kg/day) in streptozotocin (STZ)-induced diabetic rats.

Parameters		Control	SA	1WRA	*p* Value
C_{max}	μg/mL	6.29 ± 1.04	5.54 ± 1.20	7.58 ± 1.39	0.06
T_{max}	h	1.80 ± 0.45	2.40 ± 0.55	1.80 ± 0.84	0.26
AUC_{24h}	μg·h/mL	33.07 ± 6.82	41.59 ± 11.93	39.58 ± 9.50	0.37
AUC_{∞}	μg·h/mL	34.27 ± 6.63	43.49 ± 11.72	41.18 ± 10.30	0.33
$t_{1/2}$	h	4.59 ± 1.14	5.05 ± 0.64	4.53 ± 0.40	0.65
MRT	h	5.68 ± 1.28	6.63 ± 0.77	5.77 ± 0.91	0.29
Ae_{24h}	% of dose	45.14 ± 3.26	48.37 ± 5.87	41.89 ± 9.19	0.33

Data were expressed as mean ± SD from five rats of control, SA, and 1WRA groups, respectively. *p* value indicates static comparison among three groups using one-way ANOVA test. C_{max}: maximum plasma concentration; T_{max}: time to reach C_{max}. AUC_{24h} or AUC_{∞}: Area under plasma concentration–time curve from zero to 24 h or infinity. $t_{1/2}$: elimination half-life; MRT: mean residence time. Ae_{24h}: the fraction of the dose excreted in urine for 24 h as a parent form.

Similarly, the PK profiles and all the PK parameters of ginsenoside Rb1 following a single oral dose (2 g/kg) of RGE was not changed by the co-administration of metformin (50 mg/kg) (Figure 2 and Table 2).

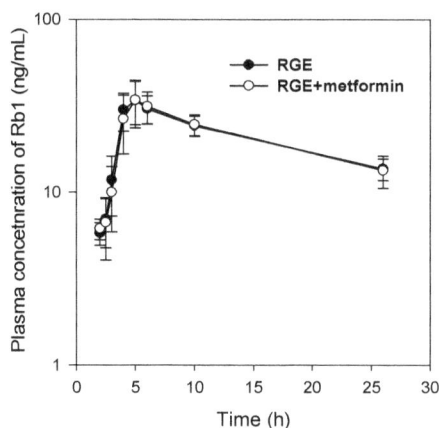

Figure 2. Plasma concentration–time profile of ginsenoside Rb1 following a single oral dose of RGE (2 g/kg) in the absence or presence of metformin (50 mg/kg) in streptozotocin (STZ)-induced diabetic rats. Data points are means ± SD of five rats.

Table 2. Plasma concentration-time profile of ginsenoside Rb1 following a single oral dose (2 g/kg) of red ginseng extract (RGE)in the absence or presence of metformin (50 mg/kg) in streptozotocin (STZ)-induced diabetic rats.

Parameters		RGE	RGE + Metformin	*p* Value
C_{max}	ng/mL	36.59 ± 7.94	35.03 ± 8.82	0.31
$AUC_{24\,h}$	ng·h/mL	512.25 ± 30.06	511.45 ± 75.26	0.98
$t_{1/2}$	h	11.88 ± 0.75	11.86 ± 0.79	0.93

Data points are means ± SD of five rats. *p* value indicates static comparison between two groups using student *t*-test.

3.2. Efficacy of Metformin with RGE in Diabetic Rats

3.2.1. Fasting Blood Glucose

The effect of oral administration of metformin, RGE, or their combinations on fasting blood glucose is shown in Figure 3. Fasting blood glucose was not elevated on day 4 after the first low dose STZ administration (30 mg/kg), but it increased to approximately 500 mg/dL after the second STZ administration (30 mg/kg) and a high fasting blood glucose level was maintained for more than 1 month. Metformin supplementation prevented the increase in fasting blood glucose level for 1 week but the second STZ administration gradually increased the value to approximately 200 mg/dL, and after 20 days of metformin administration (50 mg/kg for 5 weeks), the fasting glucose level increased to approximately 300–400 mg/dL. However, the fasting glucose levels for all periods were lower than that of the diabetic control group. RGE supplementation also gradually increased the fasting blood glucose for the 20-day supplementation and showed steady-state fasting glucose levels of approximately 300–400 mg/dL. Supplementation with metformin or RGE alone induced similar fasting blood glucose levels. The co-administration of metformin and RGE maintained the fasting blood glucose level at approximately 200 mg/dL, and it was significantly lower than that of the diabetic rats supplemented with metformin or RGE alone. The results suggest the additive effect of coadministration of RGE (2 g/kg) and metformin (50 mg/kg) for 5 weeks.

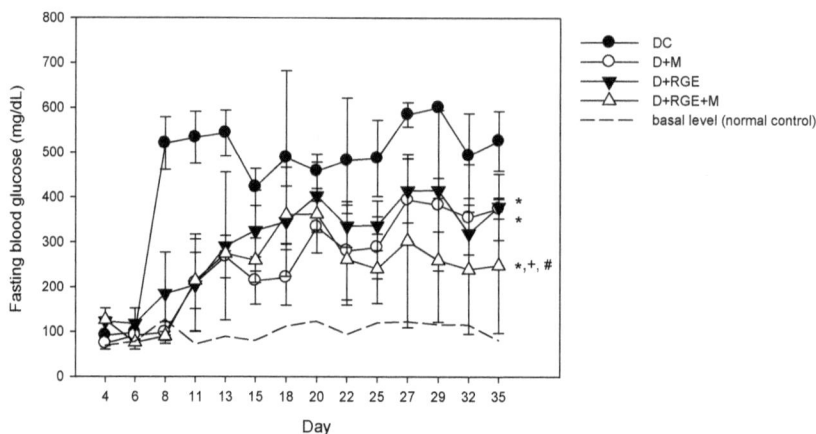

Figure 3. Effects of oral administration of metformin (M) and red ginseng extract (RGE) alone or combined on fasting blood glucose concentration of normal control (—), streptozotocin (STZ)-induced diabetic group (●, DC), diabetic rats treated with metformin (○, D + M, 50 mg/kg/day), diabetic rats supplemented with RGE (▼, D + RGE, 2 g/kg/day), and diabetic rats treated with metformin and RGE (Δ, D + RGE + M). Data points are means ± SD of four different rats per group. * $p < 0.05$ compared with DC group; + $p < 0.05$ compared with D + M group; # $p < 0.05$ compared with D + RGE group using two-way ANOVA test.

3.2.2. Body, Liver, and Pancreas Weight

There were no significant differences in the total body, liver, and pancreas tissue weights between treatment groups (Figure 4). However, the body, liver, and pancreas tissue weights of all treatment groups were lower than those of the normal control group.

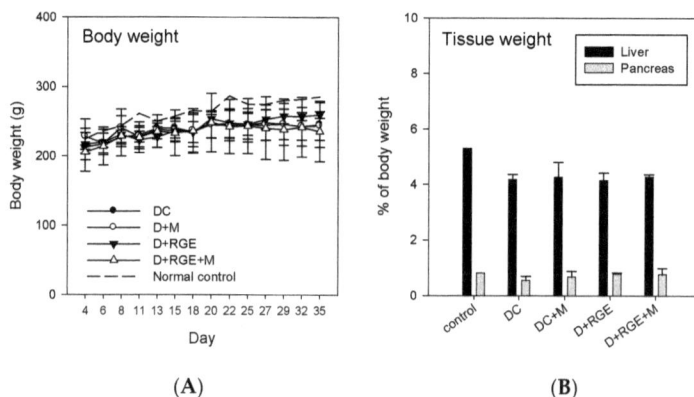

(**A**)   (**B**)

Figure 4. Effects of oral administration of metformin and red ginseng extract (RGE) alone or combined on body (**A**) and liver or pancreas (**B**) weights in normal control, streptozotocin (STZ)-induced diabetic group (DC), diabetic rats treated with metformin (D + M, 50 mg/kg/day), diabetic rats supplemented with RGE (D + RGE, 2 g/kg/day), and diabetic rats treated with metformin and RGE (D + RGE + M). Data points and bars are means ± SD of four rats per group.

3.2.3. Biochemical Results

Figure 5 shows the plasma AST and ALT levels after administration of metformin and RGE alone or in combination for 35 days. The levels of both AST and ALT in the diabetic groups increased significantly compared with that of the control group but significantly decreased by metformin and RGE alone or co-administered; however, the levels did not return to control levels. Fasting glucose level results were similar to those shown in Figure 3. The HbA1c level of the DC group increased more significantly than that of the control group, and decreased to control levels following administration of metformin and RGE alone or in combination. Likewise, the levels of free fatty acid and triglyceride were also increased in the STZ-induced diabetic group but significantly lowered by metformin and RGE alone or co-administered. However, the levels of total, HDL-, and LDL-cholesterol showed no significant difference between the STZ-induced diabetic and metformin- or RGE-treated groups.

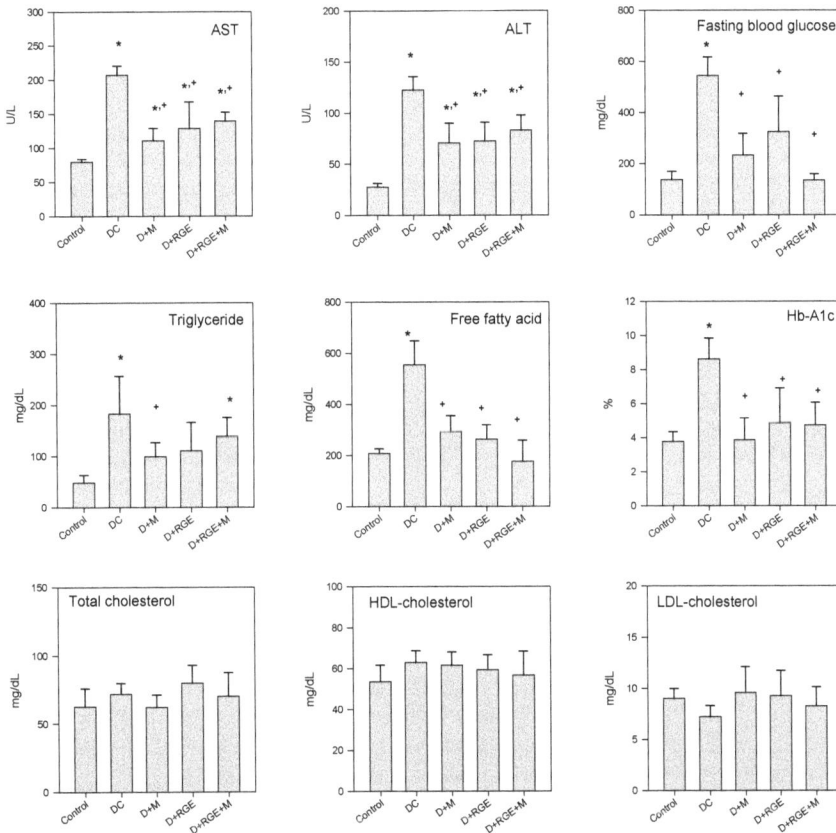

Figure 5. Biochemical parameters, alanine aminotransferase (ALT), aspartate aminotransferase (AST), fasting blood glucose, triglyceride, free fatty acid, hemoglobin-A1c (Hb-A1c), total cholesterol, high-density lipoprotein (HDL)-cholesterol, and low-density lipoprotein (LDL)-cholesterol levels in normal control, streptozotocin (STZ)-induced diabetic group (DC), diabetic rats treated with metformin (D + M), diabetic rats supplemented with RGE (D + RGE), and diabetic rats treated with metformin and RGE (D + RGE + M). Bars represent means ± SD of four rats per group; * $p < 0.05$ compared with control group using Student's *t*-test; + $p < 0.05$ compared with DC group using Student's *t*-test.

4. Discussion

STZ has been widely used to establish animal models of DM. In the present study, the administration of multiple low dose injections of STZ to rats was used to induce a mild impairment of insulin secretion and gradual autoimmune-like destruction of β-cells according to the method of Zhang et al. [14]. Moreover, they reported that STZ twice injection showed >85% success rate in development of DM, which was stable for >8 weeks [14]. In our study, the fasting glucose level was approximately 520 ± 58 mg/dL in six of the eight rats and was maintained for 4 weeks after the second STZ injection.

Since the PK of metformin could differ between diabetic and normal rats, we aimed to investigate the PK drug interaction between metformin and RGE in diabetic rats. Moreover, REG suspension (2 g/kg in 2 mL of water) has been reported to contain ginsenosides, polysaccharides, fatty acids, peptides, and polyacetylenic alcohols [19], and, therefore, metformin was administered orally 2 h after pre-treatment with RGE suspension to avoid physical interaction of both substances considering that the average gastric emptying time in rats is approximately 30 min [20,21]. The results showed that the plasma concentration, absorption, and urinary excretion of metformin were not modulated by pre-treatment of RGE to diabetic rats, suggesting that the possibility of herb–drug PK interaction between metformin and RGE is remote.

The mechanisms underlying the modulation of glucose metabolism by RGE in patients with DM would likely be perturbation of hepatic glucose production and enhancement of glucose uptake through glucose transporter 4 (GLUT4) into peripheral tissues. Recently, ginsenosides Rb1, Rb2, Rg1, Rg3, Rh2, and compound K, major pharmacological components of RGE, have been reported to suppress the hepatic gluconeogenesis via adenosine monophosphate (AMP)-activated protein kinase (AMPK) [22–24]. Importantly, enhanced GLUT4 expression mediated by activated insulin receptor substrate (IRS)/phosphatidylinositol-3,4,5-triphosphate (PI3K)/serine-threonine protein kinase signaling pathway by the treatment of RGE or ginsenosides increased glucose uptake in adipocytes or skeletal muscle cells and, thereby, decreased blood glucose or Hb-A1c levels [22,25]. In addition, enhancement of glucose uptake via GLUT4 through the upregulation of adipocytic peroxisome proliferator-activated receptor-γ also contributes to the ginsenoside-mediated glucose control mechanism [26]. The molecular mechanisms underlying the actions of metformin appear to be related to its activation of AMPK, which suppresses glucagon-stimulated glucose production, and increases glucose uptake via GLUT4 in muscles and hepatic cells [27,28]. Because of the similarity between metformin and RGE, the effects of herb–drug interaction on their efficacy seem to be important.

The levels of fasting blood glucose seemed to indicate an additive effect of the co-administration of metformin and RGE because these levels were not recovered to the normal state by the treatment of metformin (50 mg·kg^{-1}·day^{-1}) or RGE (2 g·kg^{-1}·day^{-1}) alone. However, co-treatment with metformin and RGE significantly reduced the fasting blood glucose level compared with those of monotherapy with metformin or RGE (Figure 5). Moreover, the fasting blood glucose level, which was monitored for 5 weeks after the induction of DM, showed more stability and was in the range of 200 mg/dL following co-administration of metformin and RGE. Considering the lack of PK herb–drug interaction between metformin and RGE, the additive effect of metformin and RGE on glucose control could be attributed to their similar mechanisms of action. In addition to the glucose control in STZ-induced diabetic rats, interactions of biochemical parameters including the free fatty acid level, triglyceride, AST, ALT, or cholesterol levels were not shown by the co-administration of metformin and RGE. However, we should note that, in this study, we measured fasting blood glucose level and Hb-A1c as efficacy markers for metformin and RGE treatment but not included additional corroborative hypoglycemic efficacy markers such as oral glucose test, insulin level, GLUT4 levels in the liver or skeletal muscle, and other signaling pathway markers (AMPK and IRS/PI3K) to unveil the related mechanisms by metformin and RGE interaction.

Author Contributions: Conceptualization, S.J.N. and I.-S.S.; Methodology, S.J.N., Y.J.H., W.L., and B.K.; Investigation, S.J.N., Y.J.H., W.L., B.K., and M.-K.C.; Writing-Original Draft Preparation, S.J.N.; Supervision, M.-K.C. and Y.-H.H.; Writing-Review & Editing, Y.-H.H. and I.-S.S.; Funding Acquisition, I.-S.S.

Funding: This work was supported by a grant of the Korea Institute of Planning and Evaluation for Technology in Food, Agriculture, Forestry and Fisheries (IPET) through Export Promotion Technology Development Program, funded by Ministry of Agriculture, Food and Rural Affairs (MAFRA) (No. 316017-3).

Conflicts of Interest: The authors declare no conflicts of interest.

References

1. Akbarzadeh, A.; Norouzian, D.; Mehrabi, M.R.; Jamshidi, S.; Farhangi, A.; Verdi, A.A.; Mofidian, S.M.; Rad, B.L. Induction of diabetes by streptozotocin in rats. *Indian J. Clin. Biochem.* **2007**, *22*, 60–64. [CrossRef] [PubMed]

2. Liu, Z.; Li, W.; Li, X.; Zhang, M.; Chen, L.; Zheng, Y.N.; Sun, G.Z.; Ruan, C.C. Antidiabetic effects of malonyl ginsenosides from panax ginseng on type 2 diabetic rats induced by high-fat diet and streptozotocin. *J. Ethnopharmacol.* **2013**, *145*, 233–240. [CrossRef] [PubMed]

3. Zhang, M.; Lv, X.Y.; Li, J.; Xu, Z.G.; Chen, L. The characterization of high-fat diet and multiple low-dose streptozotocin induced type 2 diabetes rat model. *Exp. Diabetes Res.* **2008**, *2008*, 704045. [CrossRef] [PubMed]

4. Al-Ali, K.; Abdel Fatah, H.S.; El-Badry, Y.A. Dual effect of curcumin-zinc complex in controlling diabetes mellitus in experimentally induced diabetic rats. *Biol. Pharm. Bull.* **2016**, *39*, 1774–1780. [CrossRef] [PubMed]

5. Srinivasan, K.; Viswanad, B.; Asrat, L.; Kaul, C.L.; Ramarao, P. Combination of high-fat diet-fed and low-dose streptozotocin-treated rat: A model for type 2 diabetes and pharmacological screening. *Pharmacol. Res.* **2005**, *52*, 313–320. [CrossRef] [PubMed]

6. Cheng, J.T.; Huang, C.C.; Liu, I.M.; Tzeng, T.F.; Chang, C.J. Novel mechanism for plasma glucose-lowering action of metformin in streptozotocin-induced diabetic rats. *Diabetes* **2006**, *55*, 819–825. [CrossRef] [PubMed]

7. Majithiya, J.B.; Balaraman, R. Metformin reduces blood pressure and restores endothelial function in aorta of streptozotocin-induced diabetic rats. *Life Sci.* **2006**, *78*, 2615–2624. [CrossRef] [PubMed]

8. Yanardag, R.; Ozsoy-Sacan, O.; Bolkent, S.; Orak, H.; Karabulut-Bulan, O. Protective effects of metformin treatment on the liver injury of streptozotocin-diabetic rats. *Hum. Exp. Toxicol.* **2005**, *24*, 129–135. [CrossRef] [PubMed]

9. Bang, H.; Kwak, J.H.; Ahn, H.Y.; Shin, D.Y.; Lee, J.H. Korean red ginseng improves glucose control in subjects with impaired fasting glucose, impaired glucose tolerance, or newly diagnosed type 2 diabetes mellitus. *J. Med. Food* **2014**, *17*, 128–134. [CrossRef] [PubMed]

10. Jung, J.H.; Kang, I.G.; Kim, D.Y.; Hwang, Y.J.; Kim, S.T. The effect of korean red ginseng on allergic inflammation in a murine model of allergic rhinitis. *J. Ginseng Res.* **2013**, *37*, 167–175. [CrossRef] [PubMed]

11. Park, T.Y.; Hong, M.; Sung, H.; Kim, S.; Suk, K.T. Effect of korean red ginseng in chronic liver disease. *J. Ginseng Res.* **2017**, *41*, 450–455. [CrossRef] [PubMed]

12. Kim, H.J.; Lee, S.G.; Chae, I.G.; Kim, M.J.; Im, N.K.; Yu, M.H.; Lee, E.J.; Lee, I.S. Antioxidant effects of fermented red ginseng extracts in streptozotocin-induced diabetic rats. *J. Ginseng Res.* **2011**, *35*, 129–137. [CrossRef] [PubMed]

13. Oh, M.R.; Park, S.H.; Kim, S.Y.; Back, H.I.; Kim, M.G.; Jeon, J.Y.; Ha, K.C.; Na, W.T.; Cha, Y.S.; Park, B.H.; et al. Postprandial glucose-lowering effects of fermented red ginseng in subjects with impaired fasting glucose or type 2 diabetes: A randomized, double-blind, placebo-controlled clinical trial. *BMC Complement. Altern. Med.* **2014**, *14*, 237. [CrossRef] [PubMed]

14. Mostafavinia, A.; Amini, A.; Ghorishi, S.K.; Pouriran, R.; Bayat, M. The effects of dosage and the routes of administrations of streptozotocin and alloxan on induction rate of type1 diabetes mellitus and mortality rate in rats. *Lab. Anim. Res.* **2016**, *32*, 160–165. [CrossRef] [PubMed]

15. Al-Khalifa, A.; Mathew, T.C.; Al-Zaid, N.S.; Mathew, E.; Dashti, H. Low carbohydrate ketogenic diet prevents the induction of diabetes using streptozotocin in rats. *Exp. Toxicol. Pathol.* **2011**, *63*, 663–669. [CrossRef] [PubMed]

16. Abunasef, S.K.; Amin, H.A.; Abdel-Hamid, G.A. A histological and immunohistochemical study of beta cells in streptozotocin diabetic rats treated with caffeine. *Folia Histochem. Cytobiol.* **2014**, *52*, 42–50. [CrossRef] [PubMed]

17. Kwon, M.; Choi, Y.A.; Choi, M.K.; Song, I.S. Organic cation transporter-mediated drug-drug interaction potential between berberine and metformin. *Arch. Pharm. Res.* **2015**, *38*, 849–856. [CrossRef] [PubMed]

18. Choi, I.D.; Ryu, J.H.; Lee, D.E.; Lee, M.H.; Shim, J.J.; Ahn, Y.T.; Sim, J.H.; Huh, C.S.; Shim, W.S.; Yim, S.V.; et al.   Enhanced absorption study of ginsenoside compound k (20-*O*-beta-(D-glucopyranosyl)-20(S)-protopanaxadiol) after oral administration of fermented red ginseng extract (hyfrg) in healthy korean volunteers and rats. *Evid. Based Complement. Altern. Med.* **2016**, *2016*, 3908142. [CrossRef] [PubMed]

19. Lee, S.M.; Bae, B.S.; Park, H.W.; Ahn, N.G.; Cho, B.G.; Cho, Y.L.; Kwak, Y.S. Characterization of korean red ginseng (panax ginseng meyer): History, preparation method, and chemical composition. *J. Ginseng Res.* **2015**, *39*, 384–391. [CrossRef] [PubMed]

20. Franklin, R.A. The influence of gastric emptying on plasma concentrations of the analgesic, meptazinol. *Br. J. Pharm.* **1977**, *59*, 565–569. [CrossRef]

21. Song, I.S.; Kong, T.Y.; Jeong, H.U.; Kim, E.N.; Kwon, S.S.; Kang, H.E.; Choi, S.Z.; Son, M.; Lee, H.S. Evaluation of the transporter-mediated herb-drug interaction potential of da-9801, a standardized dioscorea extract for diabetic neuropathy, in human in vitro and rat in vivo. *BMC Complement. Altern. Med.* **2014**, *14*, 251. [CrossRef] [PubMed]

22. Yuan, H.D.; Kim, J.T.; Kim, S.H.; Chung, S.H. Ginseng and diabetes: The evidences from in vitro, animal and human studies. *J. Ginseng Res.* **2012**, *36*, 27–39. [CrossRef] [PubMed]

23. Lee, S.; Lee, M.S.; Kim, C.T.; Kim, I.H.; Kim, Y. Ginsenoside rg3 reduces lipid accumulation with amp-activated protein kinase (ampk) activation in hepg2 cells. *Int. J. Mol. Sci.* **2012**, *13*, 5729–5739. [CrossRef] [PubMed]

24. Meng, F.; Su, X.; Li, W.; Zheng, Y. Ginsenoside rb3 strengthens the hypoglycemic effect through ampk for inhibition of hepatic gluconeogenesis. *Exp. Ther. Med.* **2017**, *13*, 2551–2557. [CrossRef] [PubMed]

25. Choi, J.; Kim, K.J.; Koh, E.J.; Lee, B.Y. Gelidium elegans extract ameliorates type 2 diabetes via regulation of mapk and pi3k/akt signaling. *Nutrients* **2018**, *10*, 51. [CrossRef] [PubMed]

26. Hwang, J.T.; Lee, M.S.; Kim, H.J.; Sung, M.J.; Kim, H.Y.; Kim, M.S.; Kwon, D.Y. Antiobesity effect of ginsenoside rg3 involves the ampk and ppar-gamma signal pathways. *Phytother. Res.* **2009**, *23*, 262–266. [CrossRef] [PubMed]

27. Zhou, G.; Myers, R.; Li, Y.; Chen, Y.; Shen, X.; Fenyk-Melody, J.; Wu, M.; Ventre, J.; Doebber, T.; Fujii, N.; et al. Role of amp-activated protein kinase in mechanism of metformin action. *J. Clin. Investig.* **2001**, *108*, 1167–1174. [CrossRef] [PubMed]

28. Abbud, W.; Habinowski, S.; Zhang, J.Z.; Kendrew, J.; Elkairi, F.S.; Kemp, B.E.; Witters, L.A.; Ismail-Beigi, F. Stimulation of amp-activated protein kinase (ampk) is associated with enhancement of glut1-mediated glucose transport. *Arch. Biochem. Biophys.* **2000**, *380*, 347–352. [CrossRef] [PubMed]

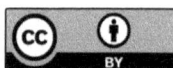

pharmaceutics

MDPI

Article

Simultaneous Determination of Five Cytochrome P450 Probe Substrates and Their Metabolites and Organic Anion Transporting Polypeptide Probe Substrate in Human Plasma Using Liquid Chromatography-Tandem Mass Spectrometry

Jae-Kyung Heo [1,2], Hyun-Ji Kim [1,2], Ga-Hyun Lee [1,2], Boram Ohk [3,4], Sangkyu Lee [1,2], Kyung-Sik Song [2], Im Sook Song [2], Kwang-Hyeon Liu [1,2,*] and Young-Ran Yoon [3,4,*]

[1] BK21 Plus KNU Multi-Omics based Creative Drug Research Team, College of Pharmacy, Kyungpook National University, Daegu 41566, Korea; anna4602@gmail.com (J.-K.H.); khj110917@nate.com (H.-J.K.); lgh2710@gmail.com (G.-H.L.); sangkyu@knu.ac.kr (S.L.)

[2] College of Pharmacy and Research Institute of Pharmaceutical Sciences, Kyungpook National University, Daegu 41566, Korea; kssong@knu.ac.kr (K.-S.S.); isssong@knu.ac.kr (I.S.S.)

[3] Clinical Trial Center, Kyungpook National University Hospital, Daegu 41566, Korea; dhrqhfka@naver.com

[4] Department of Biomedical Science, BK21 Plus KNU Bio-Medical Convergence Program for Creative Talent, College of Medicine, Kyungpook National University, Daegu 41944, Korea

* Correspondence: dstlkh@knu.ac.kr (K.-H.L.); yry@knu.ac.kr (Y.-R.Y.); Tel.: +82-53-950-8567 (K.-H.L.); +82-53-420-4950 (Y.-R.Y.); Fax: +82-53-950-8557 (K.-H.L.); +82-53-420-5218 (Y.-R.Y.)

Received: 1 June 2018; Accepted: 30 June 2018; Published: 2 July 2018

Abstract: A rapid and selective liquid chromatography-tandem mass spectrometry (LC-MS/MS) method for the simultaneous determination of organic anion transporting polypeptide 1B1 (OATP1B1) and cytochrome P450 (P450) probe substrates and their phase I metabolites in human plasma was developed. The OATP1B1 (pitavastatin) and five P450 probe substrates, caffeine (CYP1A2), losartan (CYP2C9), omeprazole (CYP2C19), dextromethorphan (CYP2D6), and midazolam (CYP3A) and their metabolites were extracted from human plasma (50 μL) using methanol. Analytes were separated on a C18 column followed by selected reaction monitoring detection using MS/MS. All analytes were separated simultaneously within a 9 min run time. The developed method was fully validated over the expected clinical concentration range for all analytes tested. The intra- and inter-day precisions for all analytes were lower than 11.3% and 8.82%, respectively, and accuracy was 88.5–117.3% and 96.1–109.2%, respectively. The lower limit of quantitation was 0.05 ng/mL for dextromethorphan, dextrorphan, midazolam, and 1′-hydroxymidazolam; 0.5 ng/mL for losartan, EXP-3174, omeprazole, 5′-hydroxyomeprazole, and pitavastatin; and 5 ng/mL for caffeine and paraxanthine. The method was successfully used in a pharmacokinetic study in healthy subjects after oral doses of five P450 and OATP1B1 probes. This analytical method provides a simple, sensitive, and accurate tool for the determination of OATP1B1 and five major P450 activities in vivo drug interaction studies.

Keywords: cytochrome P450; drug interaction; liquid chromatography-tandem mass spectrometry; organic anion transporting polypeptide; pharmacokinetics

1. Introduction

Cytochrome P450 (P450) enzymes are responsible for the oxidative metabolism of xenobiotics and endogenous substrates, and are major sources of variability in drug metabolism and pharmacokinetics [1,2]. Currently, 57 different isoforms have been characterized in humans [3]. Among them, five P450 isoforms,

CYP1A2, 2C9, 2C19, 2D6, and 3A are involved in the metabolism of more than 90% of marketed drugs [4]. Especially, CYP3A4 and CYP3A5 are major isoforms implicated in the biotransformation of macrolide antibiotics, antihistamines, benzodiazepines, calcium channel blockers, and statins [5]. In addition, CYP1A2, 2C9, 2C19, and 2D6 are implicated in the biotransformation of many drugs (CYP1A2 for caffeine, phenacetin, and tizanidine; CYP2C9 for angiotensin blockers, nonsteroidal anti-inflammatory drugs, and sulfonylureas; CYP2C19 for proton pump inhibitors and antiepileptics; and CYP2D6 for beta blockers, antidepressants, and antipsychotics) [6,7]. The modulation of P450 activities by drug interactions could affect the pharmacokinetics and pharmacodynamics of drugs. In addition to drug metabolizing enzymes, drug transporters can also cause various pharmacological consequences. Drug interactions mediated by permeability-glycoprotein (P-gp) and organic anion transporting polypeptides (OATPs) have been reported for their association with clinically important drug interactions [8]. Recent data have suggested that OATP1B1 is involved in the pharmacokinetics of some protease inhibitors (saquinavir and ritonavir [9]) and statin drugs (pravastatin and pitavastatin [10]).

The inhibition of P450s or OATPs increases plasma levels of the substrate drugs [11], whereas their induction conversely decreases plasma levels of substrate drug. These unwanted drug interactions can result in adverse drug reactions or therapeutic failure. Therefore, accurate and reliable measurements of the in vivo activity of drug-metabolizing enzymes and transporters are essential in evaluating drug interactions. For rapid and efficient evaluation of drug interactions, the cocktail (the simultaneous administration of multiple probe drugs) phenotyping method which provides information on the activities of multiple enzymes or transporters in a single experiment has been widely developed and used. It is important to develop simultaneous analytical methods for probe substrates and their metabolites in cocktail phenotyping studies. To date, there is limited data on the simultaneous analysis of probe substrates of drug metabolizing enzymes and transporters. For example, Kim et al. [12,13] reported a simultaneous analytical method for P-gp (fexofenadine) and five P450 probe substrates (caffeine for CYP1A2, losartan for CYP2C9, omeprazole for CYP2C19, dextromethorphan for CYP2D6, and midazolam for CYP3A) using liquid chromatography-tandem mass spectrometry (LC-MS/MS) in plasma. Bosilkovska et al. [14] also developed a simultaneous LC-MS/MS method for P-gp (fexofenadine) and six P450 probe substrates (caffeine for CYP1A2, bupropion for CYP2B6, flurbiprofen for CYP2C9, omeprazole for CYP2C19, dextromethorphan for CYP2D6, and midazolam for CYP3A) in plasma. However, there is no published data on the simultaneous analysis of OATP and multiple P450 probe substrates and their metabolites in plasma.

Several probe substrates have been validated to assess the activity of P450s and OATP1B1. Among them, caffeine, omeprazole, dextromethorphan, and midazolam are generally the most used as probes for CYP1A2, 2C19, 2D6, and 3A, respectively [15–17]. However, several different probe drugs have been used for CYP2C9 and OATP1B1 phenotyping studies. Flurbiprofen [14,18], losartan [15,19], tolbutamide [20], and warfarin [21] have been used for CYP2C9 phenotyping. However, tolbutamide is no longer commercially available in many countries [13], and the data for flurbiprofen and warfarin are not entirely clear [13,15]. OATP1B1 activity has been evaluated using pitavastatin [22], pravastatin [23], and rosuvastatin [24]. OATP1B1 is the most important transporter for the hepatic uptake of pitavastatin [25], while OATP1B1 and sodium-taurocholate cotransporting polypeptide (NTCP) plays an important role in rosuvastatin uptake [26]. OATP1B1 and organic anion transporter 3 (OAT3) are mainly responsible for the transport of pravastatin [27,28]. Therefore, in this study, we selected caffeine, losartan, omeprazole, dextromethorphan, midazolam, and pitavastatin as probe drugs for CYP1A2, 2C9, 2C19, 2D6, 3A, and OATP1B1, respectively. These probe drugs are commercially available for in vivo phenotyping studies, are relatively safe, and are specific for P450 isoforms and OATP1B1.

The present study, for the first time, describes an LC-MS/MS method that was developed to simultaneously analyze five P450-specific probe drugs and their metabolites as well as an OATP1B1 probe drugs in human plasma. The developed method is simpler and faster for small sample volumes than conventional models, and it uses protein precipitation method followed by LC-MS/MS analysis.

The method was validated for selectivity, sensitivity, linearity, accuracy, precision, and stability. In addition, the method was successfully used to measure the plasma concentration of the probe drugs and their metabolites in plasma samples from healthy subjects after a single oral dose of the probe drug cocktail, which contained caffeine, losartan, omeprazole, dextromethorphan, midazolam, and pitavastatin.

2. Materials and Methods

2.1. Chemicals and Reagents

Caffeine, omeprazole, and propranolol were purchased from Sigma-Aldrich (St. Louis, MO, USA). Dextromethorphan, dextrorphan, midazolam, 5′-hydroxyomeprazole, losartan, losartan carboxylic acid (EXP3174), paraxanthine, and pitavastatin were obtained from Toronto Research Chemicals Inc. (North York, ON, Canada). 1′-Hydroxymidazolam was purchased from Cayman Chemical (Ann Arbor, MI, USA). Solvents were LC-MS grade (Fisher Scientific Co., Pittsburgh, PA, USA) and the other chemicals were obtained from Sigma-Aldrich. Pooled human plasma was obtained from BioChemed Services (Winchester, VA, USA).

2.2. Preparation of Calibration Standard Samples

Stock solutions of the probe substrates, their metabolites, and propranolol (internal standard, IS) were prepared at 1 mg/mL in methanol. Paraxanthine was prepared as a 1 mg/mL solution in 50% aqueous methanol. All stock solutions were sonicated for 5 min. Working standard solutions were prepared by diluting the stock solutions in methanol. All stock and working solutions were stored at −20 °C. Calibration standards were prepared by spiking drug-free blank plasma with the working solutions to obtain concentrations within the relevant analytical ranges (5, 10, 20, 40, 100, 400, 1000, and 4000 ng/mL for caffeine and paraxanthine; 0.5, 1, 2, 4, 10, 40, 100, and 400 ng/mL for losartan, EXP3174, omeprazole, 5′-hydroxyomeprazole and pitavastatin; and 0.05, 0.1, 0.2, 0.4, 1, 4, 10, and 40 ng/mL for dextromethorphan, dextrorphan, midazolam and 1′-hydroxymidazolam) (Table 1 and Figure 1). Calibration curves for the analytes in plasma were constructed from their peak area ratios relative to that the IS using linear regression. All calibration standards samples were stored frozen at −80 °C.

Table 1. Calibration range, linearity, and limit of quantitation (LOQ) of analytes.

Analyte	Retention Time (min)	Calibration Range (ng/mL)	Correlation Coefficient (r^2)	LOQ (ng/mL)
Caffeine	2.9	5–4000	0.9982 ± 0.002	5.0
Paraxanthine	2.7	5–4000	0.9989 ± 0.001	5.0
Losartan	3.7	0.5–400	0.9989 ± 0.001	0.5
EXP3174	3.8	0.5–400	0.9978 ± 0.002	0.5
Omeprazole	3.2	0.5–400	0.9973 ± 0.002	0.5
5′-Hydroxyomeprazole	3.2	0.5–400	0.9984 ± 0.002	0.5
Dextromethorphan	3.4	0.05–40	0.9982 ± 0.002	0.05
Dextrorphan	3.1	0.05–40	0.9979 ± 0.002	0.05
Midazolam	3.4	0.05–40	0.9985 ± 0.001	0.05
1′-Hydroxymidazolam	3.4	0.05–100	0.9938 ± 0.006	0.05
Pitavastatin	3.5	0.5–400	0.9987 ± 0.001	0.5

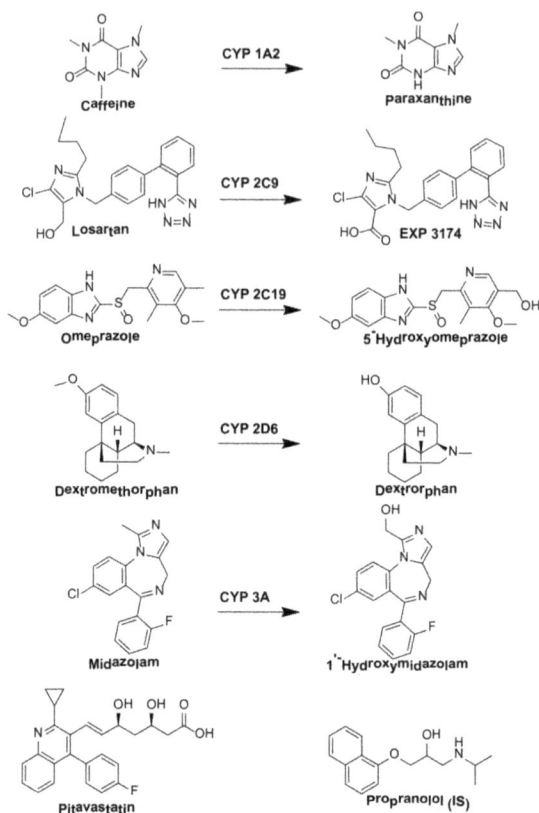

Figure 1. Chemical structure of organic anion transporting polypeptide (OATP) and cytochrome P450 (P450) probe drugs, their metabolites, and propranolol (internal standard [IS]) used in this study.

2.3. Plasma Sample Preparation

A simple protein precipitation method was used to extract the probe drugs and their metabolites from human plasma. IS solution (10 µL of 5 µg/mL propranolol) and methanol (140 µL) were added to a 50 µL of human plasma sample, which was vortexed for 10 s, and then centrifuged for 15 min (4 °C). The supernatant was transferred to an autosampler vial and 5 µL was injected into the LC-MS/MS system for the analysis.

2.4. LC-MS/MS Analysis

The probe drugs and their metabolites were analyzed using a Shimadzu LCMS-8060 liquid chromatograph-mass spectrometer system (Shimadzu, Tokyo, Japan) equipped with an electrospray ionization (ESI) interface. Analyte separation was performed using the Xbridge MS C18 column (100 × 2.1 mm, i.d., 3.5 µm; Waters, Milford, MA, USA). The mobile phase consisted of 0.1% formic acid in water (A) and 0.1% formic acid in acetonitrile (B), and was run on the following gradient: 0–1 min (5% B), 3–4 min (80% B), and 4.1–9 min (5% B). The flow rate was 0.2 mL/min. The column oven was maintained at a constant temperature of 40 °C. The electrospray ionization was conducted in the positive ion mode at 4000 V. The optimum operating conditions were as follows: vaporizer temperature, 300 °C; capillary temperature, 350 °C; and collision gas (argon) pressure 1.5 mTorr. Quantitation was performed in the selected reaction monitoring (SRM) of the [M + H]$^+$ ion and the related product ion for each drugs and its metabolites. The SRM transitions and collision energy (CE) values were determined for the drugs and their metabolites (Table 2).

Table 2. Selected reaction monitoring (SRM) transition ion and collision energy (CE) values for the analysis of analytes and internal standard (IS).

Analyte	SRM Transition Ions (*m/z*) [13,29]		CE (eV)
	Precursor Ion	Product Ion	
Caffeine	195.0	138.0	20
Paraxanthine	181.0	124.0	20
Losartan	423.0	207.0	23
EXP3174	437.0	235.0	20
Omeprazole	346.0	198.0	15
5'-Hydroxyomeprazole	362.0	214.0	15
Dextromethorphan	272.0	171.0	37
Dextrorphan	258.0	157.0	40
Midazolam	326.0	291.0	27
1'-Hydroxymidazolam	342.0	324.0	23
Pitavastatin	422.0	290.0	33
Propranolol (IS)	261.0	184.0	20

2.5. Method Validation

The developed method was validated for accuracy, linearity, precision, sensitivity, selectivity, and stability for all probe drugs and their metabolites. The selectivity was tested by analyzing human plasma samples from six different sources. The linearity of the calibration curve was examined using eight calibration points for each analyte with different concentration (Table 1). Least squares regression was used to construct the calibration curve for each analyte. To evaluate the linearity, the acceptable criteria were set at ±15% deviation of the nominal concentrations except at the lower limit of quantitation (LLOQ, ±20%), which was defined as the concentrations of the signal-to-noise ratio at 10. Quality control (QC) samples were prepared at final concentration of 20, 100, and 1000 ng/mL for caffeine and paraxanthine; 2, 10, and 100 ng/mL for losartan, EXP3174, omeprazole, 5'-hydroxyomeprazole and pitavastatin; and 0.2, 1, and 10 ng/mL for dextromethorphan, dextrorphan, midazolam, and 1'-hydroxymidazolam. The precision and accuracy were assessed by analyzing QC samples at three different concentration levels (low, middle, and high) with five replicates within one day and on six consecutive days for the intra- and inter-day validation, respectively. The precision was defined as the relative standard deviation (RSD, %), and the accuracy was calculated as follows: (mean observed concentration)/(nominal concentration) × 100. The acceptable criteria were set at ±15% deviation of the nominal concentration. The storage stability of the analytes was determined using triplicate spiked samples after 4 h at room temperature. In addition, the freeze–thaw stability of the analytes was assessed for three freeze-thaw cycles. The acceptable criteria for stability test were within a 15% loss of the initial concentrations.

2.6. Application to Pharmacokinetic Studies

Six healthy male volunteers who provided written informed consent participated in the pharmacokinetic study, which was approved (No. 2017-01-010) by the Institutional Review Board of Kyungpook National University Hospital (Daegu, Korea) and performed according to the guidelines of good clinical practice. After an overnight fast, all subjects received a single oral dose of the probe drug cocktail, which contained caffeine (100 mg), losartan (50 mg), omeprazole (20 mg), dextromethorphan (30 mg), midazolam (2 mg), and pitavastatin (2 mg). Blood samples were collected into a tube containing ethylenediaminetetraacetic acid before (0 h) and at 0.25, 0.5, 0.75, 1, 1.5, 2, 3, 4, 5, 6, 8, 10, 12, 24, and 48 h after cocktail administration. Following centrifugation at 1811× *g* for 10 min, the supernatant plasma was stored at −70 °C until the analysis. The following pharmacokinetic parameters were obtained using non-compartmental methods with Phoenix WinNonlin 7.0 (Pharsight Corporation, Certara, NJ, USA): the maximum plasma concentration (C_{max}), time to reach C_{max} (T_{max}), area under the plasma concentration-time profile (AUC), the half-life ($t_{1/2}$) in the terminal phase, and mean residence time (MRT).

3. Results and Discussion

3.1. Optimization of Analytical Conditions and Sample Preparation

To develop a reliable LC-MS/MS method suitable for the simultaneous detection of all the probe drugs and their metabolites, chromatographic and spectrometric conditions such as mobile phase, column, SRM transition ions, and collision energies were optimized. The mobile phase used had an acetonitrile content that differed slightly from that used in a previously reported method [13]. All analytes spiked into the plasma samples at 0.05–5 ng/mL, were sensitively detected and eluted within 4 min using gradient elution of 0.1% formic acid in water and acetonitrile (Table 1). For sensitive and selective analysis of the target analytes using the SRM mode, mass fragmentation patterns were investigated to select the SRM transition ions at various CE values. All analytes generated a protonated molecular ion $[M + H]^+$ in the positive ion mode. Based on the product ion scan mass spectra, the most abundant ions were selected as product ions for quantification (Table 2). All analytes were selectively separated based on retention times within 2.7 to 4 min (Figure 1).

Several sample pretreatment methods, e.g., liquid–liquid extraction [13], solid-phase extraction (SPE) [30], and on-line SPE [31] have been reported for extracting P450 probe drugs and their metabolites in plasma samples. However, previously reported extraction methods required tedious or complex extraction procedures such as double liquid-liquid extraction [13] and hybrid SPE-precipitation [30]. The protein precipitation method we established using methanol was a simple way to extract the 11 target analytes (OATP1B1 and P450 probe drugs and their metabolites) from the human plasma samples. Bosilkovska et al. [14] and Tanaka et al. [32] reported a protein precipitation method using acetonitrile; however, their method did not include pitavastatin (OATP1B1 probe drug) as the target analyte. In addition, previously reported protein precipitation methods requires large volumes (0.3 mL) of plasma [32,33]. The protein precipitation method we established using small volumes (50 μL) of plasma is a simple way to extract the eleven target analytes (OATP1B1 and P450 probe drugs and their metabolites) from the human plasma samples. Although stable isotope-labeled IS samples (such as midazolam-d4 or omeprazole-d3) are the first choices [14,34], they are relatively expensive. Therefore, we investigated several compounds including chlorpropamide [35], paracetamol [31], and terfenadine [36] to find a suitable IS, and finally chose propranolol for use in this assay.

3.2. Method Validation

Several research studies have reported the analytical method for five P450 isoform-probe drugs and their metabolites in plasma samples using LC-MS/MS. Recently, Oh et al. [13], Tanaka et al. [32], Williams et al. [16], and Zhang et al. [31] developed an LC-MS/MS method for five P450 probe drugs (caffeine, losartan, omeprazole, dextromethorphan, and midazolam) and their metabolites, which were used in an Inje cocktail [15]. Kim et al. [12] developed a simultaneous assay for four P450 probe drugs (losartan, omeprazole, dextromethorphan, and midazolam) and their metabolites as well as fexofenadine, a P-gp substrate, after protein precipitation; however, caffeine and paraxanthine were separately analyzed after liquid-liquid extraction. Bosilkovska et al. [14] also reported a simultaneous analytical method for five P450 probe drugs (including caffeine, bupropion, flurbiprofen, omeprazole, dextromethorphan, and midazolam) and their metabolites as well as fexofenadine, P-gp substrate. To date, however, there is no report for the simultaneous analysis of five P450 and OATP1B1 probe drugs. In this study, for the first time, we developed an LC-MS/MS method to simultaneously analyze five P450s specific probe drugs (caffeine, losartan, omeprazole, dextromethorphan, and midazolam) and their metabolites as well as an OATP1B1 probe drug (pitavastatin) using LC-MS/MS after protein precipitation in human plasma. The developed method was validated for selectivity, sensitivity, linearity, accuracy, precision, and stability as follows.

The selectivity of the assay was investigated by preparing and analyzing six independent blank (drug-free) samples. During the experimentation, no significant interfering peaks were observed at the retention times and SRM mass transition for all analytes. Representative SRM chromatograms for plasma samples spiked with the QC samples (100 ng/mL for caffeine and paraxanthine, 10 ng/mL for losartan, EXP3174, omeprazole, 5′-hydroxyomeprazole, and pitavastatin, and 1.0 ng/mL for dextromethorphan, dextrorphan, midazolam, and 1′-hydroxymidazolam) of all analytes and plasma collected from one subject 1 h after dosing are shown in Figure 2. For all analytes, the calibration curves were linear at 5–4000 ng/mL for caffeine and paraxanthine, 0.5–400 ng/mL for losartan, EXP3174, omeprazole, 5′-hydroxyomeprazole, and pitavastatin, and 0.05–40 ng/mL for dextromethorphan, dextrorphan, midazolam, and 1′-hydroxymidazolam (Table 1). These concentration ranges covered the expected plasma concentration for each drug after oral administration of the drug cocktail described above. A weighting factor of $1/(concentration)^2$ was applied to calibration curves for all drugs and their metabolites because of their wide calibration range. There were no interfering peaks in the blank human plasma. The coefficients of correlation (r^2) values were >0.994 for all analytes in all batches in the validation and pharmacokinetic analysis. The RSD values of the correlation coefficients were less than 0.6%. No significant differences in linear regressions were observed among the inter- and intra-day assays, indicating that the assay was reproducible [37]. The LLOQ values were 0.05 ng/mL for dextromethorphan, dextrorphan, midazolam, and 1′-hydroxymidazolam, 0.5 ng/mL for losartan, EXP3174, omeprazole, 5′-hydroxyomeprazole, and pitavastatin, and 5 ng/mL for caffeine and paraxanthine (Table 1). These LLOQ concentrations were chosen based on previously reported values for the administered doses, and they encompassed the expected concentration values of each analyte in plasma.

As shown in Table 3, the accuracy for each analyte and concentration evaluated was in the range of 88.5–114.5%, except for the middle dextromethorphan QC, which was slightly overestimated (117.3%). The intra- and inter-day assay precisions for all analytes were <11.3% and <8.8%, respectively (Table 3), suggesting that the assay had high accuracy and reliability. The data obtained satisfied the pre-defined acceptance criteria for accuracy and precision [13,14].

All analytes in plasma were stable for up to 4 h at 25 °C (Table 4). No degradation, defined as any deviation outside ±15% of the nominal concentration [13], was observed after three freeze–thaw cycles or post-treatment storage for 24 h at 4 °C (Table 4). No differences in stability occurred between the low- and high-concentration QC samples. The analytical procedure was determined to be reliable based on selectivity, sensitivity, linearity, accuracy, precision, and stability and thus, this method was applied to the plasma samples collected from subjects in the pharmacokinetic study.

Table 3. Intra- and inter-day precision and accuracy of quality control (QC) samples for all probe drugs and their metabolites in human plasma.

Analyte	Nominal Concentration (ng/mL)	Intra-Day (*n* = 5)			Inter-Day (*n* = 6)		
		Measured (ng/mL) *	RSD ** (%)	Accuracy (%)	Measured (ng/mL) *	RSD ** (%)	Accuracy (%)
Caffeine	20.0	22.2 ± 0.4	2.0	110.7	21.8 ± 0.8	3.5	109.2
	100.0	110.2 ± 2.2	2.0	110.2	103.6 ± 4.0	3.9	103.6
	1000	1071.0 ± 26.5	2.5	107.1	975.8 ± 28.0	2.8	97.6
Paraxanthine	20.0	22.2 ± 0.5	2.0	110.9	21.5 ± 0.8	3.7	107.3
	100.0	113.9 ± 0.8	0.7	113.9	102.6 ± 4.2	4.1	102.6
	1000	1073.8 ± 25.8	2.4	107.4	997.1 ± 23.9	2.4	99.7
Losartan	2.0	2.1 ± 0.0	1.5	104.8	2.1 ± 0.1	5.5	103.0
	10.0	10.7 ± 0.2	1.8	107.1	10.0 ± 0.2	1.8	100.4
	100	102.2 ± 0.8	0.8	102.2	99.0 ± 1.9	1.9	99.0

Pharmaceutics **2018**, *10*, 79

Table 3. *Cont.*

Analyte	Nominal Concentration (ng/mL)	Intra-Day (*n* = 5)			Inter-Day (*n* = 6)		
		Measured (ng/mL) *	RSD ** (%)	Accuracy (%)	Measured (ng/mL) *	RSD ** (%)	Accuracy (%)
EXP3174	2.0	2.1 ± 0.0	1.9	106.1	2.0 ± 0.1	4.0	101.1
	10.0	10.4 ± 0.2	1.7	104.3	10.0 ± 0.3	3.0	100.0
	100	99.1 ± 1.2	1.5	99.1	98.9 ± 4.6	4.7	98.9
Omeprazole	2.0	2.1 ± 0.1	3.3	104.8	2.0 ± 0.1	5.6	102.0
	10.0	11.2 ± 0.2	1.3	111.8	10.1 ± 0.7	6.5	101.4
	100	106.5 ± 1.0	1.0	106.5	96.7 ± 6.6	6.8	96.7
5′-Hydroxyomeprazole	2.0	2.0 ± 0.1	4.3	101.6	2.0 ± 0.1	2.7	102.0
	10.0	10.7 ± 0.2	1.8	106.6	10.1 ± 0.4	3.6	100.6
	100	101.2 ± 1.3	1.3	101.2	96.1 ± 3.1	3.2	96.1
Dextromethorphan	0.2	0.2 ± 0.0	7.3	97.1	0.2 ± 0.0	5.0	100.0
	1.0	1.2 ± 0.0	2.2	117.3	1.0 ± 0.0	3.1	101.8
	10	11.1 ± 0.1	1.0	111.3	10.2 ± 0.1	1.1	101.7
Dextrorphan	0.2	0.2 ± 0.0	11.3	100.2	0.2 ± 0.0	8.8	103.0
	1.0	1.1 ± 0.0	3.3	106.5	1.0 ± 0.0	2.6	103.4
	10	10.7 ± 0.3	2.5	106.5	10.2 ± 0.1	1.3	101.6
Midazolam	0.2	0.2 ± 0.0	6.3	103.1	0.2 ± 0.0	2.7	102.0
	1.0	1.1 ± 0.0	3.5	111.1	1.0 ± 0.0	1.6	100.8
	10	11.0 ± 0.1	0.6	109.9	10.1 ± 0.1	0.7	100.7
1′-Hydroxymidazolam	0.2	0.2 ± 0.0	6.3	88.5	0.1 ± 0.0	4.1	101.0
	1.0	0.9 ± 0.0	3.8	95.3	1.0 ± 0.1	6.3	99.0
	10	10.7 ± 0.1	1.2	106.9	10.0 ± 0.4	3.5	100.3
Pitavastatin	2.0	2.1 ± 0.1	2.8	105.3	2.1 ± 0.1	4.4	104.9
	10.0	11.5 ± 0.3	2.9	114.5	10.5 ± 0.5	5.1	105.3
	100	107.5 ± 1.6	1.5	107.5	99.2 ± 6.2	6.2	99.2

* Results are expressed as concentration mean ± SD. ** RSD, relative standard deviation.

Table 4. Short-term (4 h), freeze–thaw (three cycles), and post-treatment (4 °C, 24 h) stability results for all probe drugs and their metabolites in human plasma. Results are expressed as concentration mean ± SD.

Analyte	Nominal Concentration (ng/mL)	4 h Short-Term Stability (25 °C)	Freeze-Thaw Stability (−80 °C/Room Temperature)	24 h Post-Treatment Stability (4 °C)
Caffeine	100	91.8 ± 2.1	99.4 ± 3.3	96.2 ± 0.8
	1000	96.7 ± 7.6	93.9 ± 5.4	91.7 ± 2.3
Paraxanthine	100	86.1 ± 4.6	94.7 ± 1.4	96.8 ± 4.1
	1000	91.7 ± 7.5	90.0 ± 4.6	92.8 ± 1.5
Losartan	10	94.5 ± 2.1	101.9 ± 2.7	98.4 ± 3.4
	100	93.8 ± 3.8	95.6 ± 3.3	95.0 ± 2.0
EXP3174	10	90.5 ± 2.9	95.2 ± 2.6	98.8 ± 1.4
	100	91.9 ± 6.3	92.9 ± 4.0	93.1 ± 1.9
Omeprazole	10	89.8 ± 1.2	93.8 ± 1.8	94.7 ± 2.0
	100	88.9 ± 6.5	88.4 ± 3.5	94.6 ± 1.6
5′-Hydroxyomeprazole	10	99.0 ± 3.7	99.9 ± 6.6	96.5 ± 2.2
	100	91.0 ± 4.1	91.1 ± 4.8	91.0 ± 1.1
Dextromethorphan	1	107.2 ± 5.3	102.6 ± 6.4	102.5 ± 2.4
	10	100.5 ± 3.1	114.5 ± 3.6	102.5 ± 1.3
Dextrorphan	1	88.3 ± 5.2	91.0 ± 2.0	95.4 ± 12.4
	10	87.4 ± 6.3	92.1 ± 4.9	94.5 ± 4.3
Midazolam	1	105.9 ± 1.3	106.8 ± 5.3	100.5 ± 3.1
	10	104.1 ± 3.4	112.3 ± 1.3	103.6 ± 1.1
1′-Hydroxymidazolam	1	102.0 ± 5.0	99.7 ± 5.9	110.5 ± 0.3
	10	99.9 ± 7.5	107.3 ± 4.8	102.5 ± 3.0
Pitavastatin	10	91.0 ± 2.4	93.5 ± 3.6	99.1 ± 1.7
	100	93.4 ± 9.4	89.7 ± 2.6	95.4 ± 1.2

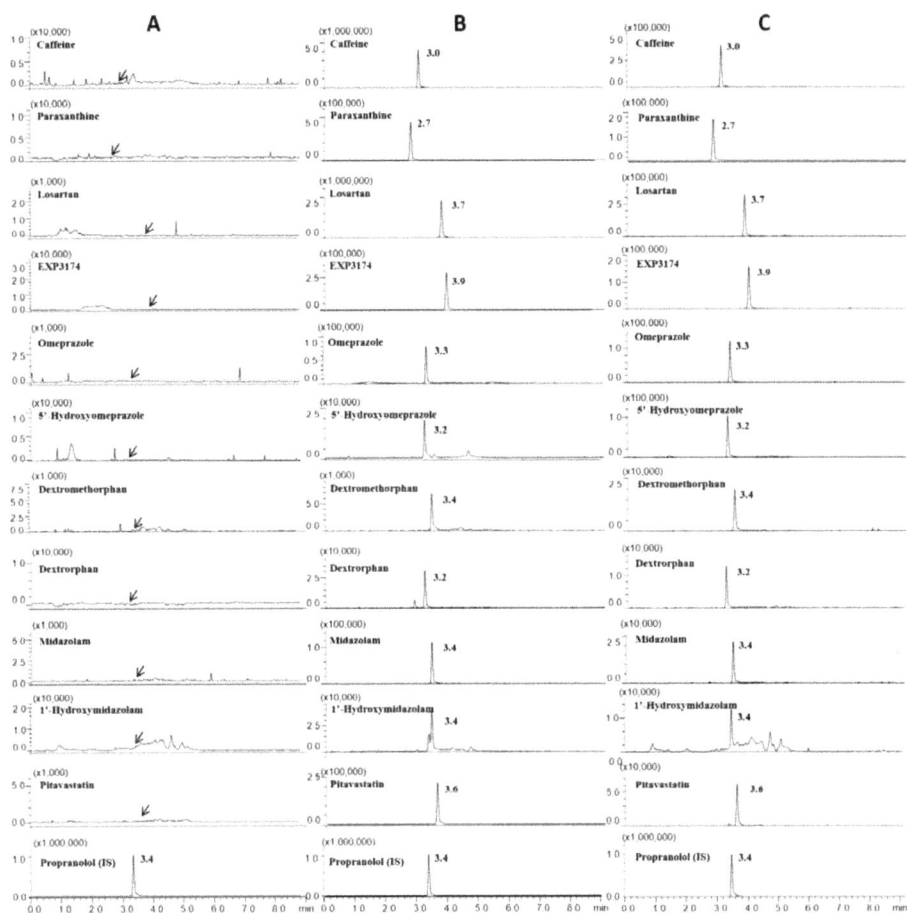

Figure 2. Selected reaction monitoring chromatograms of probe drugs, their metabolites, and internal standard (IS) in (**A**) blank plasma samples spiked with IS, (**B**) plasma samples collected from a subject 1 h after dosing and (**C**) plasma samples spiked with middle quality control (QC) concentrations.

3.3. Clinical Applications

These analytical methods were successfully used to determine concentrations of the all the probe drugs and their metabolites in human plasma samples after a single oral dose of the probe drug cocktail in six healthy volunteers. Figure 3 shows the mean plasma concentration–time profiles for OATP1B1 and five P450 probe drugs and their metabolites after the administration of cocktail drugs (Figure 3A,F). Caffeine/paraxanthine, EXP3174, dextromethorphan/dextrorphan and pitavastatin were detected over 48 h. Losartan was detected within 2 h with C_{max} and AUC from time zero to 48 h (AUC_{0-48}), values of 172.50 ng/mL and 387.50 h·ng/mL, respectively. Omeprazole and 5′-hydroxyomeprazole were detected within 4 h with C_{max}, values of 566.07 and 114.09 ng/mL, respectively. Midazolam was absorbed rapidly resulting in T_{max} of 0.5 h and C_{max} value of 7.61 ng/mL (Table 5). Therefore, the developed analytical method was sufficiently sensitive and selective for use in pharmacokinetic studies.

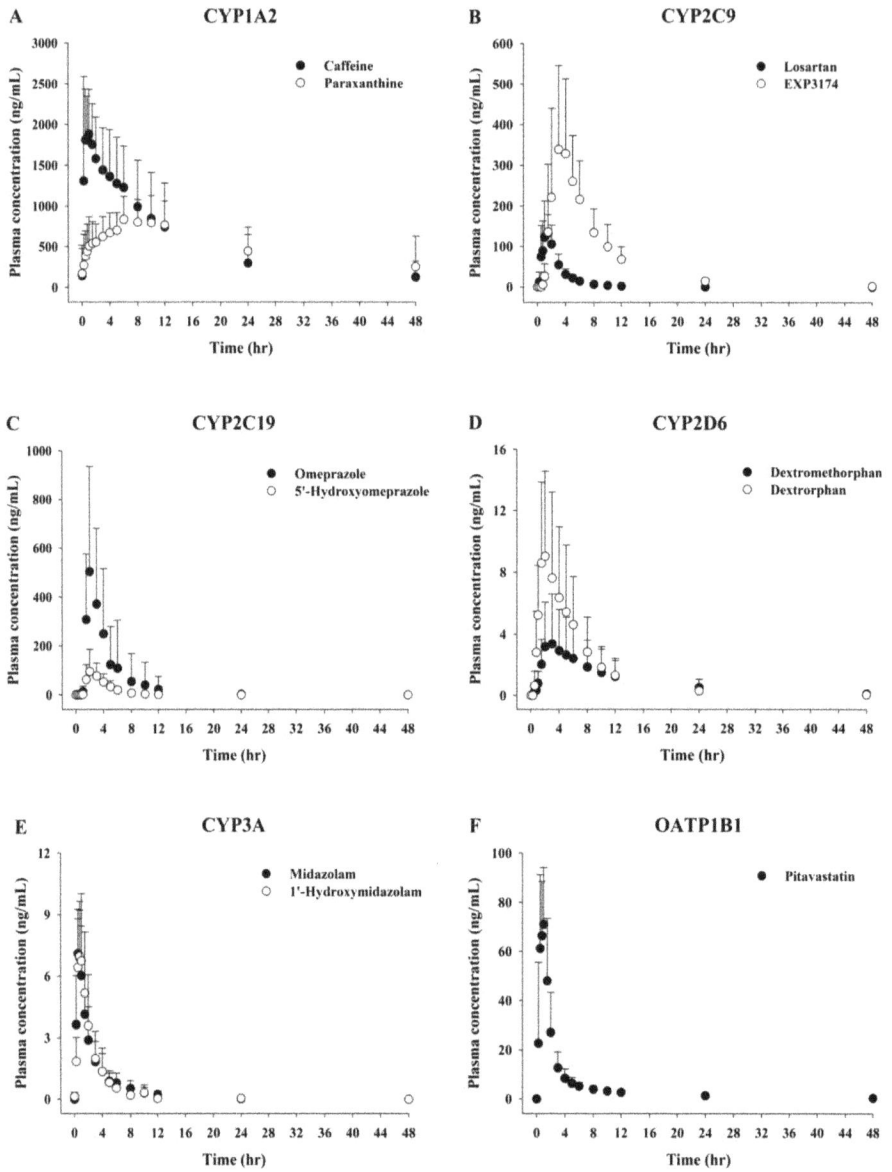

Figure 3. Mean plasma concentration-time profiles for organic anion transporting polypeptide 1B1 (OATP1B1) and cytochrome P450 probe drugs and their metabolites after administration of cocktail drugs (*n* = 6).

Table 5. Summary of pharmacokinetic parameters of organic anion transporting polypeptide 1B1 (OATP1B1) and cytochrome P450 (P450) probe drugs and their metabolites ($n = 6$). Results are expressed as mean ± SD or median (range).

Probe Drug	Pharmacokinetic Parameters	Mean ± SD
Caffeine (CYP1A2)	AUC_{0-48} (h·ng/mL)	27,327.6 ± 18,012.4
	C_{max} (ng/mL)	2350.4 ± 843.1
	T_{max} (h)	0.75 (0.25–1.50)
	$t_{1/2}$ (h)	8.84 ± 3.01
	MRT (h)	11.1 ± 4.0
Paraxanthine	AUC_{0-48} (h·ng/mL)	24,063.5 ± 13,009.8
	C_{max} (ng/mL)	925.3 ± 305.5
	T_{max} (h)	7 (5–24)
	$t_{1/2}$ (h)	12.46 ± 6.03
	MRT (h)	16.8 ± 4.7
Losartan (CYP2C9)	AUC_{0-48} (h·ng/mL)	387.5 ± 121.2
	C_{max} (ng/mL)	172.5 ± 62.6
	T_{max} (h)	1.25 (0.50–2.00)
	$t_{1/2}$ (h)	2.14 ± 0.53
	MRT (h)	2.7 ± 0.3
EXP3174	AUC_{0-48} (h·ng/mL)	2721.6 ± 1236.2
	C_{max} (ng/mL)	352.1 ± 205.6
	T_{max} (h)	3.5 (3.0–5.0)
	$t_{1/2}$ (h)	6.79 ± 0.58
	MRT (h)	8.6 ± 1.2
Omeprazole (CYP2C19)	AUC_{0-48} (h·ng/mL)	1796.2 ± 2076.3
	C_{max} (ng/mL)	566.1 ± 367.1
	T_{max} (h)	2.0 (1.5–3.0)
	$t_{1/2}$ (h)	1.34 ± 1.14
	MRT (h)	3.5 ± 1.5
5′-Hydroxyomeprazole	AUC_{0-48} (h·ng/mL)	315.6 ± 195.3
	C_{max} (ng/mL)	114.1 ± 80.9
	T_{max} (h)	2.0 (1.5–4.0)
	$t_{1/2}$ (h)	1.59 ± 1.12
	MRT (h)	3.8 ± 1.0
Dextromethorphan (CYP2D6)	AUC_{0-48} (h·ng/mL)	41.36 ± 40.33
	C_{max} (ng/mL)	3.70 ± 3.23
	T_{max} (h)	2.5 (1.0–3.0)
	$t_{1/2}$ (h)	8.50 ± 2.49
	MRT (h)	8.7 ± 4.3
Dextrorphan	AUC_{0-48} (h·ng/mL)	63.91 ± 44.51
	C_{max} (ng/mL)	10.48 ± 5.32
	T_{max} (h)	1.5 (1.0–3.0)
	$t_{1/2}$ (h)	6.44 ± 2.74
	MRT (h)	7.4 ± 1.9
Midazolam (CYP3A)	AUC_{0-48} (h·ng/mL)	18.60 ± 9.65
	C_{max} (ng/mL)	7.61 ± 2.26
	T_{max} (h)	0.5 (0.5–1.0)
	$t_{1/2}$ (h)	3.08 ± 1.43
	MRT (h)	2.8 ± 0.9
1′-Hydroxymidazolam	AUC_{0-48} (h·ng/mL)	17.65 ± 9.87
	C_{max} (ng/mL)	7.77 ± 2.77
	T_{max} (h)	0.75 (0.50–1.00)
	$t_{1/2}$ (h)	3.32 ± 3.30
	MRT (h)	2.5 ± 0.9
Pitavastatin (OATP1B1)	AUC_{0-48} (h·ng/mL)	198.1 ± 68.4
	C_{max} (ng/mL)	81.31 ± 26.04
	T_{max} (h)	0.75 (0.50–1.50)
	$t_{1/2}$ (h)	13.48 ± 5.24
	MRT (h)	9.8 ± 3.4

4. Conclusions

In this study, we have developed and validated a rapid, reliable, precise, and selective assay to determine the concentrations of five P450 isoforms (CYP1A2, CYP2C9, CYP2C19, CYP2D6, and CYP3A) probe drugs and their metabolites and the transporter OATP1B1 probe drug in human plasma using protein precipitation followed by a single LC-MS/MS run. The method was also successfully applied to a pharmacokinetic study in healthy subjects who received a cocktail of OATP1B1 and five P450 probe drugs. This method would be useful for the clinical evaluation of P450 and OATP1B1 activity, and in vivo drug–drug interactions of potential of drug candidates.

Author Contributions: S.L., K.-S.S., I.S.S., K.-H.L. and Y.-R.Y. conceived and designed the experiments; J.K.H., H.-J.K., G.-H.L., and B.O. performed the experiments; J.K.H. and B.O. analyzed the data; J.K.H., K.-H.L., and Y.-R.Y. wrote the paper. All authors approved the final manuscript.

Funding: This study was supported by the National Research Foundation of Korea, Ministry of Education [NRF-2016R1D1A1A09916782], Republic of Korea, and the Korea Institute of Planning and Evaluation for Technology in Food, Agriculture, Forestry and Fisheries (IPET) through Export Promotion Technology Development Program, funded by Ministry of Agriculture, Food and Rural Affairs (MAFRA), Republic of Korea [No 316017-3].

Conflicts of Interest: The authors declare no conflict of interest.

References

1. Zanger, U.M.; Schwab, M. Cytochrome P450 enzymes in drug metabolism: Regulation of gene expression, enzyme activities, and impact of genetic variation. *Pharmacol. Ther.* **2013**, *138*, 103–141. [CrossRef] [PubMed]
2. Michalets, E.L. Update: Clinically significant cytochrome P450 drug interactions. *Pharmacotherapy* **1998**, *18*, 84–112. [PubMed]
3. Nelson, D.R. The cytochrome P450 homepage. *Hum. Genom.* **2009**, *4*, 59–65.
4. Zhang, S.; Song, N.; Li, Q.; Fan, H.; Liu, C. Liquid chromatography/tandem mass spectrometry method for simultaneous evaluation of activities of five cytochrome P450s using a five-drug cocktail and application to cytochrome p450 phenotyping studies in rats. *J. Chromatogr. B Anal. Technol. Biomed. Life Sci.* **2008**, *871*, 78–89. [CrossRef] [PubMed]
5. Paine, M.F.; Khalighi, M.; Fisher, J.M.; Shen, D.D.; Kunze, K.L.; Marsh, C.L.; Perkins, J.D.; Thummel, K.E. Characterization of interintestinal and intraintestinal variations in human CYP3A-dependent metabolism. *J. Pharmacol. Exp. Ther.* **1997**, *283*, 1552–1562. [PubMed]
6. Indiaina University. P450 Drug Interaction Table. Available online: http://medicine.iupui.edu/clinpharm/ddis/main-table (accessed on 18 May 2018).
7. U.S. Food and Drug Administration. Drug Interactions & Labeling. Available online: https://www.fda.gov/Drugs/DevelopmentApprovalProcess/DevelopmentResources/DrugInteractionsLabeling (accessed on 18 May 2018).
8. International Transporter Consortium; Giacomini, K.M.; Huang, S.M.; Tweedie, D.J.; Benet, L.Z.; Brouwer, K.L.; Chu, X.; Dahlin, A.; Evers, R.; Fischer, V.; et al. Membrane transporters in drug development. *Nat. Rev. Drug Discov.* **2010**, *9*, 215–236. [CrossRef] [PubMed]
9. Hartkoorn, R.C.; Kwan, W.S.; Shallcross, V.; Chaikan, A.; Liptrott, N.; Egan, D.; Sora, E.S.; James, C.E.; Gibbons, S.; Bray, P.G.; et al. Hiv protease inhibitors are substrates for OATP1A2, OATP1B1 and OATP1B3 and lopinavir plasma concentrations are influenced by SLCO1B1 polymorphisms. *Pharmacogenet. Genom.* **2010**, *20*, 112–120. [CrossRef] [PubMed]
10. Yoshida, K.; Maeda, K.; Sugiyama, Y. Transporter-mediated drug–drug interactions involving oatp substrates: Predictions based on in vitro inhibition studies. *Clin. Pharmacol. Ther.* **2012**, *91*, 1053–1064. [CrossRef] [PubMed]
11. Ieiri, I.; Tsunemitsu, S.; Maeda, K.; Ando, Y.; Izumi, N.; Kimura, M.; Yamane, N.; Okuzono, T.; Morishita, M.; Kotani, N.; et al. Mechanisms of pharmacokinetic enhancement between ritonavir and saquinavir; micro/small dosing tests using midazolam (CYP3A4), fexofenadine (P-glycoprotein), and pravastatin (OATP1B1) as probe drugs. *J. Clin. Pharmacol.* **2013**, *53*, 654–661. [CrossRef] [PubMed]
12. Kim, M.G.; Kim, Y.; Jeon, J.Y.; Kim, D.S. Effect of fermented red ginseng on cytochrome P450 and P-glycoprotein activity in healthy subjects, as evaluated using the cocktail approach. *Br. J. Clin. Pharmacol.* **2016**, *82*, 1580–1590. [CrossRef] [PubMed]

13. Oh, K.S.; Park, S.J.; Shinde, D.D.; Shin, J.G.; Kim, D.H. High-sensitivity liquid chromatography-tandem mass spectrometry for the simultaneous determination of five drugs and their cytochrome P450-specific probe metabolites in human plasma. *J. Chromatogr. B Anal. Technol. Biomed. Life Sci.* **2012**, *895–896*, 56–64. [CrossRef] [PubMed]

14. Bosilkovska, M.; Deglon, J.; Samer, C.; Walder, B.; Desmeules, J.; Staub, C.; Daali, Y. Simultaneous LC-MS/MS quantification of P-glycoprotein and cytochrome P450 probe substrates and their metabolites in dbs and plasma. *Bioanalysis* **2014**, *6*, 151–164. [CrossRef] [PubMed]

15. Ryu, J.Y.; Song, I.S.; Sunwoo, Y.E.; Shon, J.H.; Liu, K.H.; Cha, I.J.; Shin, J.G. Development of the "Inje cocktail" for high-throughput evaluation of five human cytochrome P450 isoforms in vivo. *Clin. Pharmacol. Ther.* **2007**, *82*, 531–540. [CrossRef] [PubMed]

16. Williams, D.; Tao, X.; Zhu, L.; Stonier, M.; Lutz, J.D.; Masson, E.; Zhang, S.; Ganguly, B.; Tzogas, Z.; Lubin, S.; et al. Use of a cocktail probe to assess potential drug interactions with cytochrome P450 after administration of belatacept, a costimulatory immunomodulator. *Br. J. Clin. Pharmacol.* **2017**, *83*, 370–380. [CrossRef] [PubMed]

17. Streetman, D.S.; Bleakley, J.F.; Kim, J.S.; Nafziger, A.N.; Leeder, J.S.; Gaedigk, A.; Gotschall, R.; Kearns, G.L.; Bertino, J.S., Jr. Combined phenotypic assessment of CYP1A2, CYP2C19, CYP2D6, CYP3A, N-acetyltransferase-2, and xanthine oxidase with the "Cooperstown cocktail". *Clin. Pharmacol. Ther.* **2000**, *68*, 375–383. [CrossRef] [PubMed]

18. Zgheib, N.K.; Frye, R.F.; Tracy, T.S.; Romkes, M.; Branch, R.A. Validation of incorporating flurbiprofen into the pittsburgh cocktail. *Clin. Pharmacol. Ther.* **2006**, *80*, 257–263. [CrossRef] [PubMed]

19. Christensen, M.; Andersson, K.; Dalen, P.; Mirghani, R.A.; Muirhead, G.J.; Nordmark, A.; Tybring, G.; Wahlberg, A.; Yasar, U.; Bertilsson, L. The Karolinska cocktail for phenotyping of five human cytochrome P450 enzymes. *Clin. Pharmacol. Ther.* **2003**, *73*, 517–528. [CrossRef]

20. Grangeon, A.; Gravel, S.; Gaudette, F.; Turgeon, J.; Michaud, V. Highly sensitive LC-MS/MS methods for the determination of seven human CYP450 activities using small oral doses of probe-drugs in human. *J. Chromatogr. B Anal. Technol. Biomed. Life Sci.* **2017**, *1040*, 144–158. [CrossRef] [PubMed]

21. Shelepova, T.; Nafziger, A.N.; Victory, J.; Kashuba, A.D.; Rowland, E.; Zhang, Y.; Sellers, E.; Kearns, G.; Leeder, J.S.; Gaedigk, A.; et al. Effect of a triphasic oral contraceptive on drug-metabolizing enzyme activity as measured by the validated Cooperstown 5 + 1 cocktail. *J. Clin. Pharmacol.* **2005**, *45*, 1413–1421. [CrossRef] [PubMed]

22. Prueksaritanont, T.; Chu, X.; Evers, R.; Klopfer, S.O.; Caro, L.; Kothare, P.A.; Dempsey, C.; Rasmussen, S.; Houle, R.; Chan, G.; et al. Pitavastatin is a more sensitive and selective organic anion-transporting polypeptide 1b clinical probe than rosuvastatin. *Br. J. Clin. Pharmacol.* **2014**, *78*, 587–598. [CrossRef] [PubMed]

23. Maeda, K.; Ikeda, Y.; Fujita, T.; Yoshida, K.; Azuma, Y.; Haruyama, Y.; Yamane, N.; Kumagai, Y.; Sugiyama, Y. Identification of the rate-determining process in the hepatic clearance of atorvastatin in a clinical cassette microdosing study. *Clin. Pharmacol. Ther.* **2011**, *90*, 575–581. [CrossRef] [PubMed]

24. Stopfer, P.; Giessmann, T.; Hohl, K.; Sharma, A.; Ishiguro, N.; Taub, M.E.; Zimdahl-Gelling, H.; Gansser, D.; Wein, M.; Ebner, T.; et al. Pharmacokinetic evaluation of a drug transporter cocktail consisting of digoxin, furosemide, metformin, and rosuvastatin. *Clin. Pharmacol. Ther.* **2016**, *100*, 259–267. [CrossRef] [PubMed]

25. Hirano, M.; Maeda, K.; Shitara, Y.; Sugiyama, Y. Contribution of OATP2 (PATP1B1) and OATP8 (OATP1B3) to the hepatic uptake of pitavastatin in humans. *J. Pharmacol. Exp. Ther.* **2004**, *311*, 139–146. [CrossRef] [PubMed]

26. Kitamura, S.; Maeda, K.; Wang, Y.; Sugiyama, Y. Involvement of multiple transporters in the hepatobiliary transport of rosuvastatin. *Drug Metab. Dispos.* **2008**, *36*, 2014–2023. [CrossRef] [PubMed]

27. Hasegawa, M.; Kusuhara, H.; Sugiyama, D.; Ito, K.; Ueda, S.; Endou, H.; Sugiyama, Y. Functional involvement of rat organic anion transporter 3 (rOAT3; SLC22A8) in the renal uptake of organic anions. *J. Pharmacol. Exp. Ther.* **2002**, *300*, 746–753. [CrossRef] [PubMed]

28. Nishizato, Y.; Ieiri, I.; Suzuki, H.; Kimura, M.; Kawabata, K.; Hirota, T.; Takane, H.; Irie, S.; Kusuhara, H.; Urasaki, Y.; et al. Polymorphisms of OATP-C (SLC21A6) and OAT3 (SLC22A8) genes: Consequences for pravastatin pharmacokinetics. *Clin. Pharmacol. Ther.* **2003**, *73*, 554–565. [CrossRef]

29. Jindal, K.; Narayanam, M.; Singh, S. A systematic strategy for the identification and determination of pharmaceuticals in environment using advanced lc-ms tools: Application to ground water samples. *J. Pharm. Biomed. Anal.* **2015**, *108*, 86–96. [CrossRef] [PubMed]

30. Ardjomand-Woelkart, K.; Kollroser, M.; Li, L.; Derendorf, H.; Butterweck, V.; Bauer, R. Development and validation of a LC-MS/MS method based on a new 96-well hybrid-spe-precipitation technique for quantification of CYP450 substrates/metabolites in rat plasma. *Anal. Bioanal. Chem.* **2011**, *400*, 2371–2381. [CrossRef] [PubMed]

31. Zhang, Y.; Miao, L.; Lin, L.; Ren, C.Y.; Liu, J.X.; Cui, Y.M. Repeated administration of sailuotong, a fixed combination of panax ginseng, ginkgo biloba, and crocus sativus extracts for vascular dementia, alters CYP450 activities in rats. *Phytomedicine* **2018**, *38*, 125–134. [CrossRef] [PubMed]

32. Tanaka, S.; Uchida, S.; Inui, N.; Takeuchi, K.; Watanabe, H.; Namiki, N. Simultaneous LC-MS/MS analysis of the plasma concentrations of a cocktail of 5 cytochrome P450 substrate drugs and their metabolites. *Biol. Pharm. Bull.* **2014**, *37*, 18–25. [CrossRef] [PubMed]

33. Snyder, B.D.; Rowland, A.; Polasek, T.M.; Miners, J.O.; Doogue, M.P. Evaluation of felodipine as a potential perpetrator of pharmacokinetic drug-drug interactions. *Eur. J. Clin. Pharmacol.* **2014**, *70*, 1115–1122. [CrossRef] [PubMed]

34. Zhang, W.; Han, F.; Guo, P.; Zhao, H.; Lin, Z.J.; Huang, M.Q.; Bertelsen, K.; Weng, N. Simultaneous determination of tolbutamide, omeprazole, midazolam and dextromethorphan in human plasma by LC-MS/MS—A high throughput approach to evaluate drug-drug interactions. *J. Chromatogr. B Anal. Technol. Biomed. Life Sci.* **2010**, *878*, 1169–1177. [CrossRef] [PubMed]

35. Kim, M.J.; Kim, H.; Cha, I.J.; Park, J.S.; Shon, J.H.; Liu, K.H.; Shin, J.G. High-throughput screening of inhibitory potential of nine cytochrome P450 enzymes in vitro using liquid chromatography/tandem mass spectrometry. *Rapid Commun. Mass Spectrom.* **2005**, *19*, 2651–2658. [CrossRef] [PubMed]

36. Lee, B.; Ji, H.K.; Lee, T.; Liu, K.H. Simultaneous screening of activities of five cytochrome P450 and four uridine 5′-diphospho-glucuronosyltransferase enzymes in human liver microsomes using cocktail incubation and liquid chromatography-tandem mass spectrometry. *Drug Metab. Dispos.* **2015**, *43*, 1137–1146. [CrossRef] [PubMed]

37. Liu, K.H.; Lee, Y.K.; Sunwoo, Y.E.; Yu, K.S.; Kang, W.; Lee, S.S.; Yoon, Y.R.; Shin, J.G. High-performance liquid chromatographic assay of zonisamide (1,2-benzisoxazole-3-methanesulfonamide) in human plasma using a solid-phase extraction technique. *Chromatographia* **2004**, *59*, 497–500. [CrossRef]

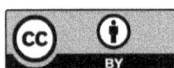

pharmaceutics

MDPI

Article

A Liquid Chromatography-Quadrupole-Time-of-Flight Mass Spectrometric Assay for the Quantification of Fabry Disease Biomarker Globotriaosylceramide (GB3) in Fabry Model Mouse

Seok-Ho Shin [1], Min-Ho Park [1], Jin-Ju Byeon [1], Byeong ill Lee [1], Yuri Park [1], Ah-ra Ko [2], Mi-ran Seong [2], Soyeon Lee [2], Mi Ra Kim [2], Jinwook Seo [3], Myung Eun Jung [3], Dong-Kyu Jin [4,*] and Young G. Shin [1,*]

[1] College of Pharmacy and Institute of Drug Research and Development, Chungnam National University, Daejeon 34134, Korea; seokho.shin.cnu@gmail.com (S.-H.S.); minho.park.cnu@gmail.com (M.-H.P.); jinju.byeon.cnu@gmail.com (J.-J.B.); byungill.lee.cnu@gmail.com (B.i.L.); yuri.park.cnu@gmail.com (Y.P.)
[2] Research Institute for Future Medicine, Samsung Medical Center, Seoul 135-710, Korea; knoxgo@hanmail.net (A.-r.K.); miran.seong@sbri.co.kr (M.-r.-S.); soyeon86.lee@sbri.co.kr (S.L.); mira0411.kim@sbri.co.kr (M.R.K.)
[3] Green Cross Research Center, Green Cross, Gyeonggi-do 446-850, Korea; jinugi1@greencross.com(J.S.); jungme@greencross.com (M.E.J.)
[4] Department of Pediatrics, Samsung Medical Center, Sungkyunkwan University School of Medicine, Seoul 06351, Korea
*   Correspondence: yshin@cnu.ac.kr (D.-K.J.); jindk@skku.edu (Y.G.S.); Tel.: +82-42-821-5931 (D.-K.J.); +82-2-3410-3525 (Y.G.S.)

Received: 16 April 2018; Accepted: 4 June 2018; Published: 7 June 2018

Abstract: Fabry disease is a rare lysosomal storage disorder resulting from the lack of α-*Gal A* gene activity. Globotriaosylceramide (GB3, ceramide trihexoside) is a novel endogenous biomarker which predicts the incidence of Fabry disease. At the early stage efficacy/biomarker study, a rapid method to determine this biomarker in plasma and in all relevant tissues related to this disease simultaneously is required. However, the limited sample volume, as well as the various levels of GB3 in different matrices makes the GB3 quantitation very challenging. Hereby we developed a rapid method to identify GB3 in mouse plasma and various tissues. Preliminary stability tests were also performed in three different conditions: short-term, freeze-thaw, long-term. The calibration curve was well fitted over the concentration range of 0.042–10 μg/mL for GB3 in plasma and 0.082–20 μg/g for GB3 in various tissues. This method was successfully applied for the comparison of GB3 levels in Fabry model mice (B6;129-Gla[tm1Kul]/J), which has not been performed previously to the best of our knowledge.

Keywords: GB3; Fabry disease; LC-QTOF-MS/MS; B6;129-Gla[tm1Kul]/J

1. Introduction

Fabry disease is an X-chromosome-linked inherited lysosomal storage disorder resulting from partial to total deficiency of the lysosomal enzyme α-galactosidase A due to the lack of α-*Gal A* gene activity [1–3]. As a result, glycosphingolipids, mainly Globotriaosylceramide (GB3) accumulates to the tissues primarily in the central nervous system, cardiovascular system, renal system (especially kidney), skin, and muscle [1,2,4,5]. The progression of the disease may affect the normal regulatory function of brain, heart, kidney, and other organs, leading to high morbidity and mortality, low quality of life [6,7]. Several methodologies on the treatment of Fabry disease has been developed including renal transplantation, somatic gene therapy, enzyme replacement using recombinant α-*Gal A* (e.g., Fabrazyme and Replagal) and the usage of small molecule pharmacological chaperone therapy (e.g., Migalastat HCl) [8–13]. With the usage of these treatments, GB3 levels in plasma and tissues dramatically decreases in Fabry patients [4,5,14–16]. These results suggest that GB3 can be used as a diagnostic biomarker and may be applied for the screening/monitoring in Fabry patients. However, the complexity of GB3 molecular structure (Figure 1) and a large number of possible GB3 isoforms made the GB3 analysis challenging [17,18].

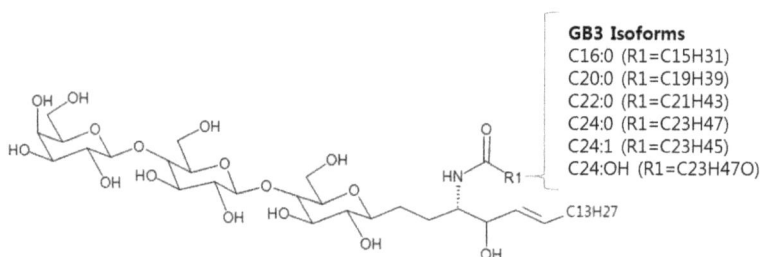

Figure 1. Structure of Globotriaosylceramide (GB3).

Early assays performed with thin layer chromatography (TLC), gas chromatography (GC), and high-performance liquid chromatography (HPLC) were time consuming and several derivatization steps were required [18–20]. With the advent of electrospray ionization tandem mass spectrometry (ESI-MS/MS) for the quantification of GB3, certain derivatization steps are not required and faster, highly sensitive analysis was achievable [17,21,22]. Recently, a nano- Liquid chromatographic mass spectrometry (LC-MS/MS) method [23] and matrix-assisted laser desorption-ionization time-of-flight (MALDI-TOF) method [24] was also developed. Several sample preparation methods have also been introduced including solid phase extraction (SPE), protein precipitation (PPT), liquid-liquid extraction (LLE), and a combined liquid extraction/protein precipitation method [16,22,25–28].

Although these methods have been well applied for in vivo studies, a quick determination of GB3 from Fabry disease model is important particularly at the early stage research. In this study, we aimed on improving the analysis throughput without compromising the data quality with very limited sample volume. As a result, we used a simple protein-precipitation method without further steps discussed in the previous studies [18–20,26–28], using a small amount of plasma/tissue samples and we have improved the throughput significantly (>300 plasma and tissue samples per day) when compared to previous methods published in the literatures [18–20,26–28].

This method was well-qualified and applied for the quantification of GB3 in various organs, including plasma, heart, liver, spleen, kidney, and brain tissues to evaluate the correlation between GB3 level and Fabry disease progression. This method was also successfully applied to evaluate new drug candidates being developed in our lab by monitoring the GB3 level change in the Fabry model mice (B6;129-Gla^{tm1Kul}/J) after dosing (data not shown).

2. Materials and Methods

2.1. Chemicals

GB3 and C17:0-GB3 were purchased from Matreya (Pleasant Gap, PA, USA). Several chemicals were obtained from Daejung Chemicals and Metals (Siheung, Gyonggi, Korea) of either GR or HPLC grade: formic acid, dimethyl sulfoxide (DMSO), methanol (MeOH), and distilled water. Bovine serum albumin was purchased from Sigma-Aldrich Chemical Corporation (St. Louis, MO, USA). Acetonitrile (ACN) from Avantor Performance Materials (3477 Corporate Parkway, Suite 200, Center Valley, PA, USA). Phosphate-buffered saline (PBS) was provided by Welgene (Dalseogu, Daegu, Korea).

2.2. Preparation of Stock Solution

GB3 stock solution was made at a concentration 1 mg/mL in DMSO. 0.2 mg/mL sub-stock solution was further prepared by spiking 0.2 mL of stock solution (1 mg/mL) into 0.8 mL of DMSO and both the stock and sub-stock solution were stored in the freezer at $-20\,^{\circ}\text{C}$. Working standard (STD) and quality control (QC) solutions were prepared by diluting the sub-stock solution. The internal standard (ISTD) *N*-heptadecanoyl ceramide trihexoside (C17:0-GB3) was made at 1 mg/mL in DMSO and stored in the refrigerator at $-20\,^{\circ}\text{C}$ until use. The final ISTD spiking solution containing 1 µg/mL of C17:0-GB3 was prepared in methanol (MeOH).

2.3. Sample Preparation-Plasma

Blank Institute of Cancer Research (ICR) mouse plasma was diluted four-fold with 4% BSA-PBS for the preparation of calibration curve STD and QC samples. For example, 1 mL blank mouse plasma was added to 4 mL of 4% BSA-PBS for STD/QC samples. For the study samples, 10 µL aliquots of study sample was added to 40 µL of 4% BSA-PBS. Ten standard working solutions of GB3 were prepared freshly in duplicate by serially diluting the standard solution at a final concentration of 10, 5, 3.33, 2.50, 1.67, 1.11, 0.83, 0.37, 0.12, and 0.042 µg/mL using DMSO. A separate weighing of the GB3 reference standard was used to make QCs. Two QC working solutions of GB3 were prepared at a final concentration of 0.4 µg/mL medium QC (MQC) and 2 µg/mL high QC (HQC) using DMSO.

Fifty microliters aliquot of the diluted plasma was added to cluster tubes. Five microliters of the corresponding standard working solution and QC solutions were also added to each cluster tubes, while 5 µL of make-up solution (DMSO) was spiked to study samples and blank samples (two blank samples with ISTD and two blank samples without ISTD (double blank)). For each sample, except for the double blanks, 200 µL of ISTD spike solution (1 µg/mL of C17:0-GB3 in MeOH) was added (200 µL of MeOH was added in the double blank as a make-up solution). All of the tubes were capped and vortexed for 1 min and centrifuged at 10,000 rpm for 5 min at $4\,^{\circ}\text{C}$. After centrifuging, 185 µL of the supernatant was transferred into LC-vial for analysis. The schematic diagram of the plasma sample preparation procedure is demonstrated in Figure 2.

2.4. Sample Preparation–Tissues (Heart, Liver, Spleen, Kidney, Brain)

A four-fold volume of 4% BSA-PBS and several zirconia beads (2 mm diameter, Lysing Matrix I®, MP Biomedicals, Solon, OH, USA) was added to blank ICR mouse tissues and the study sample tissues and then homogenized using a FastPrep®-24 tissue homogenizer (MP Biomedicals, Solon, OH, USA) for 3 min to prepare tissue homogenates. Due to the high concentration of the GB3 levels in tissues, all tissue homogenates were re-diluted 200 times (500 times for spleen tissue homogenate) with 4% BSA-PBS. Eleven standard (ten standard for heart) working solutions of GB3 were prepared freshly in duplicate by serially diluting the standard solution at a final concentration of 20, 10, 6.67, 5, 3.33, 2.22, 1.67, 1.11, 0.74, 0.25, and 0.082 µg/mL using DMSO (ten points for heart: 20, 10, 6.67, 5, 3.33, 2.22, 1.67, 0.74, 0.25, and 0.082 µg/mL). A separate weighing of the GB3 reference standard was used to make QCs. Two QC working solutions of GB3 were prepared at a final concentration of 0.8 µg/mL medium QC (MQC) and 4 µg/mL high QC (HQC) using DMSO. Fifty microliter aliquots of each diluted tissue homogenates were added to cluster tubes. The same procedure used for plasma samples was applied for tissue samples and the schematic diagram of the tissue sample preparation procedure is also demonstrated in Figure 2.

2.5. Liquid Chromatographic Mass Spectrometry (LC-MS/MS) Condition

A Shimadzu CBM-20A HPLC pump controller (Shimadzu Corporation, Columbia, MD, USA), two Shimadzu LC-20AD pumps, a CTC HTS PAL autosampler (CEAP Technologies, Carrboro, NC, USA), and a quadrupole time-of-flight TripleTOF™ 5600 mass spectrometer (Sciex, Foster City, CA, USA) equipped with a Duospray™ ion source were used for the assay development. A Phenomenex® Kinetex Phenyl-Hexyl column (2.1 × 50 mm, 2.6 µm) was used for the column separation. A binary gradient elution was employed using an aqueous mobile phase A, distilled and deionized water containing 0.1% formic acid; and an organic mobile phase B, acetonitrile containing 0.1% formic acid. The following gradient elution was used: from 0 min to 0.3 min, 35% B; from 0.3 min to 1.5 min by a linear gradient from 35% B to 95% B; 95% B was maintained for 0.8 min; and finally back to the initial condition (35% B) in 0.1 min and maintained for 1.6 min for re-equilibrium. The total run time was 4 min. The gradient was delivered at a flow rate of 0.5 mL/min and the injection volume was 10 µL. The single reaction monitoring with high sensitivity option (SRMHS) were recorded in positive ion mode. The most abundant ion was the sodium adduct $[M + Na]^+$ ion for all GB3 isoforms. Since GB3 is a glycosphingolipid, it is composed of various degrees of saturation and oxidation form of fatty acids rather than being homogenous one [25]. Due to this heterogeneous composition, the most abundant six isoforms were selected to calculate the total GB3 concentration at mass to charge ratios (m/z) of: m/z 1046.7 (C16:0), m/z 1102.7 (C20:0), m/z 1130.8 (C22:0), m/z 1156.8 (C24:1), m/z 1158.8 (C24:0), and m/z 1174.8 (C24:0-OH). The GB3 ISTD (N-heptadecanoyl ceramide trihexoside (C17:0)) peak was observed at m/z 1060 (C17:0). The total area of six major isoforms was divided by the area of GB3 ISTD to achieve response ratio (Equation (1)). The mass spectrometer conditions are summarized in Table 1.

$$\text{Response ratio} = \frac{\text{Total area of 6 major GB3 isoforms}}{\text{Area of GB3 ISTD (C17:0)}} \tag{1}$$

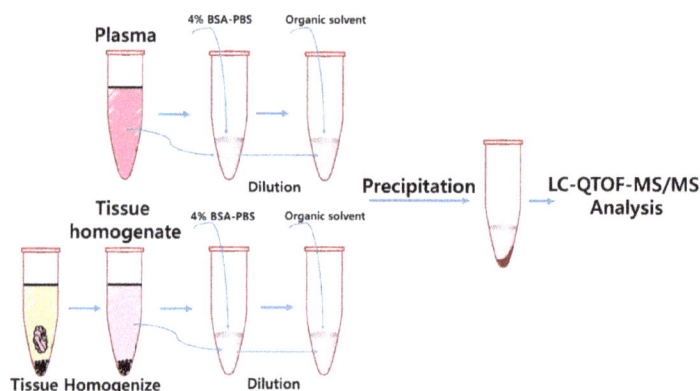

Figure 2. Sample preparation procedure.

Table 1. Mass spectrometry conditions for six Globotriaosylceramide (GB3) isoforms.

TOF-MS Condition			
GS1	50	CUR (Curtain Gas)	30
GS2	50	ISVP (Ion Spray Voltage)	5500
SRM High Sensitive Scan Mode, Positive			
GB3 Isoform	Parent-To-Parent Transition	Declustering Voltage (DP)	Collision Energy (CE)
C16:0-GB3	1046.7→1046.7	100	66
C17:0-GB3	1060.7→1060.7 (ISTD)	100	66
C20:0-GB3	1102.7→1102.7	100	66
C22:0-GB3	1130.8→1130.8	100	66
C24:1-GB3	1156.8→1156.8	100	66
C24:0-GB3	1158.8→1158.8	100	66
C24:0-OH-GB3	1174.8→1174.8	100	66

The source temperature was set to 500 °C with a curtain gas flow of 30 L/min. The ion spray voltage was set at 5500 V. The declustering potential was 100 V and the collision energy was 66 V.

High-purity nitrogen gas was used for the nebulizer/Duospray™ and the curtain gases. The mass spectrometer was automatically calibrated after the acquisition of every 20 samples using APCI positive calibration solution (Sciex, P/N 4460131) delivered by the calibration delivery system (CDS).

2.6. Method Qualification

A 'fit-for-purpose' approach was used for the method qualification. The qualification run contained duplicate calibration curves at ten concentrations for plasma and eleven concentrations for various tissues. The acceptance criteria for STDs and QCs in the qualification run were within ±30% of the precision and accuracy which is acceptable for the early stage drug discovery. Calibration was done by establishing a quadratic regression function, with an equation $y = ax^2 + bx + c$ after 1/concentration weighting. The accuracy was calculated at each QC concentration as the ratio of the measured concentration to the nominal concentration multiplied by 100%.

A preliminary stability test was conducted in mouse plasma and various tissue (heart, liver, spleen, kidney, and brain) samples under different conditions, such as short-term, long-term, and freeze-thaw stability using triplicates of high QC samples (2 μg/mL for plasma and 4 μg/mL for tissues). The short-term stability was determined at room temperature for 3 h. The long-term stability was determined after two weeks by analyzing QC samples kept frozen at −80 °C. For the freeze-thaw stability, the samples were subjected to three freeze and thaw cycles at −80 °C. The acceptance criteria for all stability tests were within ±30% of the precision and accuracy.

2.7. Software

Analyst® TF Version 1.6 (Sciex, Foster City, CA, USA) operated with Windows® (Microsoft Corp., Redmond, WA, USA) was used for the instrument control as well as the data acquisition. MultiQuant® Version 2.1.1 (Sciex, Foster City, CA, USA) was used for the peak integration. Excel 2015 (Microsoft) was used for all calculations including peak area ratios, standard curve regressions, sample concentration values, and descriptive statistics.

2.8. Application for Animal Study

Fabry disease model mice, generated on a 129SVJ X C57BL/6 background by targeted disruption of the murine α-Gal A gene (*Gla*), have been used in various studies [29,30]. These B6;129-Gla[tm1Kul]/J (also known as α-Gal A KO) mice, purchased from the Jackson laboratory (JAX stock #003535, 600 Main Street, BH, ME USA), were maintained by brother X sister mating. Male KO mice used in this study were selected by genotyping using polymerase chain reaction (PCR) analysis in tail snip DNA. Wild-type mice with the ICR strain were used as controls throughout the studies. Mice were housed in groups of 2–5 per cage under standard housing conditions. Mice were given a standard rodent diet and housed in a pathogen-free animal facility.

Mice were distributed into three different groups (four mice per group; 10, 12, and 14 weeks of age) to measure the age-related GB3 level changes in KO and WT male mice. All the KO mice were compared to WT mice for the relative GB3 levels in plasma and each of the tissues. At the study completion point, each of the mice was euthanized with CO_2. Whole blood was collected in a cluster tube and then centrifuged at 10,000 rpm for 5 min (4 °C). After centrifugation, the supernatant plasma layer was transferred to another cluster tube and stored in a deep freezer at −80 °C until analysis. Tissues (heart, liver, spleen, kidney, brain) were quickly removed, rinsed in cold phosphate-buffered saline (PBS) and stored in the deep freezer at −80 °C until analysis.

All procedures performed on the mice were reviewed and approved by the Institutional Animal Care and Use Committee (IACUC) of Samsung Biomedical Research Institute (Identification code: 20160216002, approval date: 9 March 2016) and were conducted in accord with guidelines established by the Association for Assessment and Accreditation of Laboratory Animal Care International (AAALAC International).

3. Results

3.1. Method Development: Sample Preparation and LC-MS/MS Analysis

At the early stage of biomarker research, quick identification of the GB3 level from a small amount of plasma/tissue samples from Fabry disease model is important. In the previous studies, several time-consuming sample preparation methods have been reported, including sample enrichment, such as evaporation/reconstitution steps and purification steps (LLE, SPE) [16,22,25–28]. These methods took a lot of time for sample preparation and also require a large amount (>100 μL) of study samples. In addition, none of the previous studies were done for the GB3 level in the Fabry model mice (B6;129-Gla^{tm1Kul}/J) to our knowledge in various tissues, including brains, which was developed by our own lab. Due to significantly different levels of GB3 and its analogs in plasma, as well as in various tissues, developing a method that can cover all these various study samples is very challenging. Therefore, we have focused on the development of a rapid sample preparation procedure with the usage of a less amount of plasma/tissue samples for the in vivo Fabry biomarker study. As a result, we developed a simple protein-precipitation method using minimum amount (10 μL) of samples without evaporation/reconstitution, derivatization steps or sample purification steps (solid phase extraction or liquid-liquid extraction). We also shortened the total chromatographic run time in LC-MS to 4 min and maximized sample analytical efficiency. Compared to the previous studies [18–20,26–28], our method met our throughput acceptance criteria (>300 plasma and tissue samples per day) using a small amount of study samples without further enrichment/purification for sample preparation procedure.

A liquid chromatography–quadrupole time-of-flight mass spectrometric method (LC-QTOF-MS/MS) in the positive ion mode was used to identify GB3 major isoforms. The most abundant ion in the full scan mode was the sodium adduct $[M + Na]^+$ ion for all GB3 isoforms. Due to the heterogeneous fatty acid components of GB3, the most abundant six isoforms were selected for the quantitation: m/z 1046.7 (C16:0), m/z 1102.7 (C20:0), m/z 1130.8 (C22:0), m/z 1156.8 (C24:1), m/z 1158.8 (C24:0), and m/z 1174.8 (C24:0-OH) (Figure 3). Each ion was detected using the single reaction monitoring with the high sensitivity (SRMHS) mode. The product ion showing the most abundant intensity was still the intact parent ion itself when the optimized collision energy was used. Due to the high resolution and accurate mass specificity of the TOF-MS the parent-to-parent ion transition was considered to be applicable [31], and the LC-MS chromatogram also showed good separation (Figure 4). Therefore, this parent-to-parent ion transition approach was used for the analysis of all GB3 isoforms in this study. Although the parent-daughter ion transition by the loss of 162 (except C24:0-OH) was not used for the quantitation of Gb3 isoforms, the unique transitions by the loss of 162 have been monitored as secondary transitions for the confirmation purpose of Gb3 isoforms. The broader peak width of C24:0-OH than those of other GB3 isoforms was likely due to the interaction between the hydroxyl group of C24:0-OH and the column stationary phase.

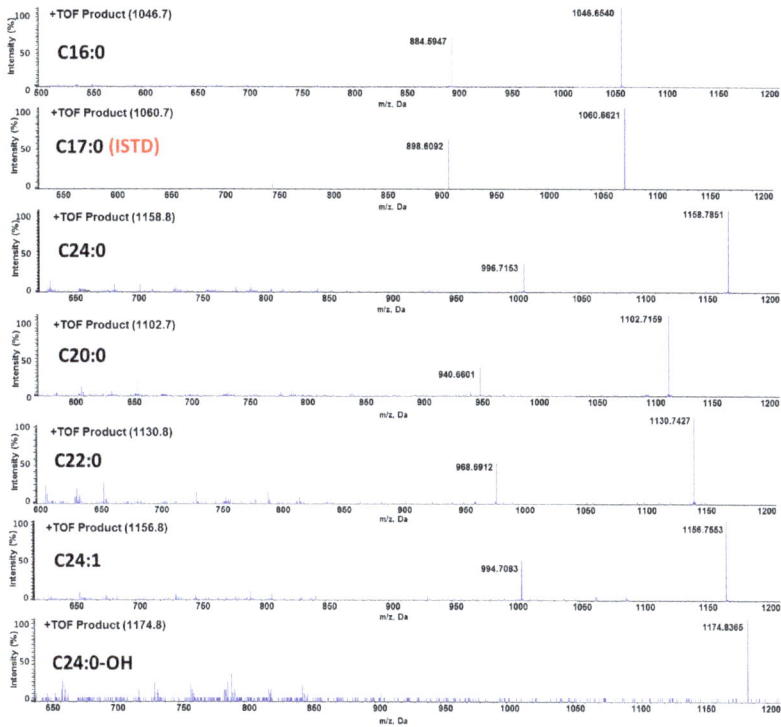

Figure 3. Product ion mass spectra of six GB3 isoforms and internal standard (ISTD).

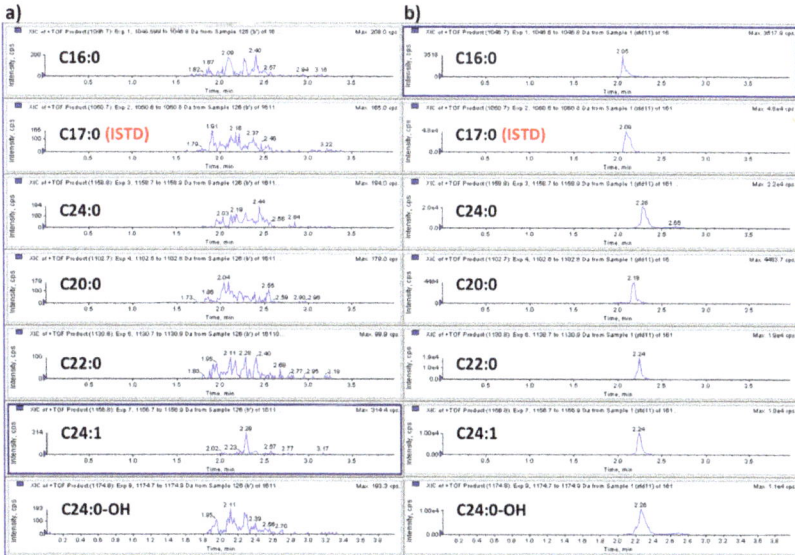

Figure 4. (**a**) LC-MS chromatograms of blank plasma, and (**b**) LC-MS chromatograms of GB3 spiked plasma.

3.2. Method Qualification

3.2.1. Calibration Curve, Accuracy, and Precision

Calibration curves with ten points (plasma, heart) and eleven points (liver, spleen, brain, kidney) were freshly prepared in duplicate for all datasets. The lower limit of quantification (LLOQ) of the assay was determined to be 0.042 µg/mL for plasma and 0.082 µg/g for all tissues based on the signal-to-noise ratio >5, respectively. The final concentration of the calibration curve range was 0.042–10 µg/mL for GB3 in plasma (10 levels) and 0.082–20 µg/g for GB3 in tissues (10 levels in heart and 11 levels in liver, spleen, kidney, and brain). One advantage of TOF mass spectrometer is the flexibility of MS data processing after acquisition. Therefore, based on the selectivity or sensitivity required for the experiment, various ion extraction width (e.g., 0.2 amu to 0.05 amu, or smaller) could be used to construct the flexible calibration curves, if needed. The quadratic regression of the curves for peak area ratios versus concentrations were weighted by 1/concentration. Calculated coefficient of determination (r) values for calibration curves were used to evaluate the fit of the curves. The correlation coefficient of the calibration curves for plasma and each of the tissues were ≥ 0.98 and are shown in Figure 5. Assay performance was determined by assessing precision (RSD (%)) and mean accuracy (%) of the QC samples and the results are shown in Table 2. Within-run accuracy and precision were evaluated using triplicates from each of the two QC concentrations. The within-run accuracy met the acceptance criteria of ±30%, ranging from 75 to 110% with precision values (RSD (%)) $\leq 30\%$ for plasma and tissue samples, which is acceptable for an early stage biomarker study.

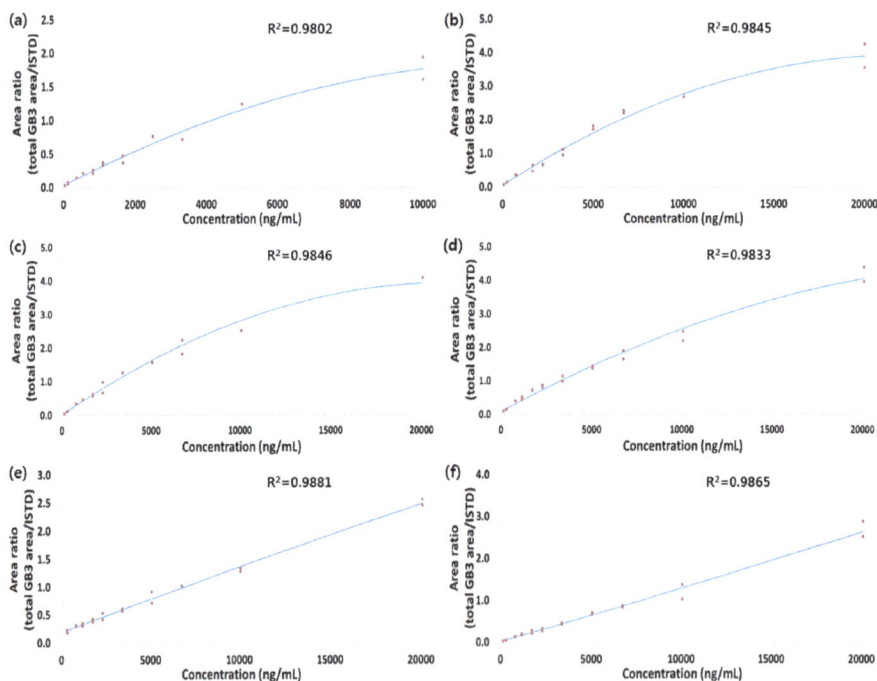

Figure 5. Calibration curve of GB3 in (**a**) plasma; (**b**) heart; (**c**) liver; (**d**) spleen; (**e**) kidney; and (**f**) brain.

Table 2. Quality control results and statistics from the qualification run for Globotriaosylceramide (GB3).

Matrix	QC Samples	Mean Concentration (ng/mL)	RSD (%)	Mean Accuracy (%)	n
Plasma	QC medium (400 ng/mL)	314.28	15.06	78.57	3
	QC high (2000 ng/mL)	2131.34	5.92	106.57	3
Heart	QC medium (800 ng/mL)	779.48	11.96	99.02	3
	QC high (4000 ng/mL)	3286.93	8.41	83.23	3
Liver	QC medium (800 ng/mL)	823.21	14.53	102.90	3
	QC high (4000 ng/mL)	3395.26	8.66	84.88	3
Spleen	QC medium (800 ng/mL)	848.22	10.64	106.03	3
	QC high (4000 ng/mL)	3861.45	25.49	96.54	3
Kidney	QC medium (800 ng/mL)	839.15	26.16	104.89	3
	QC high (4000 ng/mL)	4275.53	9.38	106.89	3
Brain	QC medium (800 ng/mL)	740.97	11.60	92.62	3
	QC high (4000 ng/mL)	3826.03	15.16	95.65	3

3.2.2. Preliminary Stability

Stability assessments were carried out to demonstrate that GB3 (either its stock solution or the spiked samples) was stable under certain sample storage and processing conditions. All of the stability tests were conducted in mouse plasma and various tissues (heart, liver, spleen, kidney, and brain) samples using triplicates of high QC samples (2 µg/mL for plasma and 4 µg/mL for tissues).

Typically three levels of QC samples (low, medium, and high) are used for the full bioanalytical method validation. However, our method is not for the full bioanalytical method validation for the IND enabling study but for the fit-for-purpose qualification method of the Gb3 biomarker at the early discovery stage for the Fabry disease mouse model. The Fabry disease model mouse normally generates very high levels of Gb3 isoforms and, therefore, one level of QCs (high) would be sufficient to demonstrate the integrity of our stability experiment. Each of the stability results are shown in Tables 3–5.

Table 3. Short-term stability results for GB3.

Matrix	Time Point (min)	Mean Area Ratio	RSD (%)	Mean Accuracy (%)	n
Plasma	0	3.78	6.54	100.00	
	60	3.27	6.02	86.66	
	120	3.64	9.04	96.49	3
	180	4.12	13.53	109.20	
Heart	0	3.06	12.10	100.00	
	60	3.09	1.70	101.09	
	120	2.88	9.98	94.34	3
	180	2.53	12.23	82.83	
Liver	0	3.14	9.73	100.00	
	60	3.07	12.30	97.80	
	120	3.17	12.58	100.97	3
	180	3.01	3.92	95.85	
Spleen	0	3.51	8.45	100.00	
	60	2.89	8.54	82.31	
	120	3.02	11.61	86.14	3
	180	2.50	3.18	71.32	
Kidney	0	2.42	10.26	100.00	
	60	3.03	2.88	125.16	
	120	2.95	14.21	121.72	3
	180	2.69	5.63	111.00	
Brain	0	1.48	3.70	100.00	
	60	1.37	16.01	92.77	
	120	1.37	16.97	92.42	3
	180	1.55	16.97	105.07	

Table 4. Freeze-thaw stability results for GB3.

Matrix	Control/FT-3 Cycle	Mean Area Ratio	RSD (%)	Mean Accuracy (%)	n
Plasma	Control	2.31	1.91	100.00	3
	FT-3 cycle	2.24	7.97	97.14	
Heart	Control	2.27	11.81	100.00	3
	FT-3 cycle	2.19	7.70	96.63	
Liver	Control	1.93	1.43	100.00	3
	FT-3 cycle	1.97	21.40	102.16	
Spleen	Control	2.23	6.15	100.00	3
	FT-3 cycle	2.12	10.07	95.20	
Kidney	Control	2.14	5.96	100.00	3
	FT-3 cycle	2.11	14.91	98.69	
Brain	Control	1.34	7.09	100.00	3
	FT-3 cycle	1.32	5.68	98.21	

Table 5. Long-term stability results for GB3.

Organ	Week	Mean Area Ratio	RSD (%)	Mean Accuracy (%)	n
Plasma	0 week	2.26	3.36	100	3
	1 week	2.29	14.55	101.46	3
	2 week	2.27	11.23	100.23	3
Heart	0 week	3.62	17.56	100	3
	1 week	3.81	8.19	105.32	3
	2 week	3.94	12.43	108.84	3
Liver	0 week	2.76	12.83	100	3
	1 week	2.52	0.73	91.18	3
	2 week	3.08	6.72	111.51	3
Spleen	0 week	4.05	4.44	100	3
	1 week	3.73	15.32	91.91	3
	2 week	3.72	5.13	91.8	3
Kidney	0 week	2.63	14.47	100	3
	1 week	2.69	10.44	102.31	3
	2 week	2.77	11.44	105.4	3
Brain	0 week	0.82	10.86	100	3
	1 week	0.8	7.71	97.46	3
	2 week	0.77	21.72	93.86	3

The stability tests for plasma were performed using triplicate of QC samples at high QC (2 μg/mL) level. The peak area ratio between total GB3 (six isoforms) and ISTD was used for the stability evaluation. The preliminary stability test showed GB3 in plasma QC sample was stable for at least 3 h at room temperature and three freeze-thaw cycles and at least two weeks of stability while storage at $-20\,^{\circ}$C with a precision value (RSD (%)) within 30% and the mean accuracy within ±30%.

The stability tests for various tissue samples were also performed using triplicate of QC samples at high QC (4 μg/mL) level. The peak area ratio between total GB3 (six isoforms) and ISTD was used for the stability evaluation. GB3 in mouse plasma and tissue QC samples were stable for at least 3 h at room temperature and three freeze-thaw cycles and at least two weeks of stability while storage at $-20\,^{\circ}$C with a precision value (RSD (%)) within 30% and the mean accuracy within ±30%.

3.3. Application for Animal Study

This LC-QTOF-MS/MS method was successfully applied for the quantification of GB3 in mouse plasma and tissue homogenate samples. We compared the average GB3 level in wild-type (WT, ICR strain) mouse (*n* = 12) to B6;129-Gla^{tm1Kul}/J (*α-Gal A* Knock Out (KO)) mouse (*n* = 12) and the results are shown in Figure 6. The results show that GB3 accumulates significantly in the Fabry model mouse (plasma: 4.85–5.35 μg/mL; heart: 2.39–3.13 μg/mg; liver: 2.53–3.58 μg/mg; kidney: 6.81–7.05 μg/mg; spleen: 8.77–14.37 μg/mg; brain: 0.36–0.54 μg/mg) when compared to that in the ICR mice tested in this experiment (plasma: 19–21 ng/mL; heart: 3.16–4.14 ng/mg; liver: 3.05–4.32 ng/mg;

kidney: 69.0–71.5 ng/mg; spleen: 4.74–7.76 ng/mg; brain: 4.70–7.05 ng/mg). Since this Fabry model mouse B6;129-Gla^tm1Kul/J was newly developed in our lab, this was the first time to report the various GB3 isoform ratios in this mouse model. A supplementary LC-MS chromatogram of GB3 in plasma and tissues are also shown in Figure 7.

The age-related GB3 level change was also monitored in this study and the results are shown in Figure 8. In general, no significant increase of GB3 was observed in plasma, heart, liver, kidney, and brain. However, approximately 63.9% increase was observed in the spleen over a four week period (aged 10 to 14 weeks). This would be an important factor to consider when designing the study protocol in the future.

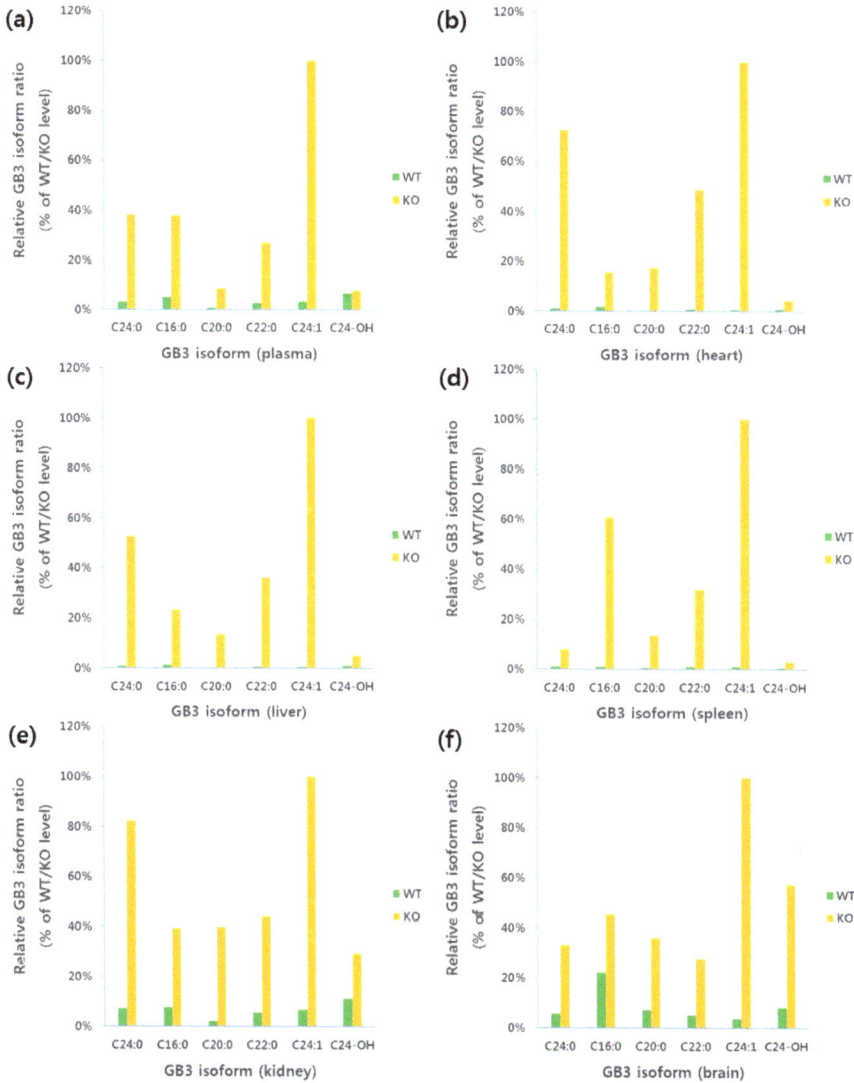

Figure 6. Relative GB3 isoform ratio in plasma and each of the tissues: (**a**) plasma; (**b**) heart; (**c**) liver; (**d**) spleen; (**e**) kidney; and (**f**) brain.

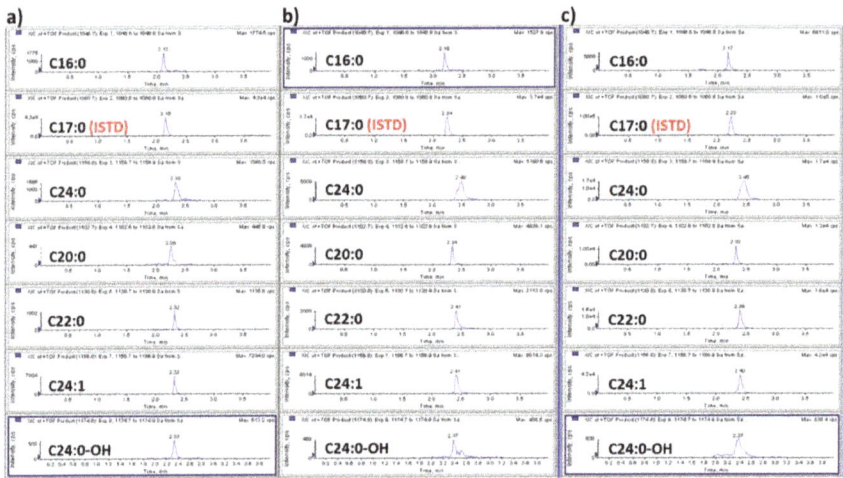

Figure 7. LC-MS chromatograms of GB3 in (**a**) plasma; (**b**) heart; and (**c**) spleen from the Fabry disease model mouse.

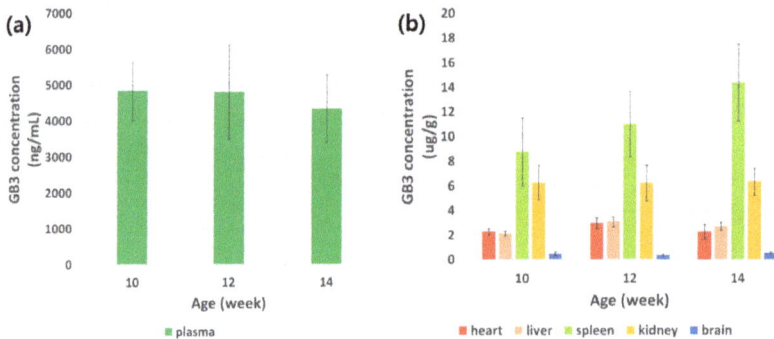

Figure 8. Age-related GB3 level changes in (**a**) plasma, and (**b**) tissues.

4. Discussion

During the early stage of Fabry disease drug discovery, it is very critical to screen the drug candidates with decent throughput. Since GB3 is an excellent biomarker which can represent the stage of Fabry disease in the Fabry model mice, we have developed a simple and robust bioanalytical method for the quantitation of GB3, particularly for the Fabry model mouse B6;129-Gla[tm1Kul]/J for the first time. This method also met our throughput criteria (>300 plasma and tissue samples per day) which were sufficient enough to cover the compounds in the screening stage.

The calibration curve was produced in plasma as well as each of the tissues separately with a final concentration of the calibration curve range was 0.042–10 µg/mL for GB3 in plasma and 0.082–20 µg/g for GB3 in tissues, respectively. For assay performance, the within-run accuracy met the acceptance criteria of ±30% which ranged from 75 to 110% with precision values ≤30% for plasma and tissue samples, which is acceptable for early drug discovery. A preliminary stability test including short-term (1, 2, and 3 h), freeze-thaw (three cycles), and long-term stability (one and two weeks) show the precision and accuracy values within the acceptance criteria of ±30%.

Pharmaceutics **2018**, *10*, 69

The assay was also applied for the quantification of GB3 in Fabry model mice (B6;129-Gla^{tm1Kul}/J) and wild-type mice (ICR strain) for the first time. The result shows that GB3 accumulates significantly in the Fabry model mouse with a relative difference in isoform ratios for each of the organs. There was no meaningful alteration of the GB3 level dependent to disease progression in plasma, heart, liver, kidney, and brain. However, GB3 level in spleen shows a meaningful age-related increase (>60% increase in four weeks) of GB3 level. Due to this method, we were able to screen many Fabry drug candidates for their efficacy of lowering GB3 levels in various tissues, as well as in plasma samples. This was particularly very important to evaluate the drug candidate's efficacy in brain which is extremely critical for the drug candidate's efficacy from the central nerve systems' perspectives.

In conclusion, this rapid LC-QTOF-MS/MS method was very useful for the screening of drug candidates to evaluate their in vivo efficacy, as well as biomarker studies in the Fabry model mice.

Author Contributions: S.-H.S., M.-H.P. and Y.G.S. designed the experiment; A.-r.K., M.-r.-S., S.L., M.R.K. and D.-K.J. developed and provided the animal model; S.-H.S., M.-H.P., J.-J.B., B.i.L. and Y.P. performed the experiments; S.-H.S. analyzed and calculated the data; J.S., M.E.J. and Y.G.S. reviewed the data; S.-H.S. wrote the paper; Y.G.S. and D.-K.J. reviewed and revised the paper.

Funding: This research received no external funding.

Acknowledgments: This research was supported by a grant of the Korea Health Technology R and D Project through the Korea Health Industry Development Institute (KHIDI), funded by the Ministry of Health and Welfare, Republic of Korea (grant number: HI13D2351).

Conflicts of Interest: The authors declare no conflict of interest.

References

1. Brady, R.O. Enzymatic abnormalities in diseases of sphingolipid metabolism. *Clin. Chem.* **1967**, *13*, 565–577. [PubMed]
2. Fabry, H. An historical overview of Fabry disease. *J. Inherit. Metab. Dis.* **2001**, *24* (Suppl. 2), 3–7. [CrossRef] [PubMed]
3. Desnick, R.J.; Allen, K.Y.; Simmons, R.L.; Woods, J.E.; Anderson, C.F.; Najarian, J.S.; Krivit, W. Fabry disease: Correction of the enzymatic deficiency by renal transplantation. *Birth Defects Orig. Artic. Ser.* **1973**, *9*, 88–96. [PubMed]
4. Desnick, R.J.; Brady, R.; Barranger, J.; Collins, A.J.; Germain, D.P.; Goldman, M.; Grabowski, G.; Packman, S.; Wilcox, W.R. Fabry disease, an under-recognized multisystemic disorder: Expert recommendations for diagnosis, management, and enzyme replacement therapy. *Ann. Intern. Med.* **2003**, *138*, 338–346. [CrossRef] [PubMed]
5. Thurberg, B.L.; Rennke, H.; Colvin, R.B.; Dikman, S.; Gordon, R.E.; Collins, A.B.; Desnick, R.J.; O'Callaghan, M. Globotriaosylceramide accumulation in the Fabry kidney is cleared from multiple cell types after enzyme replacement therapy. *Kidney Int.* **2002**, *62*, 1933–1946. [CrossRef] [PubMed]
6. MacDermot, K.D.; Holmes, A.; Miners, A.H. Anderson-Fabry disease: Clinical manifestations and impact of disease in a cohort of 98 hemizygous males. *J. Med. Genet.* **2001**, *38*, 750–760. [CrossRef] [PubMed]
7. MacDermot, K.D.; Holmes, A.; Miners, A.H. Anderson-Fabry disease: Clinical manifestations and impact of disease in a cohort of 60 obligate carrier females. *J. Med. Genet.* **2001**, *38*, 769–775. [CrossRef] [PubMed]
8. Brady, R.O.; Tallman, J.F.; Johnson, W.G.; Gal, A.E.; Leahy, W.R.; Quirk, J.M.; Dekaban, A.S. Replacement therapy for inherited enzyme deficiency. Use of purified ceramidetrihexosidase in Fabry's disease. *N. Engl. J. Med.* **1973**, *289*, 9–14. [CrossRef] [PubMed]
9. Eng, C.M.; Guffon, N.; Wilcox, W.R.; Germain, D.P.; Lee, P.; Waldek, S.; Caplan, L.; Linthorst, G.E.; Desnick, R.J.; International Collaborative Fabry Disease Study Group. Safety and efficacy of recombinant human α-galactosidase A replacement therapy in Fabry's disease. *N. Engl. J. Med.* **2001**, *345*, 9–16. [CrossRef] [PubMed]
10. Schiffmann, R.; Ries, M.; Timmons, M.; Flaherty, J.T.; Brady, R.O. Long-term therapy with agalsidase alfa for Fabry disease: Safety and effects on renal function in a home infusion setting. *Nephrol. Dial. Transplant.* **2006**, *21*, 345–354. [CrossRef] [PubMed]

11. Valenzano, K.J.; Khanna, R.; Powe, A.C.; Boyd, R.; Lee, G.; Flanagan, J.J.; Benjamin, E.R. Identification and characterization of pharmacological chaperones to correct enzyme deficiencies in lysosomal storage disorders. *Assay Drug Dev. Technol.* **2011**, *9*, 213–235. [CrossRef] [PubMed]

12. Yam, G.H.; Bosshard, N.; Zuber, C.; Steinmann, B.; Roth, J. Pharmacological chaperone corrects lysosomal storage in Fabry disease caused by trafficking-incompetent variants. *Am. J. Physiol. Cell Physiol.* **2006**, *290*, C1076–C1082. [CrossRef] [PubMed]

13. Young-Gqamana, B.; Brignol, N.; Chang, H.H.; Khanna, R.; Soska, R.; Fuller, M.; Sitaraman, S.A.; Germain, D.P.; Giugliani, R.; Hughes, D.A.; et al. Migalastat HCl reduces globotriaosylsphingosine (lyso-Gb3) in Fabry transgenic mice and in the plasma of Fabry patients. *PLoS ONE* **2013**, *8*, e57631. [CrossRef] [PubMed]

14. Kitagawa, T.; Ishige, N.; Suzuki, K.; Owada, M.; Ohashi, T.; Kobayashi, M.; Eto, Y.; Tanaka, A.; Mills, K.; Winchester, B.; et al. Non-invasive screening method for Fabry disease by measuring globotriaosylceramide in whole urine samples using tandem mass spectrometry. *Mol. Genet. Metab.* **2005**, *85*, 196–202. [CrossRef] [PubMed]

15. Whitfield, P.D.; Calvin, J.; Hogg, S.; O'Driscoll, E.; Halsall, D.; Burling, K.; Maguire, G.; Wright, N.; Cox, T.M.; Meikle, P.J.; et al. Monitoring enzyme replacement therapy in Fabry disease—Role of urine globotriaosylceramide. *J. Inherit. Metab. Dis.* **2005**, *28*, 21–33. [CrossRef] [PubMed]

16. Auray-Blais, C.; Cyr, D.; Ntwari, A.; West, M.L.; Cox-Brinkman, J.; Bichet, D.G.; Germain, D.P.; Laframboise, R.; Melancon, S.B.; Stockley, T.; et al. Urinary globotriaosylceramide excretion correlates with the genotype in children and adults with Fabry disease. *Mol. Genet. Metab.* **2008**, *93*, 331–340. [CrossRef] [PubMed]

17. Nelson, B.C.; Roddy, T.; Araghi, S.; Wilkens, D.; Thomas, J.J.; Zhang, K.; Sung, C.C.; Richards, S.M. Globotriaosylceramide isoform profiles in human plasma by liquid chromatography-tandem mass spectrometry. *J. Chromatogr. B Anal. Technol. Biomed. Life Sci.* **2004**, *805*, 127–134. [CrossRef] [PubMed]

18. Hozumi, I.; Nishizawa, M.; Ariga, T.; Miyatake, T. Biochemical and clinical analysis of accumulated glycolipids in symptomatic heterozygotes of angiokeratoma corporis diffusum (Fabry's disease) in comparison with hemizygotes. *J. Lipid Res.* **1990**, *31*, 335–340. [PubMed]

19. Kniep, B.; Muhlradt, P.F. Immunochemical detection of glycosphingolipids on thin-layer chromatograms. *Anal. Biochem.* **1990**, *188*, 5–8. [CrossRef]

20. Groener, J.E.; Poorthuis, B.J.; Kuiper, S.; Helmond, M.T.; Hollak, C.E.; Aerts, J.M. HPLC for simultaneous quantification of total ceramide, glucosylceramide, and ceramide trihexoside concentrations in plasma. *Clin. Chem.* **2007**, *53*, 742–747. [CrossRef] [PubMed]

21. Fauler, G.; Rechberger, G.N.; Devrnja, D.; Erwa, W.; Plecko, B.; Kotanko, P.; Breunig, F.; Paschke, E. Rapid determination of urinary globotriaosylceramide isoform profiles by electrospray ionization mass spectrometry using stearoyl-d35-globotriaosylceramide as internal standard. *Rapid Commun. Mass Spectrom.* **2005**, *19*, 1499–1506. [CrossRef] [PubMed]

22. Auray-Blais, C.; Boutin, M. Novel Gb(3) isoforms detected in urine of fabry disease patients: A metabolomic study. *Curr. Med. Chem.* **2012**, *19*, 3241–3252. [CrossRef] [PubMed]

23. Sueoka, H.; Aoki, M.; Tsukimura, T.; Togawa, T.; Sakuraba, H. Distributions of Globotriaosylceramide Isoforms, and Globotriaosylsphingosine and Its Analogues in an α-Galactosidase A Knockout Mouse, a Model of Fabry Disease. *PLoS ONE* **2015**, *10*, e0144958. [CrossRef] [PubMed]

24. Alharbi, F.J.; Geberhiwot, T.; Hughes, D.A.; Ward, D.G. A Novel Rapid MALDI-TOF-MS-Based Method for Measuring Urinary Globotriaosylceramide in Fabry Patients. *J. Am. Soc. Mass Spectrom.* **2016**, *27*, 719–725. [CrossRef] [PubMed]

25. Kruger, R.; Bruns, K.; Grunhage, S.; Rossmann, H.; Reinke, J.; Beck, M.; Lackner, K.J. Determination of globotriaosylceramide in plasma and urine by mass spectrometry. *Clin. Chem. Lab. Med.* **2010**, *48*, 189–198. [CrossRef] [PubMed]

26. Boutin, M.; Menkovic, I.; Martineau, T.; Vaillancourt-Lavigueur, V.; Toupin, A.; Auray-Blais, C. Separation and Analysis of Lactosylceramide, Galabiosylceramide, and Globotriaosylceramide by LC-MS/MS in Urine of Fabry Disease Patients. *Anal. Chem.* **2017**, *89*, 13382–13390. [CrossRef] [PubMed]

27. Polo, G.; Burlina, A.P.; Kolamunnage, T.B.; Zampieri, M.; Dionisi-Vici, C.; Strisciuglio, P.; Zaninotto, M.; Plebani, M.; Burlina, A.B. Diagnosis of sphingolipidoses: A new simultaneous measurement of lysosphingolipids by LC-MS/MS. *Clin. Chem. Lab. Med.* **2017**, *55*, 403–414. [CrossRef] [PubMed]

28. Boutin, M.; Gagnon, R.; Lavoie, P.; Auray-Blais, C. LC-MS/MS analysis of plasma lyso-Gb3 in Fabry disease. *Clin. Chim. Acta* **2012**, *414*, 273–280. [CrossRef] [PubMed]

29. Ioannou, Y.A.; Zeidner, K.M.; Gordon, R.E.; Desnick, R.J. Fabry disease: Preclinical studies demonstrate the effectiveness of α-galactosidase A replacement in enzyme-deficient mice. *Am. J. Hum. Genet.* **2001**, *68*, 14–25. [CrossRef] [PubMed]

30. Ohshima, T.; Murray, G.J.; Swaim, W.D.; Longenecker, G.; Quirk, J.M.; Cardarelli, C.O.; Sugimoto, Y.; Pastan, I.; Gottesman, M.M.; Brady, R.O.; et al. α-Galactosidase A deficient mice: A model of Fabry disease. *Proc. Natl. Acad. Sci. USA* **1997**, *94*, 2540–2544. [CrossRef] [PubMed]

31. Ramagiri, S.; Garofolo, F. Large molecule bioanalysis using Q-TOF without predigestion and its data processing challenges. *Bioanalysis* **2012**, *4*, 529–540. [CrossRef] [PubMed]

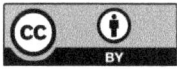

![pharmaceutics logo] *pharmaceutics*

MDPI

Article

Qualification and Application of a Liquid Chromatography-Quadrupole Time-of-Flight Mass Spectrometric Method for the Determination of Adalimumab in Rat Plasma

Yuri Park, Nahye Kim, Jangmi Choi, Min-Ho Park, Byeong ill Lee, Seok-Ho Shin, Jin-Ju Byeon and Young G. Shin

College of Pharmacy and Institute of Drug Research and Development, Chungnam National University, Daejeon 34134, Korea; yuri.park.cnu@gmail.com (Y.P.); nahye.kim.cnu@gmail.com (N.K.); jangmi.choi.cnu@gmail.com (J.C.); minho.park.cnu@gmail.com (M.-H.P.); byungill.lee.cnu@gmail.com (B.i.L.); seokho.shin.cnu@gmail.com (S.-H.S.); jinju.byeon.cnu@gmail.com (J.-J.B.)
* Correspondence: yshin@cnu.ac.kr; Tel.: +82-42-821-5931

Received: 16 April 2018; Accepted: 21 May 2018; Published: 24 May 2018

Abstract: A liquid chromatography–quadrupole time-of-flight (Q-TOF) mass spectrometric method was developed for early-stage research on adalimumab in rats. The method consisted of immunoprecipitation followed by tryptic digestion for sample preparation and LC-QTOF-MS/MS analysis of specific signature peptides of adalimumab in the positive ion mode using electrospray ionization. This specific signature peptide is derived from the complementarity-determining region (CDR) of adalimumab. A quadratic regression (weighted 1/concentration), with an equation $y = ax^2 + bx + c$, was used to fit calibration curves over the concentration range of 1–100 µg/mL for adalimumab. The qualification run met the acceptance criteria of ±25% accuracy and precision values for quality control (QC) samples. This qualified LC-QTOF-MS/MS method was successfully applied to a pharmacokinetic study of adalimumab in rats as a case study. This LC-QTOF-MS/MS approach would be useful as a complementary method for adalimumab or its biosimilars at an early stage of research.

Keywords: adalimumab; immunoprecipitation; liquid chromatography-quadrupole TOF MS; bioanalysis

1. Introduction

Since humanized and fully human monoclonal antibodies (mAbs) were approved as therapeutic pharmaceutical products, the attention for monoclonal antibody products has been growing significantly in the global pharmaceutical market [1,2].

Therapeutic mAbs offer many advantages when compared to small-molecule drugs [3]. In general, mAbs have three main characteristics: (i) target-specific binding ability to increase or decrease an important biological effect, (ii) interaction of the constant domain with cell surface receptors that causes immune-mediated effector functions, including antibody-dependent cell-mediated cytotoxicity (ADCC), complement dependent cytotoxicity (CDC) or antibody-dependent phagocytosis; and (iii) deposition of complement on multimeric immune complexes between the mAb and the target and subsequent activation of complement-dependent cytotoxicity [2,4].

Tumor necrosis factor α (TNF-α) is an inflammatory cytokine produced by activated monocytes or macrophages [5]. Therefore, TNF-α antagonist (anti-TNF) is one of the agents that has the highest affinity for TNF-α molecules and suppresses the biological activity of TNF-α [6]. One of the well-known anti-TNF drugs is adalimumab, which consists of a fully humanized monoclonal antibody and was approved by the FDA in 2002 [7]. Adalimumab is a tetramer composed of two heavy immunoglobulin G1 (IgG1) chains and two light IgG1 chains [7]. It is currently used to treat rheumatoid arthritis, psoriasis, psoriatic arthritis, ankylosing spondylitis and Crohn's disease [8].

Traditionally, pharmacokinetic evaluation of mAbs has been mainly performed by immunoassays such as enzyme-linked immunosorbent assays (ELISA), radioimmunoassay immunofluorescence assay and etc. [9]. Immunoassays have several advantages in terms of high sensitivity, robust performance and high throuput [2,10]. However, these methods also have several disadvantages such as non-specific binding as well as time-consuming and labor-intensive reagent development [8]. Immunoassays also often show cross-reactions with precursors of the target protein or with smaller metabolized fragments that are not suitable for early-stage mAbs bioanalysis [11].

Liquid chromatographic mass spectrometry (LC-MS/MS) is a complementary technique that can quantify not only small molecules or peptides but also proteins [12]. LC-MS/MS is accurate and precise and enables throughput analysis because this combines a robust separation technique with identification and quantification based on the molecular weights of the analytes [10]. In addition, LC-MS/MS is less matrix-dependent than ELISA [13].

The purpose of this paper is to explore an adalimumab quantification method using LC-QTOF-MS/MS and employing adalimumab's specific signature peptides that are involved in variable regions and produced by tryptic digestion.

2. Materials and Methods

2.1. Materials

Adalimumab was purchased from Dongwon Pharmaceutical Wholesale (Deajeon, Korea). Protein A magnetic beads were purchased from Millipore Corp (Billerica, MA, USA). RapiGest surfactant was purchased from Waters Korea (Seoul, Korea). 1,4-Dithiothreitol (DTT) was purchased from Carl Roth (Karlsruhe, Germany). Iodoacetic acid (IAA) was purchased from Wako (Osaka, Japan). The sequencing grade modified trypsin was purchased from Promega (Madison, WI, USA). All other chemicals were commercial products of analytical or reagent grade and were used without further purification.

2.2. Preparation of Stocks, Standard (STD) and Quality Control (QC) Samples

Stock solution of adalimumab was prepared at a concentration of 5000 µg/mL in a phosphate buffer solution (PBS) containing 0.1% tween 20. The stock solution was stored at 4 °C. Stock solution of adalimumab was further diluted at a concentration 500 µg/mL in PBS containing 0.1% tween 20 as sub-stock solution. Calibration working solution was prepared by serial dilution of the sub-stock solution with PBS containing 0.1% tween 20. Then, the working solution was spiked into rat plasma to yield calibration standard concentrations of 1.0, 2.0, 5.0, 10, 20, 40, 80 and 100 µg/mL. The quality control (QC) samples with final concentrations of 2.5, 25 and 50 µg/mL were also prepared in the same manner.

2.3. Preparation of Sample Digests for Quantification

Each 24 µL aliquot of plasma study samples, QCs and standards (STDs) were separately mixed with 370 µL of PBS containing 0.1% tween 20 and 30 µL of magnetic bead suspension. After gentle shaking at room temperature overnight, the magnetic bead was washed using 600 µL PBS containing 0.1% tween 20 and then was washed again using 600 µL PBS. Seventy-five microliters of RapiGest and 10 µL of DTT were added to the mixture, which was incubated for 50 min at 60 °C to denature and reduce the adalimumab bound to the magnetic beads. After a 10-min incubation at room temperature (RT), 25 µL of IAA was added and the sample was incubated in dark conditions for 30 min at RT. Ten microliters of the sequencing grade-modified trypsin were added to the sample to digest the antibody. After 1 min of shaking, the sample was incubated at 37 °C overnight. Fifteen microliters of

2 N HCl were added to the sample for quenching purposes and the sample was incubated for another 30 min at 37 °C to stop the digestion. The resulting sample was centrifuged at 7000 rpm for 5 min at 4 °C and transferred into a HPLC vial.

2.4. Liquid Chromatography–Mass Spectrometry

The liquid chromatography–mass spectrometry system consisted of a Shimadzu CBM-20A HPLC pump controller (Shimadzu Corporation, Columbia, MD, USA), two Shimadzu LC-20AD pumps, a CTC HTS PAL autosampler (CEAP Technologies, Carrboro, NC, USA) and a quadrupole time-of-flight (Q-TOF) TripleTOF^{TM} 5600 mass spectrometer (Sciex, Foster City, CA, USA). The analytical column used for this assay was a Phenomenex Kinetex Phenyl-hexyl column (50 × 2.1 mm, 2.6 μm). The mobile phase consisted of: mobile phase A, distilled and deionized water containing 0.1% formic acid; and mobile phase B, acetonitrile containing 0.1% formic acid. The gradient was as follows: from 0 min to 0.6 min, 5% B; from 0.5 min to 1.6 min by a linear gradient from 5% B to 95% B; 95% B was maintained for 0.2 min; from 1.8 min to 1.9 min by a linear gradient from 95% B to 5% B and then 5% B was maintained for 1.5 min for column re-equilibrium. The gradient was delivered at a flow rate of 0.4 mL/min and the injection volume was 10 μL.

The TOF-MS scan mass spectra and TOF-MS/MS scan mass spectra were recorded in the positive ion mode. For TOF-MS scan, m/z 100~950 with 0.2 s accumulation time was used. For TOF-MS/MS scan, the scan range was m/z 500~1000. For the quantification, doubly charged [M + 2H]$^{2+}$ ion for the specific signature peptide APYTFGQGTK (m/z 535.4) was selected and its product ion at m/z 901.8 was used for the quantitative analysis of adalimumab. High-purity nitrogen gas was used for the nebulizer/Duospray^{TM} and curtain gases. The ESI spray voltage was set at 5500 V. The source temperature was 500 °C. The curtain gas (CUR) was 30 L/min; the auxiliary gas setting (GS1 and GS2) was 50 L/min.

2.5. Method Qualification and Sample Analysis Procedure

2.5.1. Calibration Curve, Accuracy and Precision

Method qualification was carried out with a 'fit-for-purpose' approach. Quality control (QC) samples as well as standards (STDs) were used for batch acceptance. The qualification run contained duplicate calibration curves at eight concentrations and QCs at three concentrations (low, medium and high concentrations). The acceptance criterion for STDs and QCs in the qualification run was within ±25% of precision and accuracy, which is acceptable for early-stage drug discovery. Calibration curve was done by establishing a quadratic regression function, with an equation $y = ax^2 + bx + c$ after 1/concentration weighting. In addition, two blank plasma samples were in the set. QC samples (2.5, 25 and 50 μg/mL) were processed and analyzed three times in the same run (precision). The accuracy was calculated at each QC concentration as the ratio of the measured concentration to the nominal concentration multiplied by 100%.

2.5.2. Species-Dependent Matrix Effect

For species-dependent matrix effect test, three levels of QC samples were prepared in mouse and monkey plasma. Samples were quantitated with a calibration curve prepared in rat plasma. Mean accuracy and precision were also calculated.

2.5.3. Freeze and Thaw Stability

The freeze and thaw stability in rat, mouse and monkey plasma was assessed using low, medium and high QC samples (n = 3 at each concentration). For this study, the samples were subjected to three freeze and thaw cycles at −80 °C.

2.6. Software

Analyst® TF Version 1.6 (Sciex, Foster City, CA, USA) operated with Windows® (Microsoft) was used for instrument control and data acquisition. Peak integrations were operated by MultiQuant® Version 2.1.1 (Sciex, Foster City, CA, USA). Calculations including peak area ratios, standard curve regressions, sample concentration values and descriptive statistics were calculated with MultiQuant® Version 2.1.1. Pharmacokinetic calculations were performed using WinNonLin® version 6.4 (Pharsight Corporation, Mountain View, CA, USA).

2.7. Application for a Pharmacokinetic Study in Rat

Four adult male Sprague–Dawley rats (SD, 250–300 g) were purchased from the Samtako Biokorea Co. (Gyeonggi, Korea). The animals were housed in laminar flow cages that were maintained at $22 \pm 2\,^\circ$C and 50–60% relative humidity. The animals were kept in these facilities for at least a week prior to the experiment and were fasted for at least 24 h before the commencement of the experiments. Rats were cared for and treated in accordance with the Guiding Principles for the Use of Animals in Toxicology adopted by the Society of Toxicology (Reston, VA, USA) and the experimental protocols were approved by the Animal Care Committee of Chungnam National University (protocol No. CNU-00560).

Plasma samples were collected from the Sprague-Dawley rats ($n = 4$) after dosing intravenously with adalimumab at 1 mg/kg. The sampling times were 0.0014, 0.0417, 0.1667, 0.25, 1, 2, 3, 4, 7, 15, 21 and 28 days. The same set of pharmacokinetic study samples was analyzed by LC-QTOF-MS/MS.

3. Results

3.1. Method Development

3.1.1. Sample Preparation Method

In general, biological matrices such as plasma have highly abundant endogenous proteins such as albumin and immunoglobulins [14]. These endogenous proteins often interfere with the analysis of target mAb and decrease the sensitivity of the analyte. Therefore, a sample preparation method with minimal endogenous protein interference was necessary. To solve this problem, several approaches have been considered, such as albumin depletion kit, solid phase Protein A, and specific immunocapture [2,10,15]. In this study, the immunocapture using protein A magnetic beads was considered to be acceptable due to its selectivity as well as specificity. Plasma IgG and mAb were captured by a protein A magnetic bead and then washed out to remove other endogenous interference. After that, plasma IgG and mAb, bound to a protein A magnetic bead, were digested on-bead by the sequencing grade-modified trypsin. Trypsin-cleaved lysine and arginine residues in the amino acid sequence and various digested peptides from plasma IgG and mAbs were released into the supernatants. The supernatants were then analyzed by LC-QTOF-MS/MS for the target-specific signature peptide of adalimumab.

Generally, it would be ideal if trypsin digestion was carried out after acid dissociation and elution. However, one big challenge of this approach would be recovery from the protein A bead after binding. In addition, trypsin digestion efficiency is another challenge to consider due to lower pH after acid dissociation. Other matrix interference from endogenous immunoglobulins and etc. is another factor to carefully evaluate from this conventional trypsin digestion after acid dissociation followed by elution. Our approach, using on-bead digestion with trypsin, could have some disadvantages such as a large excess of tryptic peptide matrices derived from the protein A ligand, which might interfere with our assay. However, this method is very fast and robust and the interference from these endogenous matrix peptides could be minimized by selecting a specific signature peptide as well as its unique parent ion-product ion transition combination in the next section.

3.1.2. Selection of Target-Specific Signature Peptide

A couple of specific signature peptides were sought that would be applicable and specific to adalimumab using freeware software 'Skyline' (MacCoss Lab Software, https://skyline.ms/). As a result, three peptides out of various digested peptides were selected from the complementarity-determining region (CDR) of adalimumab. The three specific peptide sequences are as follows: NYLAWYQQKPGK, APYTFGQGTK and GLEWVSAITWNSGHIDYADSVEGR.

During the LC-QTOF-MS/MS analysis, two out of three peptides were detected (APYTFGQGTK and NYLAWYQQKPGK), while the GLEWVSAITWNSGHIDYADSVEGR peptide was not, possibly due to poor ionization. Although both APYTFGQGTK and NYLAWYQQKPGK peptides looks acceptable, APYTFGQGTK showed better peak intensity and better signal-to-noise ratio than NYLAWYQQKPGK in our experimental conditions (Figure 1). APYTFGQGTK was not detected in rat blank plasma or any other source during sample preparation and therefore was proven to be quite a unique signature peptide representing adalimumab. Therefore, APYTFGQGTK was chosen as the specific signature peptide for the quantitation of adalimumab in our experiment.

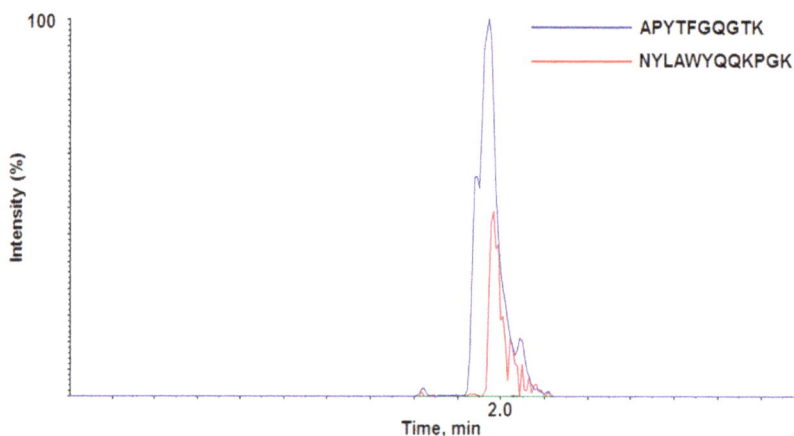

Figure 1. LC-QTOF-MS/MS chromatogram of the two proposed signature peptides.

Figure 2 shows the MS/MS spectrum of the adalimumab-specific signature peptide (APYTFGQGTK). From the doubly charged parent ion observed at m/z 535.27, several product ions were observed and the ion at m/z 901.45 showed the best sensitivity and selectivity.

3.1.3. Liquid Chromatography–Mass Spectrometry Analysis Using Quadrupole Time-of-Flight mass spectrometer

Conventionally, triple quadrupole mass spectrometers (low-resolution instrument) have been used for the quantitative analysis of small molecules. Recently, a Q-TOF mass spectrometer has been introduced to quantify large molecules such as proteins for pharmacokinetic studies [16]. In the past, Q-TOF had drawbacks in terms of sensitivity, linear dynamic range and speed, which meant it was unlikely to fill the need for reliable quantification in bioanalysis when compared to triple quadrupole mass spectrometer. However, the latest Q-TOF is good enough to overcome these shortcomings and shows good sensitivity and selectivity for the analysis of large molecules or peptides in single injection. In this study, the lower limit of quantification (LLOQ), accuracy, precision and linear dynamic range using LC-QTOF-MS/MS were good enough for our discovery non-GLP PK studies in rats.

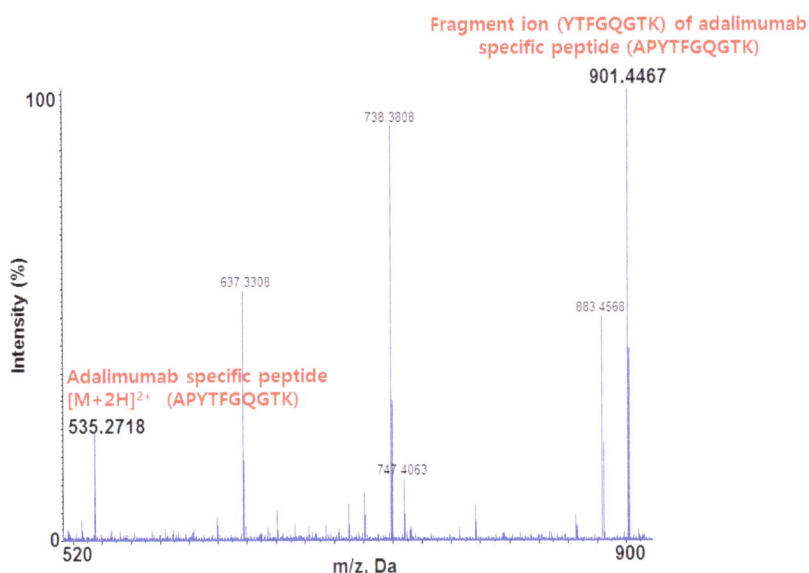

Figure 2. MS/MS spectrum of adalimumab specific peptide [M + 2H]$^{2+}$ and its fragment peptide.

3.2. Method Qualification

3.2.1. Calibration Curve, Linearity and Sensitivity

LC-QTOF-MS/MS analysis using the specific signature peptide in high-resolution mode was used for the quantitation of adalimumab. Calibration curves consisting of eight points in duplicate were prepared fresh for all datasets in rat plasma. The calibration curve range was 1–100 µg/mL. A representative chromatogram at the LLOQ (signal-to-noise ratio: ~9) is shown in Figure 3. This sensitivity was significant enough for most preclinical studies with a dose level ≥1 mg/kg to cover the expected concentration range throughout the PK time course. With a larger volume (~40 µL) of sample (or trypsin), more optimized conditions of LC-QTOF-MS/MS or a more sensitive mass spectrometer, we were also able to improve the LLOQ below 1 µg/mL in the preclinical species plasma, if needed (data not shown). The quadratic regression of the curves using peak area versus concentrations was weighted by 1/concentration. The calculated correlation coefficient value (r) for calibration curve was used to evaluate the linearity of the curve. The correlation coefficient of the calibration curve was ≥0.9931 and the LLOQ of 1 µg/mL was easily achieved in this method.

3.2.2. Accuracy, Precision and Species-Dependent Matrix Effect

Assay performance was determined by assessing inter/intra-day accuracy (%) and precision (%CV) of the QC samples (Table 1). Inter/intra-day accuracy and precision for rat plasma were performed using QC samples (*n* = 9) at low, medium and high QC levels. Accuracy (%) was defined as the calculated concentration, expressed as a percent deviation from nominal concentration. Precision was expressed as the percent coefficient of variation (%CV). The qualification run met the acceptance criteria of ±25% accuracy and precision for all QC samples.

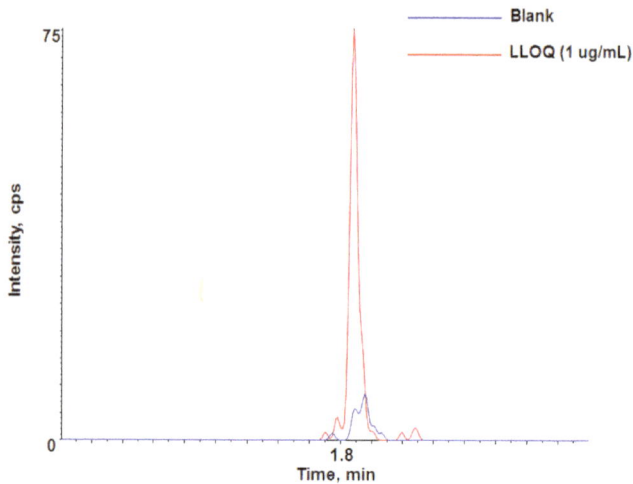

Figure 3. Representative chromatogram of lower limit of quantification (LLOQ, 1 µg/mL) for adalimumab-specific signature peptide in rat plasma.

Table 1. Inter/intra-day accuracy and precision of adalimumab in quality control samples.

Run No.	Statistics	QC Low (2.5 µg/mL)	QC Med (25 µg/mL)	QC High (50 µg/mL)
1	Mean	2.53	25.3	52.3
	Precision (%CV)	13.1	1.76	3.54
	n	3	3	3
	Accuracy (%)	101	101	105
2	Mean	2.73	23.9	56.3
	Precision (%CV)	2.6	11.13	11.55
	n	3	3	3
	Accuracy (%)	109	95	113
3	Mean	2.57	25.1	47.3
	Precision (%CV)	17.3	10.54	4.44
	n	3	3	3
	Accuracy (%)	103	100	95
Inter-day	Mean	2.61	24.77	51.97
	Precision (%CV)	11	7.81	6.51
	n	9	9	9
	Accuracy (%)	104	99	104

This assay developed for rat plasma samples was also evaluated for plasma samples from other species (mouse and monkey). If there are no/few species-dependent matrix effects between species, the rat plasma calibration curve should be able to quantitate adalimumab in other preclinical species as well. Table 2 shows no significant species-dependent matrix effects between rat plasma and other species. Also, Figure 4 shows that the selected signature peptides are unique in the plasma of several preclinical species. Although all three levels of the QC samples were passed, the interference from the blank monkey plasma appeared to be slightly higher than in rat or mouse blank plasma. Therefore, if this method was to be applied to monkey plasma PK samples, a slightly higher LLOQ (e.g., 2 µg/mL) would be helpful for the calibration curve in monkey plasma. Overall, the rat plasma calibration curve should be applicable to analyze adalimumab in mouse and monkey plasma samples if needed.

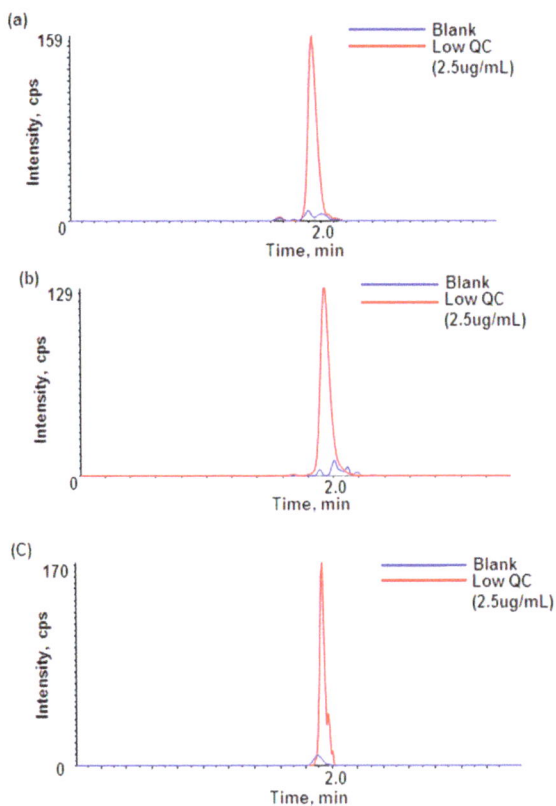

Figure 4. Comparison of peak intensities between blank and QC low in plasma: (**a**) blank and QC low in rat plasma; (**b**) blank and QC low in mouse plasma; (**c**) blank and QC low in monkey plasma.

Table 2. Various species-dependent matrix effects in mouse and monkey plasma. (a) Quality control result in mouse plasma; (b) quality control result in monkey plasma.

(a)					
Mouse	Theoretical Concentration (µg/mL)	Mean Concentration (µg/mL)	Precision (%CV)	*n*	Accuracy (%)
QC low	2.5	2.85	13.2	3	114
QC medium	25	29.4	5.74	3	118
QC high	50	57	1.43	3	114

(b)					
Monkey	Theoretical Concentration (µg/mL)	Mean Concentration (µg/mL)	Precision (%CV)	*n*	Accuracy (%)
QC low	2.5	2.09	4.9	3	84
QC medium	25	23.4	11.19	3	94
QC high	50	48.1	5.12	3	96

3.2.3. Freeze and Thaw Stability

Freeze and thaw stability assessments were carried out to demonstrate that adalimumab in plasma samples was stable under freeze and thaw conditions. The freeze and thaw stability experiments for rat, mouse and monkey plasma were performed using QC samples ($n = 3$) at low, medium and high QC levels. The mean values of the freeze and thaw stability QC samples at each level were compared with the nominal concentrations. The results are summarized in Table 3. The acceptance criterion for the freeze and thaw stability samples was within ± 25% precision and accuracy, which is acceptable for early drug discovery studies, and the results all met the acceptance criteria. As a result, adalimumab in rat, mouse and monkey plasma QC samples was stable through three freeze and thaw cycles.

Table 3. Freeze and thaw stability assessment in preclinical species (three cycles) (a) Freeze and thaw stability in rat plasma; (b) freeze and thaw stability in mouse plasma; (c) freeze and thaw stability in monkey plasma.

(a)					
Rat	Theoretical Concentration (µg/mL)	Mean Concentration (µg/mL)	Precision (%)	*n*	Accuracy (%)
QC low	2.5	2.58	10.5	3	103
QC medium	25	25.6	13.67	3	102
QC high	50	57.3	8.73	3	115

(b)					
Mouse	Theoretical Concentration (µg/mL)	Mean Concentration (µg/mL)	Precision (%)	*n*	Accuracy (%)
QC low	2.5	2.62	16.7	3	105
QC medium	25	28	3.26	3	112
QC high	50	60.2	0.94	3	120

(c)					
Monkey	Theoretical Concentration (µg/mL)	Mean Concentration (µg/mL)	Precision (%)	*n*	Accuracy (%)
QC low	2.5	2.26	2.8	3	91
QC medium	25	19.5	12.42	3	78
QC high	50	40.3	8.52	3	81

3.2.4. Application to a Pharmacokinetic Study in Rats

The qualified LC-QTOF-MS/MS method was successfully applied to a pharmacokinetic study of adalimumab in Sprague–Dawley (SD) rats. Plasma samples obtained after intravenous administration of 1 mg/kg were analyzed by LC-QTOF-MS/MS for the quantification of adalimumab concentrations. To assure acceptance of study sample analytical runs, at least two-thirds of the QC samples had to be within ±25% accuracy, with at least half of the QC samples at each concentration meeting these criteria. When 1 mg/kg of adalimumab was administered to the rats, the drug concentrations in rat plasma were all within the calibration curve range. The time–concentration profile is shown in Figure 5. Although no head-to-head comparison for the PK profiles was carried out between this LC-QTOF-MS/MS method and other conventional methods, the PK profile produced by LC-QTOF-MS/MS looked comparable to the reference adalimumab human PK profile published in studies using conventional methods. Unlike the PK profiles of small molecules, most monoclonal antibody drugs typically show bi-phase elimination PK profiles, which consist of a short half-life alpha-phase distribution followed by a beta-phase elimination with a long half-life. Therefore, a two-compartment model was used for the PK parameters of adalimumab in this experiment. (Table 4) [17]. The time-concentration graph of adalimumab in Figure 5 also showed typical two-compartment monoclonal antibody PK characteristics with a short alpha-phase and a long beta-phase half-life (~10 days).

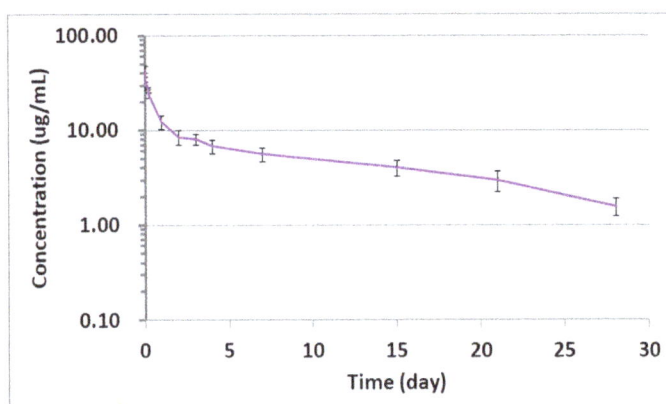

Figure 5. Time-concentration profile of adalimumab in rat plasma from the study subjects receiving 1 mg/kg adalimumab by intravenous administration. The data represent the mean ± standard deviation (SD, $n = 4$).

Table 4. Pharmacokinetic parameters of adalimumab after 1 mg/kg intravenous injection in rats.

Compound	PK parameters							
	AUC (μg·Day/mL)	Cl (mL/Day/kg)	Alpha Half Life (Day)	Beta Half Life (Day)	C_{max} (μg/mL)	V_1 (mL/kg)	V_{ss} (mL/kg)	Compartment Model
Adalimumab	155.29	6.68	0.2	9.82	41.64	24.1	85.83	2

4. Discussion

Immunoassay has been used for over 50 years and has traditionally been used to quantify large molecules. However, this method has some disadvantages [18]. The main disadvantages are that it is time-consuming and requires labor-intensive reagent development [8]. Immunoassays also often show cross-reaction with precursors of the target protein or with smaller metabolized fragments that are not suitable for early-stage mAbs bioanalysis [11]. LC-MS/MS can overcome the disadvantages of immunoassay. Compared to traditional immunoassay, LC-MS/MS technique does not require the preparation of time-consuming and high-cost reagents for specific antibody detection. Combined with LC-MS/MS and immunocapture methods, analytes can be selectively extracted without interferences such as anti-drug antibodies (ADA), which interfere with protein drug targets in the biological matrix [19].

Adalimumab is a recombinant human IgG1 monoclonal antibody [20]. Therefore, human IgG1 is also detected when quantifying adalimumab in the human matrix, making it difficult to distinguish it from the target drug. Therefore, the specific signature peptide of adalimumab was selected because it was distinguishable from human IgG1.

A LC-QTOF-MS/MS method was developed for the determination of adalimumab in rat plasma using a specific signature peptide (APYTFGQGTK) to demonstrate the feasibility of this method for adalimumab or its biosimilars. The calibration curve was acceptable over a concentration range from 1 to 100 μg/mL for adalimumab using quadratic regression with 1/concentration weighting. This LC-QTOF-MS/MS method was sensitive, selective, accurate and reproducible for the determination of adalimumab concentration and has been applied successfully to an adalimumab rat PK study. There was no significant species-dependent matrix effect between rats and other preclinical species, which means this method would be applicable to other preclinical sample analyses without developing new reagents for sample preparation. In conclusion, this method was useful for the analysis of adalimumab and could also be used as a complementary method for adalimumab or its biosimilars in early-stage research and development.

Author Contributions: Y.P., M.-H.P. and Y.G.S. designed the experiment; Y.P., N.K., J.C., M.-H.P., B.i.L., S.-H.S. and J.-J.B. performed the experiments; Y.P., N.K. and J.C. analyzed the data; Y.P. wrote the paper; Y.G.S. reviewed and revised the paper.

Acknowledgments: This research was supported by a research fund of Chungnam National University.

Conflicts of Interest: The authors declare no conflict of interest.

References

1. Ecker, D.M.; Jones, S.D.; Levine, H.L. The therapeutic monoclonal antibody market. *MAbs* **2015**, *7*, 9–14. [CrossRef] [PubMed]
2. Park, M.H.; Lee, M.W.; Shin, Y.G. Qualification and application of a liquid chromatography-quadrupole time-of-flight mass spectrometric method for the determination of trastuzumab in rat plasma. *Biomed. Chromatogr.* **2016**, *30*, 625–631. [CrossRef] [PubMed]
3. Breedveld, F.C. Therapeutic monoclonal antibodies. *Lancet* **2000**, *355*, 735–740. [CrossRef]
4. Catapano, A.L.; Papadopoulos, N. The safety of therapeutic monoclonal antibodies: Implications for cardiovascular disease and targeting the pcsk9 pathway. *Atherosclerosis* **2013**, *228*, 18–28. [CrossRef] [PubMed]
5. Voller, A.; Bartlett, A.; Bidwell, D.E. Enzyme immunoassays with special reference to elisa techniques. *J. Clin. Pathol.* **1978**, *31*, 507–520. [CrossRef] [PubMed]
6. Balkwill, F. Tnf-alpha in promotion and progression of cancer. *Cancer Metastasis Rev.* **2006**, *25*, 409–416. [CrossRef] [PubMed]
7. Azevedo, V.F.; Troiano, L.D.C.; Galli, N.B.; Kleinfelder, A.; Catolino, N.M.; Martins, P.C.U. Adalimumab: A review of the reference product and biosimilars. *Biosimilars* **2016**, *6*, 29–44. [CrossRef]
8. Sandborn, W.J.; Hanauer, S.B.; Rutgeerts, P.; Fedorak, R.N.; Lukas, M.; MacIntosh, D.G.; Panaccione, R.; Wolf, D.; Kent, J.D.; Bittle, B.; et al. Adalimumab for maintenance treatment of crohn's disease: Results of the classic ii trial. *Gut* **2007**, *56*, 1232–1239. [CrossRef] [PubMed]
9. Darwish, I.A. Immunoassay methods and their applications in pharmaceutical analysis: Basic methodology and recent advances. *Int. J. Biomed. Sci.* **2006**, *2*, 217–235. [PubMed]
10. Liu, H.; Manuilov, A.V.; Chumsae, C.; Babineau, M.L.; Tarcsa, E. Quantitation of a recombinant monoclonal antibody in monkey serum by liquid chromatography-mass spectrometry. *Anal. Biochem.* **2011**, *414*, 147–153. [CrossRef] [PubMed]
11. Becher, F.; Pruvost, A.; Clement, G.; Tabet, J.C.; Ezan, E. Quantification of small therapeutic proteins in plasma by liquid chromatography-tandem mass spectrometry: Application to an elastase inhibitor epi-hne4. *Anal. Chem.* **2006**, *78*, 2306–2313. [CrossRef] [PubMed]
12. Domon, B.; Aebersold, R. Mass spectrometry and protein analysis. *Science* **2006**, *312*, 212–217. [CrossRef] [PubMed]
13. Heudi, O.; Barteau, S.; Zimmer, D.; Schmidt, J.; Bill, K.; Lehmann, N.; Bauer, C.; Kretz, O. Towards absolute quantification of therapeutic monoclonal antibody in serum by lc-ms/ms using isotope-labeled antibody standard and protein cleavage isotope dilution mass spectrometry. *Anal. Chem.* **2008**, *80*, 4200–4207. [CrossRef] [PubMed]
14. Roopenian, D.C.; Akilesh, S. Fcrn: The neonatal fc receptor comes of age. *Nat. Rev. Immunol.* **2007**, *7*, 715–725. [CrossRef] [PubMed]
15. Li, H.; Ortiz, R.; Tran, L.; Hall, M.; Spahr, C.; Walker, K.; Laudemann, J.; Miller, S.; Salimi-Moosavi, H.; Lee, J.W. General lc-ms/ms method approach to quantify therapeutic monoclonal antibodies using a common whole antibody internal standard with application to preclinical studies. *Anal. Chem.* **2012**, *84*, 1267–1273. [CrossRef] [PubMed]
16. Shen, H.W.; Yu, A.M. Conference report: New analytical technologies for biological discovery. *Bioanalysis* **2010**, *2*, 181–184. [CrossRef] [PubMed]
17. Ferri, N.; Bellosta, S.; Baldessin, L.; Boccia, D.; Racagni, G.; Corsini, A. Pharmacokinetics interactions of monoclonal antibodies. *Pharmacol. Res.* **2016**, *111*, 592–599. [CrossRef] [PubMed]

18. Cross, T.G.; Hornshaw, M.P. Can lc and lc-ms ever replace immunoassays? *J. Appl. Bioanal.* **2016**, *2*, 108–116. [CrossRef]
19. Wilffert, D.; Bischoff, R.; van de Merbel, N.C. Antibody-free workflows for protein quantification by lc-ms/ms. *Bioanalysis* **2015**, *7*, 763–779. [CrossRef] [PubMed]
20. Kaymakcalan, Z.; Sakorafas, P.; Bose, S.; Scesney, S.; Xiong, L.; Hanzatian, D.K.; Salfeld, J.; Sasso, E.H. Comparisons of affinities, avidities, and complement activation of adalimumab, infliximab, and etanercept in binding to soluble and membrane tumor necrosis factor. *Clin. Immunol.* **2009**, *131*, 308–316. [CrossRef] [PubMed]

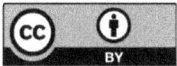

pharmaceutics

MDPI

Article

Simultaneous Determination of Procainamide and *N*-acetylprocainamide in Rat Plasma by Ultra-High-Pressure Liquid Chromatography Coupled with a Diode Array Detector and Its Application to a Pharmacokinetic Study in Rats

Anusha Balla [1], Kwan Hyung Cho [2], Yu Chul Kim [3,*] and Han-Joo Maeng [1,*]

[1]   College of Pharmacy, Gachon University, Incheon 21936, Korea; aanushaballa@gmail.com
[2]   College of Pharmacy, Inje University, Gimhae 50834, Korea; chokh@inje.ac.kr
[3]   Department of Pharmaceutical Engineering, Inje University, Gimhae 50834, Korea
*   Correspondence: yckim@inje.ac.kr (Y.C.K.); hjmaeng@gachon.ac.kr (H.-J.M.);
    Tel.: +82-55-320-3399 (Y.C.K.); +82-32-820-4935 (H.-J.M.)

Received: 9 March 2018; Accepted: 27 March 2018; Published: 30 March 2018

Abstract: A simple, sensitive, and reliable reversed-phase, Ultra-High-Pressure Liquid Chromatography (UHPLC) coupled with a Diode Array Detector (DAD) method for the simultaneous determination of Procainamide (PA) and its major metabolite, *N*-acetylprocainamide (NAPA), in rat plasma was developed and validated. A simple deproteinization method with methanol was applied to the rat plasma samples, which were analyzed using UHPLC equipped with DAD at 280 nm, and a Synergi™ 4 μm polar, reversed-phase column using 1% acetic acid (pH 5.5) and methanol (76:24, v/v) as eluent in isocratic mode at a flow rate 0.2 mL/min. The method showed good linearity ($r^2 > 0.998$) over the concentration range of 20–100,000 and 20–10,000 ng/mL for PA and NAPA, respectively. Intra- and inter-day accuracies ranged from 97.7 to 110.9%, and precision was <10.5% for PA and 99.7 to 109.2 and <10.5%, respectively, for NAPA. The lower limit of quantification was 20 ng/mL for both compounds. This is the first report of the UHPLC-DAD bioanalytical method for simultaneous measurement of PA and NAPA. The most obvious advantage of this method over previously reported HPLC methods is that it requires small sample and injection volumes, with a straightforward, one-step sample preparation. It overcomes the limitations of previous methods, which use large sample volume and complex sample preparation. The devised method was successfully applied to the quantification of PA and NAPA after an intravenous bolus administration of 10 mg/kg procainamide hydrochloride to rats.

Keywords: procainamide; *N*-acetylprocainamide; ultra-high-pressure liquid chromatography; rat; plasma; pharmacokinetics

---

1. Introduction

Procainamide (PA, *p*-amino-*N*-[2-(diethylamino)ethyl]benzamide monohydrochloride; 4-amino -*N*-[2-(diethylamino)ethyl]benzamide) (Figure 1A) is a type IA cardiac antiarrhythmic drug, which has been widely used to treat supraventricular or ventricular arrhythmia for more than 60 years [1,2], and is the drug of choice for the treatment of hemodynamically-tolerated, sustained, monomorphic ventricular tachycardia [3–5]. In addition to the above-mentioned therapeutic aspects, it has been shown that PA has other pharmacological effects, for example, it reduces the hepatotoxic and nephrotoxic effects of cisplatin and has been reported to have anti-inflammatory effects in a rat model of sepsis [6,7]. However, PA has potentially-serious adverse effects, such as, hypotension, polymorphous ventricular tachycardia, lupus-like syndrome, or agranulocytosis, and its applicability is limited by its narrow therapeutic window [2,8,9].

PA is predominantly metabolized to N-acetylprocainamide (NAPA) (Figure 1B) by N-acetyltransferase II in liver, and NAPA has similar pharmacologic activity to PA [10,11]. The metabolic activity for PA to NAPA shows high inter-subject variation due to a genetic polymorphism in N-acetyltransferase II. It has been shown that the systemic exposure ratio of NAPA/PA in rapid acetylators is higher than that of slow acetylators [10–12]. Because NAPA is an active metabolite, the pharmacological and adverse effects observed after PA administration might be due to both PA and NAPA. For these reasons, the determination of the concentrations of PA and NAPA in the systemic circulation is likely to be necessary to investigate the Pharmacokinetic/Pharmacodynamic (PK/PD) and/or Toxicokinetic/Toxicodynamic (TK/TD) properties, and the development of an analytical method for simultaneous determination of PA and NAPA levels in plasma is required.

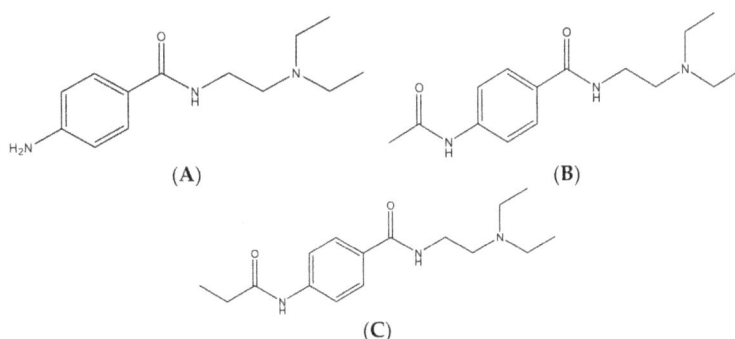

(A) (B)

(C)

Figure 1. Chemical structures of (A) procainamide; (B) N-acetylprocainamide; and (C) N-propionylprocainamide (the Internal Standard, IS).

A small number of methods has been devised to quantitate PA and NAPA simultaneously in plasma by Thin Layer Chromatography (TLC) [13,14], Gas-Liquid Chromatography (GLC) [15], and HPLC [16–26], but most lack sensitivity and/or specificity. Although several UV-HPLC methods achieved sensitivity and specificity improvements, they require multistep sample preparations that involve Liquid–Liquid Extraction (LLE), evaporation, and reconstitution. In addition, large sample volumes (0.2–2.5 mL) and injection volumes (10–100 μL) are required [16–26] (Table S1). To our knowledge, no method for the simultaneous determination of PA and NAPA by Ultra-High-Pressure Liquid Chromatography (UHPLC) has been described to focus on the analytical application of preclinical studies. UHPLC systems utilize small particle sizes in columns, which increases separation efficiencies and leads to better resolutions and sensitivities, and reduces the times required for analysis [27,28]. In the present study, a UHPLC-Diode Array Detector (DAD)-based method requiring simple protein precipitation for sample preparation was developed and validated for the simultaneous determinations of PA and NAPA in plasma, and successfully applied to a pharmacokinetic study in rats.

2. Materials and Methods

2.1. Chemicals and Reagents

Procainamide hydrochloride (HCl) (M_W 271.79 g/mol, purity $\geq$ 98.0%), NAPA (M_W 277.36 g/mol, purity $\geq$ 99.0%) and N-propionylprocainamide (NPPA, M_W 291.39 g/mol, purity $\geq$ 99.0% and the Internal Standard (IS) used) (Figure 1C) were purchased from Sigma-Aldrich (St. Louis, MO, USA). Methanol was purchased from Honeywell Burdick and Jackson (Muskegon, MI, USA). Acetic acid and triethylamine were from Sigma-Aldrich (St. Louis, MO, USA). Water was purified using the aquaMAX™, ultra-pure water purification system (YL Instruments, Anyang, Korea). All other chemicals and solvents were of reagent or HPLC grade and used without further purification.

2.2. UHPLC System and Chromatographic Condition

The analysis was performed using the Agilent 1290 Infinity II UHPLC system (Agilent Technologies, Santa Clara, CA, USA), equipped with an auto-sampler (G7167B), a flexible pump (G7104A), a Multicolumn Thermostat (MCT) (G7116B), and a DAD detector (G7117A). A Synergi™ 4 µm polar, Reversed-Phase (RP) 80A column (150 × 2.0 mm, Phenomenex, Torrance, CA, USA) was used for separation. Isocratic elution was employed with a mobile phase consisting of 1% acetic acid, pH 5.5 (containing 0.01% triethylamine), and methanol (76:24, v/v) at a flow rate 0.2 mL/min. Before use, the mobile phase was adjusted to pH 5.5, filtered, and degassed. The injection volume was set at 2 µL, and the DAD detector to 280 nm. The column and autosampler tray were maintained at 25 °C and 4 °C, respectively.

2.3. Preparation of Calibration Standards and Quality Control (QC) Samples

Stock solutions of PA, NAPA, and NPPA (IS) were prepared separately at 1 mg/mL by dissolving accurately-weighed amounts of the compound in Double-Distilled Water (DDW). A series of working standard solutions of each compound were prepared by serial dilution of the respective stock solutions with DDW. A working internal standard solution of 200 ng/mL was prepared by diluting the IS stock solution in methanol. Calibration curve standard samples of PA and NAPA were prepared by spiking 90 µL of drug-free rat plasma with 10 µL of working standard solutions to give final concentrations of 10, 20, 50, 100, 200, 500, 1000, 2000, 5000, 10,000, and 100,000 ng/mL for PA, and 10, 20, 50, 100, 200, 500, 1000, 2000, 5000, and 10,000 ng/mL for NAPA. QC samples were prepared in the same way to final concentrations of 20 (Lower Limit of Quantification (LLOQ)), 60 (low QC), 8000 (mid QC), and 80,000 ng/mL (high QC) for PA, and 20 (LLOQ), 60 (low QC), 800 (mid QC), and 8000 ng/mL (high QC) for NAPA. All stock and working solutions were stored at −20 °C until required for analysis.

2.4. Sample Preparation

A simple protein-precipitation method was used for the analysis. Plasma samples (100 µL) were transferred into separate Eppendorf tubes and an aliquot of 200 µL of IS (200 ng/mL of NPPA in methanol) was added. After vortex-mixing for 1 min and centrifugation at 15,000 rpm for 15 min at 4 °C, 2 µL aliquots of the methanolic supernatants were injected into the UHPLC system.

2.5. Method Validation

The devised method was validated for selectivity, sensitivity, linearity, accuracy, precision, recovery, and stability. The selectivities for PA and NAPA were evaluated to determine possible interference by endogenous substances. Blank plasma samples from six randomly-selected Sprague-Dawley (SD) rats were used, and the UHPLC chromatograms of blank plasma, blank plasma spiked with PA (100 ng/mL), blank plasma spiked with NAPA (100 ng/mL), and blank plasma spiked with IS (200 ng/mL) were compared. Linearity was assessed by plotting the peak area ratios of each analyte to IS versus the nominal concentrations ranging from 20–100,000 and 20–10,000 ng/mL for PA and NAPA, respectively. Least squares regression with a weighting factor of 1/x was used to construct five calibration curves and to determine the correlation coefficient. Intra-day and inter-day precision and accuracy for PA and NAPA were evaluated by analyzing six replicates of QC samples (20, 60, 8000, and 80,000 ng/mL for PA and 20, 60, 800, and 8000 ng/mL for NAPA) over 5 consecutive days. Accuracies were calculated as mean ratios of observed and nominal concentrations. The precision was defined as Relative Standard Deviation (RSD). Six sets of QC samples were prepared on five different days, and each set of samples was analyzed within 24 h. Limits of Detection (LODs) and LLOQs for PA and NAPA were determined by visual evaluation and using Signal-to-Noise ratios (S/N) of 3:1 and

5:1, respectively. The acceptance criteria for precision and accuracy at LLOQ are within 20% RSD for precision and between 80% and 120% for accuracy.

The percentage recoveries of PA and NAPA in plasma after deproteinization with methanol were calculated. UHPLC peak areas of PA and NAPA in plasma after deproteinization with methanol were compared with those obtained from four nominal concentrations in methanol. Percentage IS recovery was determined at a concentration of 200 ng/mL.

The stabilities of PA, NAPA, and IS were evaluated under different conditions. To determine the stabilities of stock solutions of analytes and the IS, three replicate stock solutions (100 ng/mL for PA and NAPA, and 200 ng/mL for IS) were analyzed and peak areas were compared with a stock solution after storage for 6 h at room temperature and 4 weeks at −20 °C. To determine the stabilities of analytes and IS in rat plasma, short-term stability, long-term stability, freeze-thaw stability, and autosampler stability were assessed at four concentrations of PA and NAPA (20, 60, 8000, and 80,000 ng/mL for PA and 20, 60, 800, and 8000 ng/mL for NAPA), with three replicates for each concentration. The short-term stability was assessed by allowing QC samples to stand at room temperature for 4 h prior to analysis; long-term stability by storing QC samples at −20 °C for 4 weeks; freeze-thaw stability cycle by subjecting QC samples to three cycles of freezing at −20 °C for 24 h; and thawing at room temperature. In addition, the analysis was repeated after 24 h to determine auto-sampler stability at 4 °C.

2.6. Application to Pharmacokinetic Studies of Procainamide HCl

The animal experiment was performed in accordance with the Guidelines for Animal Care and Use issued by Gachon University. Experimental protocols involving the animals used in this study were reviewed and approved by the Animal Care and Use Committee of the Gachon University (#GIACUC-R2017011, approval date on 25th May 2017). Sprague-Dawley (SD) rats (7–8 weeks old, 220–280 g) were purchased from Nara Biotech (Pyeongtaek, Korea). Food and water were freely provided, and animals were allowed a week to adjust to the laboratory environment before commencing the experiment and maintained under a 12:12 h light/dark cycle.

To evaluate the relevance of the analysis method, an Intravenous (IV) pharmacokinetic study of PA was performed in SD rats. Rats were anesthetized (with a mixture of Zoletil and Rompun) and then a femoral vein and artery were cannulated for drug administration and blood sample collection, respectively [29]. PA HCl in saline (10 mg/kg) was then administered ($n = 5$) via the cannulated femoral vein. Blood was then collected at 0 (blank), 1, 5, 15, 30, 60, 120, 180, 240, 360, and 480 min after drug administration. After each blood sampling, the volume of blood collected was replaced with an equal volume of saline to compensate for blood loss. Collected blood was immediately centrifuged at 14,000 rpm for 15 min at 4 °C, and plasma was then separated and stored at −20 °C until analysis.

The plasma concentration–time profiles of PA and NAPA were plotted and analyzed using the non-compartmental method using WinNonlin (Ver. 5.0.1) [29]. For PA, the Area Under the plasma Concentration–time curve (AUC) was calculated using the linear trapezoidal method. AUC_{last} (from time zero to last time point), AUC_{inf} (from time zero to infinity), total body Clearance (CL), Volume of distribution at steady state (V_{ss}), Mean Residence Time (MRT), and elimination half-life ($t_{1/2}$), of PA were determined individually. Similarly, the pharmacokinetic parameters of the major metabolite, NAPA, were obtained including peak Concentration (C_{max}) and Time to reach C_{max} (T_{max}). In addition, the AUC ratio of PA and NAPA (AUC_{NAPA}/AUC_{PA}) was calculated using AUC_{inf} values for each rat.

3. Results and Discussion

3.1. Optimization of Chromatographic Analysis

To develop a simple method suitable for the simultaneous determination of PA and NAPA, chromatographic conditions, such as, eluent, column, and column conditions, were optimized. The mobile phase used had a methanol content that differed slightly from that used in a previously-reported method [20]. Namely, a slight increase in methanol content in the mobile phase improved the peak shapes and shortened the total run time. A polar-RP column was found to provide suitable retention times and better peak shapes than other columns (e.g., C-8 and C-18 columns). For example, tested C-8 and C-18 columns generated peak tailing, with a poor quantitation limit, or required a long retention time of IS (i.e., more than 30 min).

To obtain the highest recovery using a straightforward method, we selected deproteinization by methanol over liquid-liquid or solid-phase extraction. The deproteinization method was further optimized in terms of organic solvent. We tested acetonitrile and methanol, and subsequently selected methanol because it provided better peak shapes and sensitivity.

3.2. Selectivity

UHPLC chromatograms of blank rat plasma samples verified the absence of interference at the retention times of PA, NAPA, and IS, which were 6.8, 9.9, and 15.6 min, respectively. Figure 2 shows representative chromatograms of blank plasma (Figure 2A), plasma spiked with IS (Figure 2B), plasma spiked with PA and IS (Figure 2C,E), and plasma spiked with NAPA and IS (Figure 2D,F).

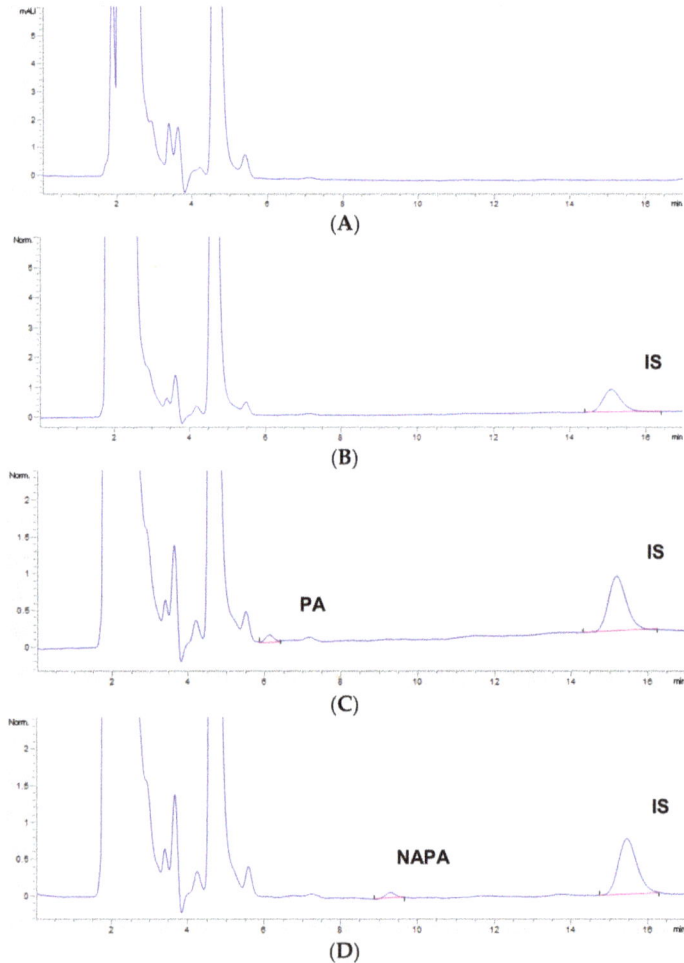

Figure 2. *Cont.*

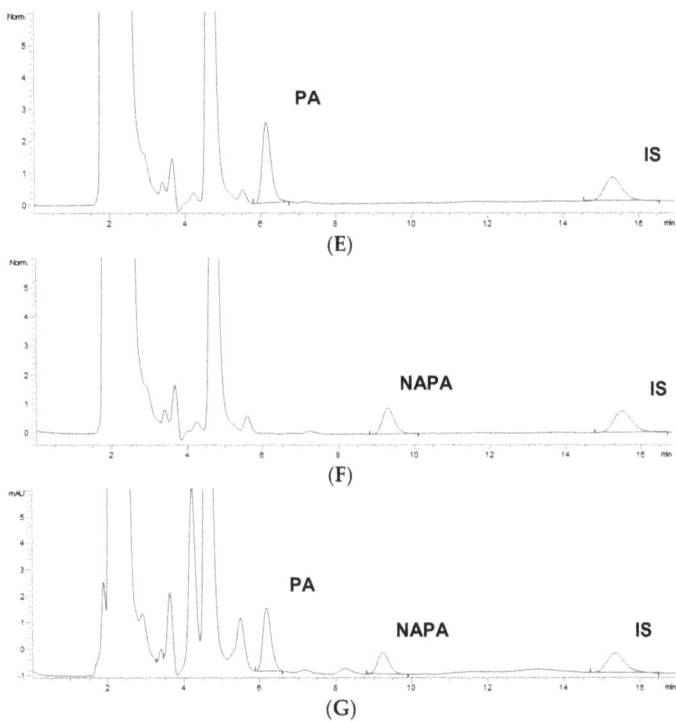

Figure 2. Chromatograms of (**A**) blank rat plasma; (**B**) plasma spiked with IS (200 ng/mL); (**C**) plasma spiked with procainamide (20 ng/mL, lower limit of quantification (LLOQ)) and IS (200 ng/mL); (**D**) plasma spiked with *N*-acetylprocainamide (20 ng/mL, LLOQ) and IS (200 ng/mL); (**E**) plasma spiked with procainamide (1000 ng/mL) and IS (200 ng/mL); (**F**) plasma spiked with *N*-acetylprocainamide (500 ng/mL) and IS (200 ng/mL) and (**G**) 30 min after intravenous administration of procainamide hydrochloride (10 mg/kg). PA: procainamide, NAPA: N-acetylprocaiamide, IS: internal standard.

3.3. Linearity

The calibration curve (*n* = 5) for PA was linear over the concentration range 20–100,000 ng/mL, and that for NAPA was linear over the range 20–10,000 ng/mL. Least squares regression with a weighting factor of 1/x was used to determine the calibration curves of PA and NAPA. The calibration equation for PA was y = (0.00198 ± 0.00007) x + (0.00804 ± 0.00391) with a coefficient of determination (r^2) of 0.9995 ± 0.0004, the calibration equation for NAPA was y = (0.00262 ± 0.00015) x + (0.03151 ± 0.01200) with a coefficient determination (r^2) = 0.9984 ± 0.0012. The results indicate that UHPLC-DAD response for both analytes was directly proportional to analyte concentration in plasma, and that assays were linear and reliable.

3.4. Precision and Accuracy

To determine intra- and inter-day accuracies and precisions, QC samples of PA and NAPA were prepared at concentrations of 20, 60, 8000, and 80,000 ng/mL and 20, 60, 800, and 8000 ng/mL, respectively. Six replicates were analyzed at each concentration. A summary of intra- and inter-day accuracies and precisions of PA and NAPA is provided in Table 1. Intra-day accuracies for PA ranged from 98.6 to 110.9% and RSDs from 2.0 to 7.5%, and inter-day accuracies ranged from 97.7 to 100.1%

and RSDs from 5.2 to 10.5%. Similarly, intra-day accuracies for NAPA ranged from 99.7 to 109.2% and RSDs from 1.0 to 6.1%, and inter-day accuracies ranged from 100.8 to 106.3% and RSDs from 4.6 to 10.5%. Hence, intra- and inter-day accuracies and precisions for both analytes were within the ranges of standard FDA guidelines [30].

Table 1. Accuracy and precision of procainamide and *N*-acetylprocainamide in plasma.

Analytes	Nominal Concentration (ng/mL)	Intra-day (*n* = 6)			Inter-day (*n* = 30)		
		Measured Concentration (ng/mL)	Precision (RSD %)	Accuracy (%)	Measured Concentration (ng/mL)	Precision (RSD %)	Accuracy (%)
PA	20	22.1	2.0	110.3	19.5	10.5	97.7
	60	60.5	7.5	110.9	59.9	7.1	99.8
	8000	7890	4.2	98.6	8011	5.2	100.1
	80,000	79,079	4.0	98.9	78,994	6.0	98.7
NAPA	20	20.0	6.1	99.7	20.9	10.5	104.3
	60	62.1	3.3	103.4	60.5	9.1	100.8
	8000	873.2	1.0	109.2	850.1	4.6	106.3
	80,000	8031	5.1	100.4	8238	6.1	103.0

PA: procainamide; NAPA: *N*-acetylprocainamide; RSD: relative standard deviation.

3.5. Sensitivity

Initially, LODs and LLOQs of PA and NAPA were determined by visual evaluation and found to be 10 and 20 ng/mL, respectively. LOD and LLOQ values were also determined using S/N ratios with acceptability of ≥3 for LOD and ≥5 for LLOQ. The S/N ratios for the LOD and LLOQ of PA were 3.7 and 6.7, respectively, and for NAPA were 3.5 and 5.9, respectively. Further, the LLOQ values for both analytes were confirmed to meet specified precision and accuracy values. The LLOQs for PA and NAPA were confirmed at 20 ng/mL, with accuracies less than 113.7% and 117.3% for PA and NAPA, respectively, and percent RSD of 10.5% for both PA and NAPA. The representative UHPLC chromatograms at LLOQ of PA and NAPA are shown in Figure 2C,D. Compared to LLOQs from previous literatures, it is indicated that our LLOQs for PA and NAPA using UHPLC-DAD are highly sensitive, without condensation in rat plasma. Although a previously-reported HPLC method with LLE provided better sensitivity for both PA and NAPA, this method is unlikely accessible for the preclinical pharmacokinetic studies due to the large sample volume required (i.e., 500 μL) [20].

3.6. Recovery

PA recovery was determined at concentrations of 20, 60, 8000, and 80,000 ng/mL and NAPA recovery at concentrations of 20, 60, 800, and 8000 ng/mL. IS recovery was determined at 200 ng/mL. Mean PA recovery values ranged from 95.6 to 103.3% and RSDs from 0.4 to 8.3%, while mean NAPA recovery values ranged from 93.7 to 100.0% and RSDs from 0.4 to 10.8%. Thus, recoveries for both analytes were near 100% and reproducible.

3.7. Stability

To determine the stock solution stabilities of PA, NAPA, and IS (100 ng/mL for PA and NAPA, and 200 ng/mL for IS), analytes were analyzed in triplicate after standing at room temperature for 6 h or at −20 °C for 4 weeks. As compared with fresh stock solutions, the determined stability values (%) of PA, NAPA, and IS were 103.3, 99.8, and 101.3%, respectively, after standing at room temperature for 6 h, and 104.6, 103.4, and 102.0%, respectively, after storage for 4 weeks at −20 °C. The stabilities of PA and NAPA in rat plasma were determined at four concentrations of PA and NAPA (20, 60, 8000, and 80,000 ng/mL for PA and 20, 60, 800, and 8000 ng/mL for NAPA) in triplicate. As compared with freshly-prepared QC samples, the stability (%) of PA in plasma QC samples allowed to stand at room temperature for 4 h was 91.6–108.1%, and that of samples stored at −20 °C for 4 weeks was 91.6–107.8 %. The stability (%) of PA after three freeze-thaw cycles, and after storage at 4 °C in an autosampler for 24 h, were 95.6–103.6% and 94.4–104.6%, respectively. Similarly, short-term, long-term, freeze-thaw, and autosampler stability ranges of NAPA were 95.3–102.0%, 92.4–102.6%, 96.3–102.7%, and 98.3–102.7%, respectively. The results of stability studies for PA and NAPA are listed in Table 2. These results show that PA and NAPA were stable under these storage and processing conditions.

Table 2. Stability of procainamide and *N*-acetylprocainamide in plasma [1].

Concentration (ng/mL)	Stability (%)	
	PA	NAPA
Freeze-thaw stability (3 cycles)		
20	103.6 ± 7.9	97.3 ± 6.5
60	98.9 ± 1.5	96.3 ± 2.0
8000	99.8 ± 1.0	102.7 ± 1.8
80,000	95.6 ± 0.8	100.3 ± 2.2
Auto-sampler stability (24 h at 4 °C)		
20	104.6 ± 6.0	102.7 ± 0.9
60	103.1 ± 2.2	98.3 ± 1.2
8000	103.4 ± 2.2	101.1 ± 3.0
80,000	94.4 ± 1.5	100.2 ± 1.7
Short-term stability (4 h at room temperature)		
20	108.1 ± 6.7	97.2 ± 9.4
60	103.5 ± 11.1	99.0 ± 1.6
8000	104.0 ± 2.3	102.0 ± 2.7
80,000	91.6 ± 4.6	95.3 ± 2.4
Long-term stability (4 week at −20 °C)		
20	107.8 ± 1.1	92.4 ± 2.5
60	106.1 ± 12.1	102.6 ± 2.5
8000	101.5 ± 2.4	96.4 ± 1.1
80,000	91.6 ± 4.6	97.3 ± 3.2

[1] Results are presented as Mean $\pm$ SD (n = 3); PA: procainamide; NAPA: *N*-acetylprocainamide.

3.8. Application to Pharmacokinetic Studies of Procainamide HCl

The validated analytical method was applied to a pharmacokinetic study of PA HCl in SD rats that were administered a single dose of 10 mg/kg IV. Representative chromatograms from plasma samples collected 30 min after IV administration are shown in Figure 2G. PA concentrations in plasma were measurable for up to 4 h after injection, whereas NAPA was measurable for up to 8 h, as shown in Figure 3. The pharmacokinetic parameters determined were as follows: $t_{1/2}$, AUC_{last}, AUC_{inf}, MRT, CL, V_{ss}, C_{max}, and T_{max}. The results are summarized in Table 3. The AUC_{inf}, CL, V_{ss}, and $t_{1/2}$ of PA were 136 ± 12.1 μg·min/mL, 73.8 ± 6.51 mL/min/kg, 2070 ± 316 mL/kg, and 52.4 ± 2.20 min, respectively. The AUC_{inf} and $t_{1/2}$ of NAPA were 177 ± 29.5 and 131 ± 31.7, respectively. The mean AUC_{NAPA}/AUC_{PA} ratio (based on AUC_{inf} values) was 1.30 ± 0.191. The pharmacokinetic parameters of PA were comparable to those reported by previous studies [31–33]. Namely, CL, V_{ss}, and $t_{1/2}$ were 61.94–119 6 mL/min/kg, 3720 4860 mL/kg, and 47.4–55 min, respectively, after IV administration of PA (50 mg/kg) in rats [31–33]. The pharmacokinetic parameters of NAPA were also similar to a previous report [32]. The terminal half-life of NAPA after IV administration of PA (50 mg/kg) in rats was 104 min [32]. Collectively, these observations indicate that the devised UHPLC-DAD method can be employed to assay plasma samples and perform pharmacokinetic studies on PA and NAPA.

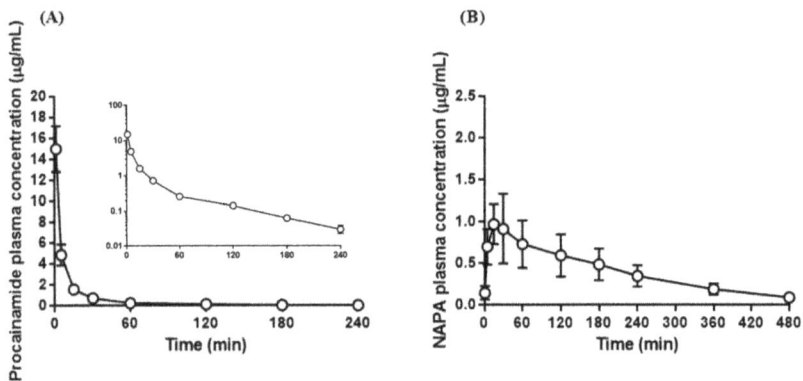

Figure 3. Application of the developed method to a pharmacokinetic study of procainamide; Plasma concentration-time profile of (**A**) procainamide and (**B**) *N*-acetylprocainamide after intravenous administration of procainamide hydrochloride (10 mg/kg) in rats (mean ± SD, *n* = 5).

Table 3. Pharmacokinetic parameters of procainamide and its metabolite, *N*-acetylprocainamide after intravenous administration of procainamide hydrochloride (10 mg/kg) in rats (mean ± SD, *n* = 5).

Parameter	Procainamide	*N*-acetylprocainamide
AUC_{last} (µg·min/mL)	134 ± 12.5	156 ± 36.8
AUC_{inf} (µg·min/mL)	136 ± 12.1	177 ± 29.6
$t_{1/2}$ (min)	52.4 ± 2.20	131 ± 31.7
MRT (min)	28.5 ± 2.99	181 ± 38.3
V_{ss} (mL/kg)	2070 ± 316	-
CL (mL/min/kg)	73.8 ± 6.51	-
C_{max} (µg/mL)	-	0.949 ± 0.124
T_{max} (min)	-	21.0 ± 8.22
AUC_{NAPA}/AUC_{PA} ratio	1.30 ± 0.191	

4. Conclusions

In the current study, we devised a UHPLC-DAD-based method for the simultaneous quantification of PA (a commonly-used antiarrhythmic agent) and its major metabolite, NAPA. The developed method has advantages over previously-reported HPLC methods. Namely, it requires only a single protein precipitation step to prepare plasma samples, and is straightforward, rapid, and cheap. In addition, it requires a relatively small volume (100 µL) of plasma for pharmacokinetic studies, which invariably involve the testing of large numbers of samples, and the small injection volume (2 µL) used minimizes carryover. The method exhibits good linearity and precision across the concentration ranges 20–100,000 ng/mL for PA and 20–10,000 ng/mL for NAPA. In conclusion, the technique used could be applied to determine concentrations of PA and NAPA simultaneously in preclinical studies.

Supplementary Materials: The following are available online at http://www.mdpi.com/1999-4923/10/2/41/s1, Table S1: Summary of HPLC bioanalytical method for simultaneous determination of procainamide and *N*-acetylprocainamide in the previous literatures.

Acknowledgments: This work was supported by Basic Science Research Program through the National Research Foundation of Korea (NRF) funded by the Ministry of Science, ICT & Future Planning (2016R1D1A1B03931470).

Author Contributions: Han-Joo Maeng and Yu Chul Kim conceived and designed the experiments; Anusha Balla performed the experiments; Han-Joo Maeng, Yu Chul Kim and Anusha Balla analyzed the data; Han-Joo Maeng and Kwan Hyung Cho contributed reagents/materials; Han-Joo Maeng and Yu Chul Kim wrote the paper.

Conflicts of Interest: The authors declare no conflict of interest.

References

1. Ellenbogen, K.A.; Wood, M.A.; Stambler, B.S. Procainamide: A perspective on its value and danger. *Heart Dis. Stroke* **1993**, *2*, 473–476. [PubMed]
2. Giardina, E.V. Procainamide: Clinical pharmacology and efficacy against ventricular arrhythmias. *Ann. N. Y. Acad. Sci.* **1984**, *432*, 177–188. [CrossRef] [PubMed]
3. Bauer, L.A. *Applied Clinical Pharmacokinetics*, 2nd ed.; McGrow-Hill: New York, NY, USA, 2008.
4. Gorgels, A.P.M.; van den Dool, A.; Hofs, A.; Mulleneers, R.; Smeets, J.L.; Vos, M.A.; Wellens, H.J. Comparison of procainamide and lidocaine in terminating sustained monomorphic ventricular tachycardia. *Am. J. Cardiol.* **1996**, *78*, 43–46. [CrossRef]
5. American Heart Association. Guidelines 2000 for Cardiopulmonary Resuscitation and Emergency Cardiovascular Care. Part 6: Advanced cardiovascular life support: Section 5: Pharmacology I: Agents for arrhythmias. *Circulation* **2000**, *102*, I112–I128.
6. Fenoglio, C.; Boncompagni, E.; Chiavarina, B.; Cafaggi, S.; Cilli, M.; Viale, M. Morphological and histochemical evidence of the protective effect of procainamide hydrochloride on tissue damage induced by repeated administration of low doses of cisplatin. *Anticancer Res.* **2005**, *25*, 4123–4128. [PubMed]
7. Shih, C.C.; Liao, M.H.; Hsiao, T.S.; Hii, H.P.; Shen, C.H.; Chen, S.J.; Ka, S.M.; Chang, Y.L.; Wu, C.C. Procainamide inhibits DNA methylation and alleviates multiple organ dysfunction in rats with endotoxic shock. *PLoS ONE* **2016**, *11*, e0163690. [CrossRef] [PubMed]
8. Roden, D.M.; Reele, S.B.; Higgins, S.B.; Wilkinson, G.R.; Smith, R.F.; Oates, J.A.; Woosley, R.L. Antiarrhythmic efficacy, pharmacokinetics and safety of N-acetylprocainamide in human subjects: Comparison with procainamide. *Am. J. Cardiol.* **1980**, *46*, 463–468. [CrossRef]
9. Strasberg, B.; Sclarovsky, S.; Erdberg, A.; Duffy, C.E.; Lam, W.; Swiryn, S.; Agmon, J.; Roden, K.M. Procainamide-induced polymorphous ventricular tachycardia. *Am. J. Cardiol.* **1981**, *47*, 1309–1314. [CrossRef]
10. Karlsson, E. Clinical pharmacokinetics of procainamide. *Clin. Pharmacokin.* **1978**, *3*, 97–107. [CrossRef]
11. Campbell, T.J.; Williams, K.M. Therapeutic drug monitoring: Antiarrhythmic drugs. *Br. J. Clin. Pharmacol.* **1998**, *46*, 307–319. [CrossRef]
12. Okumura, K.; Kita, T.; Chikazawa, S.; Komada, F.; Iwakawa, S.; Tanigawara, Y. Genotyping of N-acetylation polymorphism and correlation with procainamide metabolism. *Clin. Pharmacol. Ther.* **1997**, *61*, 509–517. [CrossRef]
13. Kark, B.; Sistovaris, N.; Keller, A. Thin-layer chromatographic determination of procainamide and N-acetylprocainamide in human serum and urine at single-dose levels. *J. Chromatogr.* **1983**, *277*, 261–272. [CrossRef]
14. Wesley-Hadzija, B.; Mattocks, A.M. Quantitative thin-layer chromatographic method for the determination of procainamide and its major metabolite in plasma. *J. Chromatogr.* **1977**, *143*, 307–313. [CrossRef]
15. Kessler, K.M.; Ho-Tung, P.; Steele, B.; Silver, J.; Pickoff, A.; Narayanan, S.; Myerburg, R. Simultaneous quantitation of quinidine, procainamide, and N-acetylprocainamide in serum by gas-liquid chromatography with a nitrogen-phosphorus selective detector. *Clin. Chem.* **1982**, *28*, 1187–1190. [PubMed]
16. Butterfield, A.G.; Cooper, J.K.; Midha, K.K. Simultaneous determination of procainamide and N-acetylprocainamide in plasma by high-performance liquid chromatography. *J. Pharm. Sci.* **1978**, *67*, 839–842. [CrossRef] [PubMed]
17. Carr, K.; Woosley, R.L.; Oates, J.A. Simultaneous quantification of procainamide and N-acetylprocainamide with high-performance liquid chromatography. *J. Chromatogr.* **1976**, *129*, 363–368. [CrossRef]
18. Coyle, J.D.; Mackichan, J.J.; Boudoulas, H.; Lima, J.J. Reversed-phase liquid chromatography method for measurement of procainamide and three metabolites in serum and urine; percent of dose excreted as deemethyl metabolites. *J. Pharm. Sci.* **1987**, *76*, 402–405. [CrossRef] [PubMed]
19. Lai, C.M.; Kamath, B.L.; Look, Z.M.; Yacobi, A. Determination of procainamide and N-Acetylprocainamide in biological fluids by high pressure liquid chromatography. *J. Pharm. Sci.* **1980**, *69*, 982–984. [CrossRef] [PubMed]
20. Lessard, E.; Fortin, A.; Coquet, A.; Bélanger, P.M.; Hamelin, B.A.; Turgeon, J. Improved high-performance liquid chromatographic assay for the determination of procainamide and its N-acetylated metabolite in plasma: Application to a single-dose pharmacokinetic study. *J. Chromatogr. Sci.* **1998**, *36*, 49–54. [CrossRef] [PubMed]

21. Patel, C.P. Improved liquid chromatographic determination of procainamide and *N*-acetylprocainamide in serum. *Ther. Drug. Monit.* **1983**, *5*, 235–238. [CrossRef] [PubMed]

22. Raphanaud, D.; Borensztejn, M.; Dupeyron, J.P.; Guyon, F. High performance liquid chromatography of procainamid and *N*-scetylprocainamide in human blood plasma. *Ther. Drug. Monit.* **1986**, *8*, 365–367. [CrossRef] [PubMed]

23. Stearns, F.M. Determination of procainamide and *N*-acetylprocainamide by "high-performance" liquid chromatography. *Clin. Chem.* **1981**, *27*, 2064–2067. [PubMed]

24. Su, S.C.; Au, W.Y.W. An improved microanalytical procedure for the quantitationof procainamide and *N*-acetyl procainamide in serum by high-performance liquid chromatography. *J. Liq. Chromatogr.* **1978**, *1*, 783–794. [CrossRef]

25. Weddle, O.H.; Mason, W.D. Rapid determination of procainamide and its *N*-acetyl derivative in human plasma by high-pressure liquid chromatography. *J. Pharm. Sci.* **1977**, *66*, 874–875. [CrossRef] [PubMed]

26. Wesley, J.F.; Lasky, F.D. High performance liquid chromatographic analysis of the antiarrhythmic drugs procainamide, disopyramide, quinidine, propranolol and metabolites from serum extracts. *Clin. Biochem.* **1981**, *14*, 113–118. [CrossRef]

27. Nováková, L.; Matysová, L.; Solich, P. Advantages of application of UPLC in pharmaceutical analysis. *Talanta* **2006**, *68*, 908–918. [CrossRef] [PubMed]

28. Dong, M.W.; Zhang, K. Ultra-high-pressure liquid chromatography (UHPLC) in method development. *Trends Analyt. Chem.* **2014**, *63*, 21–30. [CrossRef]

29. Kim, Y.C.; Kim, I.B.; Noh, C.K.; Quach, H.P.; Yoon, I.S.; Chow, E.C.Y.; Kim, M.; Jin, H.E.; Cho, K.H.; Chung, S.J.; et al. Effects of 1α,25-dihydroxyvitamin D3, the natural vitamin D receptor ligand, on the pharmacokinetics of cefdinir and cefadroxil, organic anion transporter substrates, in rat. *J. Pharm. Sci.* **2014**, *103*, 3793–3805. [CrossRef] [PubMed]

30. US Food Drug Administration. Guidance for Industry, Bioanalytical Methods Validation. 2013. Available online: https://www.fda.gov/downloads/Drugs/Guidances/ucm368107.pdf (accessed on 5 March 2018).

31. Basseches, P.J.; DiGregorio, G.J. Pharmacokinetics of procainamide in rats with extrahepatic biliary obstruction. *J. Pharm. Sci.* **1982**, *71*, 1256–1259. [CrossRef] [PubMed]

32. Liu, L.L.; Knowlton, P.W.; Svensson, C.K. Effect of amiodarone on the disposition of procaiamide in the rat. *J. Pharm. Sci.* **1988**, *77*, 662–665. [CrossRef] [PubMed]

33. Schneck, D.W.; Grove, K.; Dewitt, F.O.; Shiroff, R.A.; Hayes, A.H., Jr. The quantitative disposition of procainamide and *N*-acetylprocainamide in rat. *J. Pharm. Exp. Ther.* **1978**, *204*, 219–225.

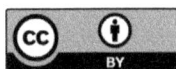

MDPI

St. Alban-Anlage 66

4052 Basel

Switzerland

Tel. +41 61 683 77 34

Fax +41 61 302 89 18

www.mdpi.com

Pharmaceutics Editorial Office

E-mail: pharmaceutics@mdpi.com

www.mdpi.com/journal/pharmaceutics

www.ingramcontent.com/pod-product-compliance
Lightning Source LLC
Chambersburg PA
CBHW051839210326

41597CB00033B/5706